Fantasies of Ito Michio

THEATER: THEORY/TEXT/PERFORMANCE

Series Editors: David Krasner, Rebecca Schneider, and Harvey Young

Founding Editor: Enoch Brater

Recent Titles:

Readying the Revolution: African American Theater and Performance from Post-World War II to the Black Arts Movement
by Jonathan Shandell

Fantasies of Ito Michio
by Tara Rodman

Racing the Great White Way: Black Performance, Eugene O'Neill, and the Transformation of Broadway
by Katie N. Johnson

Chocolate Woman Dreams the Milky Way: Mapping Embodied Indigenous Performance
by Monique Mojica and Brenda Farnell

Democracy Moving: Bill T. Jones, Contemporary American Performance, and the Racial Past
by Ariel Nereson

Moving Islands: Contemporary Performance and the Global Pacific
by Diana Looser

Scenes from Bourgeois Life
by Nicholas Ridout

Performance Constellations: Networks of Protest and Activism in Latin America
by Marcela A. Fuentes

Interchangeable Parts: Acting, Industry, and Technology in US Theater
by Victor Holtcamp

Ruins: Classical Theater and Broken Memory
by Odai Johnson

Gaming the Stage: Playable Media and the Rise of English Commercial Theater
by Gina Bloom

Immersions in Cultural Difference: Tourism, War, Performance
by Natalie Alvarez

Performing the Intercultural City
by Ric Knowles

Microdramas: Crucibles for Theater and Time
by John H. Muse

Fantasies of Ito Michio

Tara Rodman

University of Michigan Press
Ann Arbor

Copyright © 2024 by Tara Rodman
Some rights reserved

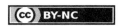

This work is licensed under a Creative Commons Attribution-NonCommercial 4.0 International License. *Note to users:* A Creative Commons license is only valid when it is applied by the person or entity that holds rights to the licensed work. Works may contain components (e.g., photographs, illustrations, or quotations) to which the rightsholder in the work cannot apply the license. It is ultimately your responsibility to independently evaluate the copyright status of any work or component part of a work you use, in light of your intended use. To view a copy of this license, visit http://creativecommons.org/licenses/by-nc/4.0/

For questions or permissions, please contact um.press.perms@umich.edu

Published in the United States of America by the
University of Michigan Press
Manufactured in the United States of America
Printed on acid-free paper
First published October 2024

A CIP catalog record for this book is available from the British Library.

Library of Congress Cataloging-in-Publication data has been applied for.

ISBN 978-0-472-07683-3 (hardcover : alk. paper)
ISBN 978-0-472-05683-5 (paper : alk. paper)
ISBN 978-0-472-90448-8 (open access ebook)

DOI: https://doi.org/10.3998/mpub.12781398

The University of Michigan Press's open access publishing program is made possible thanks to additional funding from the University of Michigan Office of the Provost and the generous support of contributing libraries.

For Jesse

CONTENTS

List of Illustrations	ix
Acknowledgments	xi
Introduction	1
1 Japanese Exemplarity and Exceptionalism: Germany, 1912–1914	36
2 Modernist Mythologizing: London, 1914–1916	62
3 Japoniste Collections: New York, 1916–1929	91
4 Japanese America and Fantasies of Integration: California, 1929–1941	124
5 Cosmopolitanism, Masculinity, and National Embodiment in the Borderless Empire: Japan, 1931; Mexico, 1934; Japan, 1939–1940; Japan, 1940–1941	161
6 Pan-Asianism between Internment and Propaganda: The Asia-Pacific War, 1941–1945	185
7 Being Watched: Making New Bodies for a New Japan, 1945–1955	214
Conclusion	253
Notes	259
Bibliography	289
Index	305

Digital materials related to this title can be found on the Fulcrum platform via the following citable URL: https://doi.org/10.3998/mpub.12781398

ILLUSTRATIONS

Figure 1: Toyo Miyatake, "Ito Michio in *Blue Danube* Costume," 1937.   21

Figure 2: Toyo Miyatake, "Ito Michio in Javanese Dance."   23

Figure 3: Arnold Gente, "Ito Michio," 1921.   48

Figure 4: Jeff Watts for DTSBDC, Sarah Halzack performs *Ave Maria*
(Itō, 1914).   49

Figure 5: Alvin Langdon Coburn, "Dancer Michio Ito" (Ito with
namahage mask), ca. 1916.   58

Figure 6: Ito Michio, drawing of Pizzicati.   63

Figure 7: Alvin Langdon Coburn, "Michio Itō performing his
Fox Dance," ca. 1916.   73

Figure 8: Alvin Langdon Coburn, "Dancer Michio Ito" (Ito with
ukiyo-e), ca. 1916.   83

Figure 9: Alvin Langdon Coburn, "Michio Itō as the Guardian of the
Well from W. B. Yeats's play *At the Hawk's Well*," 1916.   89

Figure 10: Toyo Miyatake, "Ito Michio in *Tango*."   92

Figure 11: Alfred J. Frueh, "Manhattan Nights and Exotic Entertainers,"
1917.   106

Figure 12: Nickolas Muray, "Michio Ito," ca. 1922–1930.   118

Figure 13: "Welcoming the Imperial Naval Exercises" ("Kangei teikoku
renshū kantai"). *Rafu Shimpo*, August 23, 1929.   130

Figure 14: Toyo Miyatake, Nisei girls dancing.   145

Figure 15: Toyo Miyatake, *Etenraku*, 1937.   154

Figure 16: Toyo Miyatake, *Blue Danube*, 1937.   156

Figure 17: Hollywood Bowl Publicity Collage, 1937, Sixth Week,
August 17-19-20.   157

Figure 18: Ito Michio, *Echiketto*, 11.   219

Figure 19: *Fantasy Japonica*, 1946.   224

Figure 20: *Fantasy Japonica* (?), 1946.   225

Figure 21: *Sakura Flowers*, 1947.   228

Figure 22: *Rhapsody in Blue*, 1947. 230

Figure 23: *Tabasco*, 1947. 232

Figure 24: *Rhapsody in Blue*, rehearsal, 1947. 236

Figure 25: Erniettes practicing with Ito, 1947 (?). 239

Figure 26: Jack K. Ohi, "Ito Pro Model First Round Auditions,"
August 1954. 248

Figure 27: "Sumire Models First Generation Training." 251

ACKNOWLEDGMENTS

Finishing up a book is an experience of sitting with the knowledge that I have been helped, supported, and taught by so many, far beyond reason. I offer here an insufficient expression of my thanks, and a promise to carry it forward.

My teachers have most forcefully inspired and shaped me. To Cindylisa Muñiz, who called me "Dr. Rodman" when I was just an earnest high school English student—the questions you taught me to ask are, fundamentally, the ones that guide this book. At Yale, both John Rogers and Nigel Alderman modeled how to analyze a text until it opens up, miraculously, into an entire, interconnected world. David Krasner made me a better writer and introduced me to performance theory—and made me realize I could do it too. Deb Margolin encouraged us to create a theater of desire; that simple, powerful, idea haunts this book. And my advisor, Joseph Roach, whose deft way of placing just the right book in your hands, of asking one disarming but penetrating question, and of letting his students' ambitions take them far beyond their own expectations, stands as a model for my own teaching. His continued generosity and encouragement have meant so much.

At Northwestern, I learned from professors whose teaching and research opened my eyes to what was possible in creative, deep scholarship. Dassia Posner's clear-eyed advice and firm encouragement have calmed me many times over. Elizabeth Son's sincere investment in me, and our joyful conversations, have meant so much. Tracy Davis's zeal for historical inquiry and analysis is the model I keep myself to. Harvey Young taught me that rigorous scholarship goes best with deep collegiality; he has been one of the lodestars of my academic journey. My dissertation committee's feedback then, and continued support now, forms the foundation of my work as a scholar. Andrew Leong's suggestions of citations, of interpretive paths, and of historical details has kept me busy, and expanded the possibilities for what this book could be. Christopher Bush always seemed to understand what I was trying to say, long before I knew it myself. And Susan Manning—the gift of being your advisee is hard to articulate and impossible to repay. You made it possible for me to do a seemingly impracticable project, asked the questions that continued to make it grow, and modeled how to be an innovative and conscientious scholar, teacher, colleague, friend, and parent, all at once.

A very special thanks goes to Junko Sato and Phyllis Lyons at Northwestern. Kushida Kiyomi taught me at the Inter-University Center in Yokohama; she has since become an extraordinary colleague, and it was, without a doubt, due to her interventions and support that this project was able to come to fruition, despite the pandemic and other challenges. I give you my deepest thanks.

I arrived at University of California, Irvine, to find wonderful colleagues in the Department of Drama. I am so grateful to all of you, especially Andrew Borba, Juliette Carrillo, Zach Dietz, Mike Hooker, Vinnie Olivieri, Jaymi Lee Smith, and Joel Veenstra. The department chairs, first Gary Busby and now Don Hill, have done so much to support me at UCI. The administrative staff who power our department have given me much assistance—and many laughs: Marcus Beeman, Leslie Blough, Charmayne Durham, and Ciara Holbach. My colleagues in the PhD group have modeled what it is to pursue wide-ranging academic research with curiosity, enthusiasm, and rigor; I feel lucky that you are the group I am stuck in meetings with: Ketu Katrak, Tony Kubiak, Ian Munro, Zachary Price, Bryan Reynolds, and especially Daphne Lei, who has been such a dedicated mentor. That I also get to work with the inspiring Julie Burelle, Jade Power-Sotomayor, Hentyle Yapp, Rishika Mehrishi, and Mysia Anderson at UCSD has been the icing on the cake. Thank you to my wonderful undergraduate and graduate students, especially my remarkable advisees, Chengyuan Huang, Diana Fathi, and An-Ru Chu. Colleagues in Dance—S. Ama Wray, Jennifer Fisher, Ariyan Johnson, and Alan Terricciano—have provided a special sense of connection. I am grateful for the support of first Dean Stephen Barker and now Dean Tiffany López, who have created in the Claire Trevor School of the Arts a space for artistic and academic inquiry to meet. Thanks to my fantastic colleagues in the humanities: Emily Baum, Chris Fan, David Fedman, Joe Jeon, Susan Klein, Julia Lee, Mimi Long, Theodore Martin, Annie McClanahan, Jeanne Scheper, and Bert Winther-Tamaki. A special shout-out to my festival co-conspirators, Judy Wu and Charlotte Griffin. And to Jenny Fan who rounds out our group as Women Who Eat. Amanda Swain helped me navigate the world of fellowships. And Scott Stone, who is the world's most amazing librarian: thank you

Acknowledgments

for every mislabeled news item, rare book, and historical oddity that you have tracked down for me.

Writing a book on Ito Michio has given me the chance to connect with members of his family, other Ito scholars, and dancers in his lineage. Thank you to Mary-Jean Cowell, Kevin Riordan, Carol Sorgenfrei, Yutian Wong, Emi Yagishita, and especially Carrie J. Preston who has always offered encouragement. Satoru Shimazaki gave permission to watch films of his masterclasses. Dana Tai Soon Burgess enthusiastically shared his experiences and insights into Ito's technique; our conversations became a cherished part of this work. Alan Miyatake has been so generous in sharing his grandfather's work and offered such support for this project; every photograph makes me smile with appreciation. And an immense thanks to Michele Ito, who has done so much to preserve and share her grandfather's legacy, and has been so willing to answer questions, provide resources, and encourage this work.

It has been the dream of an academic lifetime to get to work with LeAnn Fields at University of Michigan Press; I am so grateful for her faith in the project. Haley Winkle has been ready to answer every question, while Marcia LaBrenz crucially moved the book through production. Many thanks go to Sarah Berg, Sara Cohen, Danielle Coty-Fattal, and Daniel Otis. Jessica Hinds-Bond insightfully prepared the index. The manuscript's reviewers expanded and made precise the book's interventions; I am grateful for their thoughtfulness and attentiveness. David Krasner and Harvey Young were instrumental in placing the book at Michigan; thank you for your ongoing support; and to Rebecca Schneider, as well. Ellen Tilton-Cantrell saved me months by clarifying some of the book's core ideas. Maggie Lipinski, Sariel Golumb, and Mana Yamagiwa provided crucial research assistance. The incomparable Asako Katsura took charge of securing illustrations and permissions; she provided the perfect mix of enthusiasm and steely resolve that we would get this done.

Support for the research and writing of this book was provided by grants from the National Endowment for the Humanities/Japan-U.S. Friendship Commission and the NEH Open Book Program, the Fulbright Commission, the Nippon Foundation, the American Society for Theatre Research, Northwestern University, and the University of California, Irvine, which provided COVID-relief research funds, and the UCI Humanities Center, which provided a publication subvention. Librarians and archivists aided my work: Kiyoyo Pipher and Cameron Penwell at the Asian Division, Library of Congress; Yukako Tatsumi and Kara Jenkins at the Gordon W. Prange Collection, University of Maryland; Mary Khasmanyan at University of California, Santa

Barbara; the staff of the New York Public Library for the Performing Arts, and of Special Collections of Northwestern University; Steve Lacoste at the Archives of the Los Angeles Philharmonic; and Kazuno Moegi and Hasegawa Rie at the Tsubouchi Memorial Theatre Museum at Waseda University.

This book's research was also carried out during a Selected Research Project: "Foundational Research on the Ernie Pyle Theater based on the Senda Collection: A Record of Michio Ito's Dance Practice and Genre-Crossing Performances from 1946 to 1948," at the Collaborative Research Center for Theatre and Film Arts, a Joint Usage/Research Center for Theatre and Film Arts, Theatre Museum, Waseda University. It is thanks to this project that I am able to use the photographs seen in illustrations 19, 20, 22, 25, 26, and 27. The publication of these images is my responsibility; copyright owners are unknown. If readers know who owns the copyright, please contact me.

My ideas developed through the invitations to share my work and the thoughtful feedback I received over the years. Thank you to Jacqueline Shea Murphy and Linda Tomko, to Aragorn Quinn, to Elliot Mercer and SanSan Kwan, to Emily Wilcox and Katherine Mezur, and to the Japanese Arts and Globalization Works-in-Progress Retreat run by the amazing Bill Marotti. Thank you to the University of Michigan Press for permission to use portions of my earlier essay: "Imagined Choreographies: Itō Michio's Philippine's Pageant and the Transpacific Performance of Japanese Imperialism," in *Corporeal Politics: Dancing East Asia* (2020).

It's possible that my favorite part of this whole thing was the manuscript workshop, at which my all-time academic crushes gathered together and filled my brain with their brilliance, humor, and care. To Rosemary Candelario, Andrew Leong, Joshua Takano Chambers-Letson, and Satoko Shimazaki: the ways in which this book grew under your attentive suggestions cannot be overstated; your thoughts are in so many of its lines.

I owe much to the mentorship, encouragement, and help I've been given by people whose own work inspired me long before: Bruce Baird, Penny Farfan, Reginald Jackson, Anthea Kraut, SanSan Kwan, Katherine Mezur, Amy Stanley, Julia Walker, and Emily Wilcox, who has been such a champion of new work in our field. Christopher Reed sent an encouraging email out of the blue, which kept me going for months. Robin Bernstein provided career and writing advice at many crucial junctures.

Some of the deepest joys of this project were the experiences I had in Japan. Sincere thanks to Takemoto Mikio for hosting me at Waseda University; to Kodama Ryūichi for welcoming me to his seminar and providing

Acknowledgments

xv

warm support ever since; to Aoki Arisa for so many kind explanations; to Oyamada Yūki, for hours of conversation; to Karube Noriko for such meaningful help and friendship; to David Ewick for fascinating discussions and shared enthusiasms; to Misha and Jenn Kapranov and to Daniel Sternheimer for generous meals; and, from the bottom of my heart, thanks to Kazui and Takato Yabe for taking me under their wing and giving me so many precious experiences.

Academia has gifted me incredible friendships, sustaining conversations, and inspiration. I'd like to thank AB Brown, Beth Carter, Rebecca Chaleff, Emma Chubb, Tarryn Chun, Amanda Culp, Jessica Friedman, Ellen Gerdes, Lisa Kelly, Kareem Khubchandani, Hayana Kim, So-Rim Lee, Lizzie Leopold, Laura Lodewyk, Shi-Lin Loh, Jasmine Mahmoud, Patrick McKelvey, Eliot Mercer, Christine Mok, Jessica Nakamura, Ariel Nereson, VK Preston, Amy Swanson, Grace Ting, Nikki Yeboah, Soo Ryon Yoon, and Ji Hyun (Kayla) Yuh.

Life in Irvine has been—if a bit surprisingly—utterly wonderful, and that is due to the people who make this a joyful community. Thank you to the Chen-Fan Pack, who were the first to welcome us to Irvine. Mackenzie and Willie Chase, Jenn Fang and James Lamb, and the people who eat all the pancakes: Phoebe, Juniper, Selene, and James. Wine Club: Shira and Chang Liu, and James Weatherall and Cailin O'Connor, and the wine apprentices: Evenstar, Vera, wee James, Ayelet, and Noa. Allie Harrison and Russell and Remy Vernon, for the best conversations. The Chen family: Albert, Caroline, Robert, Jackson, and Emma; you are our rocks here. Beth Lopour and Dan and Nathan Shrey for outdoors adventures and silly backyard hangs. Jade, Brian, Juliet, and Rose Jenkins for garbage-truck walks and general outrage. Lee Cabatigan, and Leif and Hesper Hanson, for skiing, biking, and skateboarding escapades. Kristen, Josh, Wyatt, and Max Taylor for making us feel so much more rooted. Our unbelievable Turing Street neighbors—most especially Larisa Castillo who takes such good care of us, and Constance Steinkuehler and Kurt Squire, who are there with compassion, advice, and rounds of laughter. And to Annie and Lulu McClanahan and Theodore Martin; you've always been there, for shared dinners, commiseration, celebration, wise words, great stories, and all-around friendship.

None of this, absolutely none of it, would have been possible without the care given to our children—and to us!—by the people who have taught me how to see the whole person: Kandi Boag, Sherri Embry, Marcherie Brooks Bey, Neli Iotzova, Crystal Poole, Darlene Tsai, Rakhee Parekh, Paula Todini, Nika Vicqueneau, Yun Liao, and Julie Bookwalter. Melanie Smith has been

xvi   Acknowledgments

steadfast and inspiring to us. And the biggest thanks to April Odulio, who has cared for our family, and made such a difference, every day.

To the people who make up the rest of life and make it so full of joy: Nate Loewentheil, Michelle Bayefsky, and Sophie; Santiago Suarez, Catalina Garcia, and Tomas; Javier Puig, Holly Bui, Cinco, and Warren; Ted Fertik, Sochie Nnaemeka, Obi, and Udo; Joshua Batson; Harvey Lederman; Mark Steitz; Reggie Wilson; Justin Trigg; Paulo Uribe and Emilio; Ken Bernard, Lila, Wesley, and Vivian; and Marco Zappacosta, Fiona, Hugo, and Linguini and Parmesan. To Joanna Linzer, without whom I would not have made it through IUC. Ron Wilson stretches time and shows me all the places there are for joy. Jyana Browne, who has answered every tearful call and frantic text with a knowing laugh and wise words. Michelle Liu Carriger, who has been there every step of the way, with friendship, advice, and keen social analysis, and who, at the eleventh hour, battled UCLA's microfilm machines to get me one last image. Anndrea Mathers puts things in perspective and, with incisive humor, reminds me it's going to be okay. Dwayne Mann always makes me laugh and remember that people are the most important. Faye Gleisser put aside her own work to read so many different drafts; her belief in this project, and her friendship, have kept me going. Jordana Cox always knows the right thing to say, will drop everything for a chat, and thrills at a good stumble. Aileen Robinson will decipher everything with me late into the night; she will drive for hours and be up for anything, especially a good hug. Isabelle Smeall, Kelly Conron, Rebecca Levi, Kathryn Doyle: your calls, texts, postcards, and visits have run alongside all of this and kept me whole. Thank you for laughing at me when I get too serious, for always having a glass of wine ready, for piling onto the nearest couch for a snuggle, for breaking into dance parties at any hour of the day, for keeping track of this weird career and project, for knowing me best.

Right around when I started this project, I also gained a second family. Thank you to Paul Wolfson, Margie Peteraf, Sarah Peteraf, Ben Zlotoff, and Emma and Noah. You have put up with me working through vacations; you are the first to be indignant on my behalf whenever something goes wrong; and you have cheered me on at every step. I am beyond lucky to have your support and love.

Max, you've taught me to be game for new adventures and open to people, in all their variety. Mom and Dad, everything starts with, and has been made possible, by you. Mom: you gave me a never-ending gift—my love of books; Dad: you taught me to love poetry, but not to fall for the sound of

Acknowledgments   xvii

words if they didn't also mean something. You have both believed in me without fail, and every day, I appreciate your love more and more.

Leo and Naomi: you are the source of my deepest joy, and wildest wonder. You have begun to ask about this book, about Japan, about dance, with a tender curiosity that makes it all worth it, and makes me so excited for all that you will become. And Jesse, who has read countless drafts, talked over every point, wiped away tears, cheered at each insight and step forward, found connections and arguments I didn't know were there, taken on extra loads of housework, childcare, and errands, moved to France, moved to Japan, and who is cutting words for me as I write this . . . and that is just the book. Our life outside of it is more than I could ever have imagined; I feel so lucky and so grateful for every day. Thank you.

Introduction

The 1964 Tokyo Olympics offered a comeback—for Japan, and for the choreographer Ito Michio. In this final decade of his five-decade-long career, Ito had slipped into relative obscurity from his fame in the '20s and '30s as an internationally successful dancer and choreographer. Tapped in 1960 to direct the torch relay and opening ceremonies, for Ito the Tokyo Olympics was a chance for him to again choreograph his vision of dance as a form of embodied cosmopolitanism, and to do so for a global audience. Ito's personal goals matched those of the Olympic planning committee: the 1964 Games, the first held in Asia, were understood as Japan's chance to reintroduce itself postwar as a peaceful, modern, and cosmopolitan nation.

In Ito's plan, the torch relay—a tradition invented only for the 1936 Berlin games—would begin on Greece's Mount Olympus.[1] Athletes on foot, on camel, and on horseback would physically trace the historic Silk Road as, one after another, they carried the flame from Turkey to Syria, through Iraq, Iran, and Afghanistan. Continuing across the continent, the torch would travel down into India, to Burma and Thailand, and then proceed north through Vietnam and China, to then curve down through North and South Korea to finally arrive at Japan. Each passing of the torch would be celebrated with a recital of regional folk music and dance. Rich local histories of performance would thus complement the event's emphasis on athleticism. These presentations would culminate in the grand opening ceremony at Tokyo's Yoyogi Stadium, where massed dancing youth would direct their bodies to the arrival of the torch, inaugurating the XVIII Olympic Games.

In this vision, Ito framed dance as a mediating form of internationalism. By bringing many dance traditions together, and by encouraging these traditions to be transmitted from one body to another, and from one nation to another, Ito's plan situated dance as a practice that enables cosmopolitanism. The expansiveness of Ito's plan—the transport of performance and fire over 10,000 kilometers—produced a geography unified through the passage of moving bodies: a cohesive Asia, a joined East and West, and a Japan situated as both endpoint and mediator of this journey. Even as it proclaimed a new role for Japan on the world stage, Ito's vision was also a palimpsest of Olympic and Japanese history, reviving choreographies and ideologies of imperialism and fascism that the 1964 Games meant to leave behind.

The Silk Road theme mined an influential intellectual tradition from the early twentieth century that sought to determine the origins of the Japanese people. Today, it is common to hear that Japan is an island nation, isolated and homogenous. This commonplace, in fact, only became an accepted truth in the postwar period, as a rationalization for reducing the country's territory to its four main islands following its defeat in World War II. But during Ito's lifetime, and even well before, in the Meiji Era (1868–1912), the question of Japan's essential character was an actively debated issue, and one that was crucial to the nation's growing imperial agenda. In this period, two competing theories emerged.[2] The "mixed-nation theory" (*kongō minzoku kokka-ron*) originated in the mid-1800s with Western historians and anthropologists describing the Japanese as an immigrant/conquering nation; this perspective was soon absorbed by Japanese intellectuals as the primary model to argue for Japan's assimilative capacities. In the 1880s, an anti-Western backlash precipitated the birth of a competing "homogenous-nation theory" (*tan'itsu minzoku kokka*), which said that the Japanese nation was coterminous with "Japanese people"—who were understood as the original inhabitants of the archipelago and the direct ancestors of contemporary Japanese. Even as the homogenous-nation theory gained adherents, the mixed-nation theory remained predominant throughout much of the first half of the twentieth century, even as Japan moved into its totalitarian period. Indeed, one appeal of the mixed-nation theory was its utility in justifying imperialism and the incorporation of other Asian nations under Japanese rule.

In support of the mixed-nation theory, many intellectuals took the Silk Road as historic evidence that Japan's fundamental essence was syncretic and intercultural, rather than isolated and homogenous. Writers such as Okakura Tenshin (Kakuzō) and Watsuji Tetsurō turned to the eighth-century capital of Nara, which they identified as the Silk Road's endpoint. Nara is a city of innumerable Buddhist temples and statuary, all revealing material and stylistic influence from across Asia. Nara thus represented the paradigmatic cosmopolitan city, a site of collection and recombination of the innumerable goods, cultural practices, and languages that traveled along the passage connecting Europe and Asia.[3] As an ancient capital, Nara represented Japan's

Introduction 3

broader, historic capacity as the storehouse of Asian heritage—as Okakura famously termed it, "a museum of Asiatic civilization."[4] For these early
twentieth-century intellectuals, the Silk Road thus connected their contemporary desires to understand Japan as a syncretic nation to an authorizing,
cosmopolitan past.

The ongoing persuasiveness of the mixed-nation theory was its assertion
that Japan's internationalist periods were never new, but rather, a recurring
part of the nation's history and essence. By mining a particular moment
of Japan's regional history (the Nara period), it produced a "tradition" that
could be called on to justify many different constructions of Japan's modern
national character. Thus, when Japan began its breakneck project of modernization following its forcible opening to US trade by Commodore Perry
in 1854, the syncretic argument suggested that in absorbing new Western
technologies and practices, Japan was actually being faithful to an essential
"Japan-ness." And when Japan embarked on its imperial project of conquest
and administration of other Asian nations, the mixed-nation theory justified
this agenda, and argued for the assimilation of Japan's colonized subjects. Ito's
use of the Silk Road theme for the 1964 Olympics resuscitated this tradition
to conjure a Japan that had risen from its wartime isolation and defeat to
recover its cosmopolitan essence.

Even as Ito's Olympic plan turned to Japan's distant past in order to break
with its recent militarism, it nevertheless evoked the canceled 1940 Olympics
and Japan's alignment with the Axis powers. The very ritual of the torch relay
was a still-fresh innovation: it had originated at the 1936 Berlin Olympics as
part of the effort to choreograph Hitler's legitimacy and Germany's mytho-
historic ties to Greece. The designer of the relay, Carl Diem, was invested
in perpetuating it as an ongoing Olympic tradition. The next Games were
scheduled to be held in Tokyo in 1940, and Diem offered his assistance to
the Tokyo Olympic Organizing Committee. The plan he presented was for
a torch relay along the historic Silk Road. The planning committee eagerly
adopted Diem's proposal, even though the war with China meant that his
proposed route would already be unfeasible. Indeed, in July 1938, the Tokyo
Games were canceled, as Japan's government chose to devote all available
resources to the war in China.[5] Ito's plan, which hewed closely to Diem's
original scheme, thus recycled an explicitly imperialist, if not fascist, vision,
even as it claimed to patch a rupture in Japanese history. Ito's adoption of the
Silk Road theme thus linked Japan's postwar present to multiple moments of
the nation's past—the cosmopolitanism of the Nara period, the era of early

twentieth-century modernization, and the years of Japanese imperialism during the Asia-Pacific War.

This book begins with Ito's 1964 Olympic plans because they exemplify several themes that will continue to appear: cosmopolitanism as a practice of performance; the relationship between choreographic aesthetics and imperial histories; and the way that Ito's self-promotion was frequently achieved through promotion of "Japan"—itself a mutable and contested idea. Ito's Olympic proposal also highlights the necessity of engaging plans and ideas, even when, or especially when, they do not come to fruition. Indeed, one more thing should be said about Ito's Olympic plans: they never happened. On November 6, 1961, Ito Michio died of a cerebral hemorrhage. When the Olympics took place three years later, instead of Ito's relay of human bodies and cultural performances, an airplane flew the torch from Athens to Tokyo, a journey that was both cheaper and usefully symbolic of Japan's technological and industrial capabilities, an insistence that the nation would now fling itself into the future, rather than re-perform the bodies of its past. Ito's plan—unrealized, and probably impossible to have been carried out in any case—was thus a fantasy, the first of many that this book will consider.

Accounting for Fantasy

A trip to Egypt, a friendship with Vaslav Nijinsky, a meeting with President Harding—such stories have bedeviled scholars seeking to pin down an "accurate" narrative of Ito's life. Indeed, Ito's younger brother Senda Koreya ultimately wrote a corrective biographical preface for the Japanese publication of the first book written about Ito, by his student Helen Caldwell. And as Ito's Japanese biographer, Fujita Fujio, wrote, "In publishing this book, the most challenging aspect was distinguishing between Michio's dreams and reality."[6] Rather than pushing these stories and schemes to the side as false leads, I foreground these fabrications and unrealized activities as *fantasies*—as the creative acts of imagination that sustained Ito's life and career.

Ito is important. We seem to know that much. He has been the subject of articles, book chapters, and popular publications in English and Japanese. Whether because of the people he knew, the people he taught, the projects he contributed to, or the phenomena he can be made to stand for, he has become a subject of increasing interest, both within academia and outside of it. "Recovered" to American modern dance history first by one of his dance

Introduction 5

students, Helen Caldwell, and then by Mary-Jean Cowell and Satoru Shimazaki, within an "East-West" rubric, he has since been identified as a figure who might be claimed as central to multiple disciplines: transnational modernism by Carrie Preston and Kevin Riordan, Asian American dance studies by Yutian Wong, and Japanese theater and dance studies by Carol Sorgenfrei, Midori Takeishi, and Emi Yagishita.[7] But generic, linguistic, and disciplinary boundaries have partitioned his career, precluding a fuller appreciation of the continuities that persist across these divides, and of the ways in which all these terms—"East"/ "West"/ "the Orient," "modernism," "modern dance," "Asian American," and "Japan"—were being actively constructed during his life, a fluxity in which he played a part. This book is indebted to all of this previous scholarship, and rather than looking to supersede this tradition of a many-faceted Ito with a "comprehensive" account, I want to suggest that we take this fracturing as symptomatic of Ito's fundamental elusiveness; he is a figure, in both his life and many afterlives, who evades being pinned down. I propose here that one reason for this is the substantial role that fantasy played in his life—and as I will offer later in this introduction, that fantasy might also be a powerful method for engaging this elusiveness.

Fantasy threads together the personal, the collective, and the theatrical, and it is in these conjunctions that I find it a productive framework for thinking about Ito. As Jacqueline Rose observes in her book *States of Fantasy*, people usually first think of fantasy as the licentious flights that a mind takes in private, into uninvited and impermissible territories. In common speech, fantasy suggests the illicit and the personal. In fact, writes Rose, fantasy is deeply intertwined with "the question of how subjects tie themselves ethically to each other and enter a socially viable world."[8] That is, fantasy is how we construct a sense of self within the actual material world of social and political relations, and it is, therefore, an activity in which the personal and the collective are intimately tied. How this mooring takes place is a question addressed by Jean Laplanche and Jean-Bertrand Pontalis, who characterize fantasy not as the *object* of desire, but as the theatrical scenario or setting for an exploration of desire: "But the fantasm is not the object of desire, it is a scene. In the fantasm, the fantasm itself, the subject does not aim at an object or its sign, he figures himself in the sequence of images."[9] Crucial here is the sense of being watched, and watching oneself being watched. These ideas, of fantasy as that which binds the individual to their social world, and as a theatrical scene in which the individual performs themself, are central to how I think about Ito.

Theater is not only a metaphor for the stagedness of fantasy. It also helps us understand fantasy's relationship to what is usually meant by "reality." While some may think of the theater as a world of imagination, operating at a remove, those who work in and study the theater know that it is intimately and intricately enmeshed with the world it seems to offer an escape from. So too, with fantasy, as Rose, following Freud, explains: in contrast to dreams, which disintegrate in the unconscious, "fantasy is always heading for the world it only appears to have left behind."[10] Fantasy, like the theater, only *seems* to be a world apart. The importance of both of these practices is articulated by Rose: "we build in fantasy our claim to solidity in the world."[11] Fantasy is how we know ourselves, how we perform ourselves and come to think of those performances as constitutive of ourselves. Ito's fantasies—his invented anecdotes, unrealized projects, and quixotic affiliations—though perhaps not the "real" or the "what happened" of his life, were the things that made it solid.

Another way of saying this is: in common parlance, fantasy often means escapism. Like fantasy, escapism offers solace and delusion, two things that can keep people going—for better or worse. But what I want to delineate with fantasy is an aspect of likeliness. While escapism offers the pleasure of imagining the impossible, fantasy involves a belief in its attainability, and fantasy takes place amid conditions that make its realization feel possible. Ito's fabrications, unrealized projects, political associations, and performances of self are fantasies because they hovered, tantalizingly, near to the "real,"—and indeed, sometimes were indistinguishable from the "real." In this likeliness, fantasy provided the ground of his artistic career, and perhaps, his survival.

I think of Ito's fantasies as forming into a few distinct strands. The stories Ito invented make up one strand of my focus. In their imaginative richness, we see Ito as he wanted to see himself. Moreover, as compensatory stories, by which Ito wrote himself into various histories, we get a sense of the contours of his own sense of isolation and loss. A second strand consists of the unrealized or failed artistic projects that exist only on the pages of his notebooks. Working in the medium of live performance, Ito was always hampered by budgets, deadlines, talent, political situations, and the grandeur of his own ambitions. But if these projects are subjected to the same process of performance reconstruction that is a primary method for historical research in performance-related fields, then they fill out important aspects of his artistic oeuvre.

Third, Ito's fantasies offer us a glimpse into his affiliations, and the affiliations he desired. By affiliation, I mean something between individual and

Introduction 7

group identity; these are concepts that describe a particular stance or way of relating to the world, such as modernism, Pan-Asianism, or cosmopolitanism. These are abstract terms, usually thought of as ideologies. I want us to think of them instead as fantasies, not because they describe chimerical desires, but because recognizing them as fantasies allows us to understand why so many people have invested in these and related abstractions. Affiliative fantasies provide a sense of belonging; they articulate personal desires through channels of camaraderie and collectivity. This use of fantasy, then, is in line with Neferti Tadiar's use of the term, building on Slavoj Žižek, to highlight the "subjective dimension" and "desiring or libidinal character" of the actual practices "that determine as well as comprise much of the social life and modern history of nations."[12]

And finally, the work of dance-making involves fantasy. Several of Ito's pieces were explicitly dramaturgical fantasies—pieces are set in faraway imagined places, such as courtly Europe, or "Lotus Land"; they depict storybook characters, such as the "Little Shepherdess"; and they imagine, frequently on a large scale, triumphant national histories. But dance-making, both in process and performance, is also a particular form of fantasy-making, where the act of choreography and embodiment offers a vision of an alternative world. This aspect of fantasy has much in common with the concept of "world-making"—in its reparative dimensions, but also in its equally possible hegemonic permutations. Ito's dances often imagined various utopic visions; but they also provided opportunities for the embodiment and reproduction of racial stereotypes, national-imperial mythologies, and the mixture of aestheticism and entertainment that frequently allows for a plausible deniability of the consequences of such representations.

If Ito produced numerous fantasies, he was also, in ways both compelling and disturbing, the object of many fantasies. As a Japanese subject living and working across Europe, the US, and Japan, during a period in which Japan was the prompt for romanticized and dehumanizing imaginaries, Ito was the screen for his collaborators', patrons', and spectators' many desires—desires in which his own body and work could never be teased apart from the national, racial, and imperial significations assigned it. Fantasy helps us understand the complex oscillation of Ito's reception, because it both recognizes him as the objectified object of others' desires, and invites us to consider the desires he pursued, and satisfied, in the process of engaging those around him.

Some may connect my attention to fantasy with psychoanalysis and the work of Freud, Lacan, Žižek, and Laplanche and Pontalis. Certainly, some of the most generative theorizations of fantasy have come from that field, because, as Leslie Bow observes, part of psychoanalysis's value has been its "theorizing from the individual to the collective."[13] Bow's gloss highlights how fantasy has illuminated understandings of national imaginaries, as in the works of Lauren Berlant and Jacqueline Rose, but also points to its centrality in Asian American literary analysis, where it has served as a more or less explicit framework in the psychoanalytic readings carried out by theorists such as Bow, Juliana Chang, Anne Anlin Cheng, David Eng, and Karen Shimakawa.[14] In my engagement with Asian American studies scholarship in particular, this book builds on the foundational work of these engagements with psychoanalysis, though it does not, ultimately, pursue it as a line of inquiry.

Instead, I want to shift out of the head and into the body; I want to think about how the body fantasizes. When Ito stretched his arms out from his body, again and again, like a whirling vortex in his famous dance *Pizzicati*, what longings are carried from his torso, across his shoulders, arms, elbows, wrists, and tensely reaching hands? When Ito walked down New York's Fifth Avenue, what fantasies were elaborated in his jaunty steps, in his gently swaying shoulders, and eyes that only seemed to be directed ahead, but were always achingly, minutely aware of the looks he drew from those around him? Across this book, I insist that the body is not merely a reflection of people's private fantasies; it is not simply an object on which fantasies are projected. Instead, I insist, the body might also be a powerful site of fantasy. Following Susan Foster, Randy Martin, André Lepecki, and Rebekah Kowal, among many others in dance studies, the body *does* things. But here, instead of thinking about this doing as a kind of performativity, an effecting of a change, I suggest that what the body does is to become, itself, the "setting for the elaboration of desire." The body realizes the fantasy, physically, if fleetingly, in the motions, poses, tensions, and slacknesses it assumes.

Constructing a Biography

Although I will spend much of this book thinking about Ito Michio's fantasies, it is worth observing that a simple outline of his life already reads as a kind of fantastical narrative of international border-crossing, political maneuvering, and artistic hustling. Ito's background reveals that his eager engagement with the West, his attraction to the arts, and his comfort moving in elite circles

Introduction   9

were all proclivities patterned by his family. Ito's father, Tamekichi, was born in Isematsusaka to a line of doctors, and studied physics and architecture in San Francisco in the mid-1880s, where he also converted to Christianity. When he returned to Japan in 1888, he specialized in Western architecture, made Western-style furniture, and also worked as a dry cleaner. Tamekichi made a name for himself as the first designer of earthquake-resistant houses in Japan, by inventively merging Japanese house design and techniques of joinery with the American technology of nails and bolts.[15] Just as ingenious was his self-presentation as the "American Architect Itō Tamekichi," demonstrating the same flair for self-promotion that his son Michio was to exhibit. Ito's mother, Kimie, née Iijima, came from an elite family. Kimie's older brother, Iijima Isao, had studied physiology at Tokyo University, the nation's premier institution, and then spent three years studying at Leipzig University. He saw in Tamekichi a fellow Western-educated, "modern" Japanese youth, and so set the couple up.

Tamekichi and Kimie had nine children; first a daughter, Yoshiko (1889), then in 1891 a son, Kōichi, who died a month after birth. Michio, the third child, was born on April 13, 1893. Three boys followed: Kanae (1895), Yūji (1897), and Kisaku (1899). Next came another girl, Nobuko (1902), and then Kunio (1904), who is best known by his professional name, Senda Koreya. Another boy, Tadao, arrived in 1907. In the early 1900s, Tamekichi had an affair with another woman, Tanaka Namiji, who bore three children who were given the Itō family name: a girl, Aiko (1905), and two boys, Teiryō (1908) and Ousuke (1911). The entire family was remarkably oriented toward the arts; all of the male children who survived into adulthood went into the theater, music, or architecture professions; with the exception of Yoshiko, who married a prominent army general, the other female children also married artists and performers.

From a young age, Ito demonstrated notable musical talent. When he graduated from the private mission school Aoyama Gakuin, his eldest sister's husband, the army general Furushō Motō, invited Ito to stay with him in Germany to pursue his musical studies. In preparation for this opportunity, Kimie determined that Ito should attend the Tokyo Music School in Ueno, Tokyo. The family purchased a piano and hired the famous Japanese opera soprano Miura Tamaki of *Madame Butterfly* fame, as well as the foreign music teachers Welkmeister and Junger. Ito read *Hedda Gabler* and *When We Dead Awaken* with his German teacher, and met with Chiba Shūho, a scholar of German literature who had recently been in Germany and seen numerous theater performances during his stay. Miura Tamaki also invited Ito, along with Ishii Baku, Shimizu Kintarō, and Komori Toshi, to take *nihon buyō* (traditional Japanese dance) lessons from Wakayagi Kichitoyo. These peers, especially Ishii Baku and Komori Toshi, were to become future collaborators with Ito, as they made their own trips to Europe and the US.

Ito's period of preparation plunged him into Tokyo's contemporary theater world; with hindsight, it is evident that he was working in the milieu that would be recognized as the heart of Japan's emerging modern theater movement. In July of 1911, Miura Tamaki left her position at the Tokyo Music School to join the newly organized opera section of the Imperial Theatre as a lead actress. Miura secured roles for Ito in a few of the theater's opera productions. These were *Cavaliera Rusticana* in December 1911, *Yuya* in February 1912, and Welkmeister's *Shakka* (Siddhartha) in June 1912. Just before he left, Ito helped found the *shingeki* troupe Toridesha with friends from the Tokyo Higher Normal School. The group included Murata Minoru, Kishida Tatsuya, and Uno Shirō. On October 15, 1912, they gave a trial performance of Maurice Maeterlinck's *L'interieur* and Nagata Mikihiko's *Maihime Dariā* (The Dancing Girl Dahlia) at the Seiyōken in Tsukiji, attended by important figures of Japan's modern theater movement, such as the translator, critic, and playwright Tsubouchi Shoyō and the director Osanai Kaoru.[16] Ito later described the performance as a "youthful effort"—they paired Maeterlinck's story with staging heavily influenced by Edward Gordon Craig, whose theater essays they had been reading. The group members had also just seen Gerhart Hauptmann's *Lonely Lives* and Maeterlinck's *Death of Tintagiles*; they felt their production was an effort to clear similar stylistic ground for Japanese modern theater. Ito's Toridesha experience upends common assumptions that his arrival in Europe was the moment of exposure to an entirely new world of modern performance. The group's fluency with the works of modern dramatists and Craig's emerging stage theories reveal the familiarity of early twentieth-century Japanese artists with European modernist experiments, and the vibrancy of the Tokyo modern theater scene. And yet, drawn by the excitement and cultural capital of training in Europe, Ito felt compelled to leave, and on November 6, 1912, he sailed from Yokohama.

Ito landed in Marseilles on December 23, 1912, and arrived in Berlin five days later. At this chronological point, Ito's accounts of his own activities begin to include his narrative fantasies. These will be discussed in detail in chapter 1, but here I want to stress that while his memoirs give the impression that he was alone in Europe, making his way as the sole and exceptional

Introduction

Japanese artist, in fact he had the company of many other Japanese youths throughout his European period. On his way to Europe, he traveled with Saitō Kazō and Ishibashi Katsurō; the latter had been a middle school classmate.[17] Saitō, a graduate of the design department of the Tokyo Art School, was traveling to Europe with the express purpose of joining the composer Yamada Kōsaku to visit the new Jaques-Dalcroze Institute for Eurythmics at Hellerau. Yamada, also a graduate of the Tokyo Music School, was just finishing his studies at Berlin's National Music Conservatory, and he was at the center of a group of young Japanese men all studying music there. Saitō introduced Ito to Yamada, who became a lifelong friend, and whose own interest in Jaques-Dalcroze effectively changed the course of Ito's career. While in Berlin, Ito saw a performance of the Ballets Russes, at which Anna Pavlova—though not Vaslav Nijinsky—performed. After a brief stay in Leipzig, where he studied vocalization and German pronunciation, Ito enrolled at the Institute, and began his studies there on August 12, 1913.

Ito studied for a year in Hellerau, learning the fundamentals of the eurythmic method and enjoying the school's idyllic mix of internationalism and artistic collaboration. This experience served as the basis not only for his own dance method, but for his abiding belief in art as a utopic force for remaking societies and for achieving world peace. Ito's time at the Institute was interrupted by World War I; he escaped Germany on August 14, 1914, a week before Japan joined the Allied bloc, and traveled to London in the company of other fleeing Japanese. On August 16, he arrived in London.

Ito's two years in London gave him the artistic and social cachet that undergirded the rest of his career. Early on, he booked some performances at the popular Coliseum theater, and also caught the attention of elite hostesses, such as Lady Ottoline Morrell and Lady Maud Cunard, for whom he provided dinner party entertainment. Then the American poet Ezra Pound, who was working on a set of translations of noh plays begun by Ernest Fenollosa, sought out Ito and induced him to perform some noh dances. Again, Ito was not alone in this, but put together a demonstration with the painter Kume Tamijurō and the writer Kōri Torahiko, two out of the good number of young Japanese men carrying out artistic and educational sojourns in London at the time. It was Ito alone, however, who joined Pound and the Irish poet W. B. Yeats in mounting a production of Yeats's play *At the Hawk's Well*. With two salon performances on April 2 and 4, 1916, this production became one of the signal events in histories of Anglo-modernism, and it gave Ito, who created the role of the Hawk, a lasting cultural imprimatur.

As war encroached on life in London, Ito again moved, arriving in New York on August 13, 1916. There, Ito developed a repertoire of "oriental" and interpretive dances, consolidated his dance method, and taught in studios across the city. He also participated in several Broadway productions, ranging from the 1923 *Greenwich Village Follies, The Mikado* (1927), and *Madame Butterfly* (1928), to his own *Pinwheel Revel* (1922) and his debuting the role of the Witch Doctor in Eugene O'Neill's *Emperor Jones* (1920). Alongside these endeavors, he was joined by friends from Japan in the spring and summer of 1918: the dancer Komori Toshi, and his friend Yamada Kōsaku, who collaborated with Ito on productions of the noh *Tamura* at the Neighborhood Playhouse, a staging of *At the Hawk's Well* with new music written by Yamada at the Greenwich Village Theatre, and a series of dance concerts experimenting with the Japanese modern dance form, the "dance poem."

Ito's personal life developed alongside and intertwined with his professional work. In 1921, he was joined by one of his younger brothers, the singer Yūji, who took part in many of Ito's projects, and also established his own career in production, costumes, and props at Radio City Music Hall. Yūji would later, in 1934, marry Teiko Ono, an important American-born dancer in her own right, who then collaborated with Michio in Los Angeles, and also trained Yuriko Kikuchi, who was to become an important figure in Martha Graham's company (with whom Ito also worked in New York). Ito further rooted himself in the US when, on April 6, 1923, he married one of his troupe's dancers, Hazel Wright, and on October 10, 1923, their first son, Donald was born; Gerald (Jerry) was born July 12, 1927. In 1929, Ito carried out a cross-country tour with his troupe and family, and once in California, they decided to stay.

Ito spent the 1930s in Los Angeles, where he took advantage of the region's bid to become a cultural center by advocating for modern dance as a force for community and art. He established a series of dance studios across Southern California, and staged several large-scale "dance symphonies" at the Hollywood and Rose Bowls, while continuing to offer smaller dance concerts. He also worked in film, playing roles in *Dawn of the East* (1921), *Booloo* (1938), *Spawn of the North* (1938), and consulting and choreographing for *No, No, Nanette* (1930), *Madame Butterfly* (1932), and *The Sunset Murder Case* (1941). Meanwhile, Ito built a relationship with the Japanese immigrant community in Southern California, working in tandem with local elites to foster experiences of integration for the Nisei (second generation) through his dance lessons and productions. While in Califor-

Introduction   13

nia, Ito facilitated the visits of other Japanese artists: his brother Kisaku came in 1929; Ito organized the US tour of Tsutsui Tokujirō's *shimpa* troupe in 1930; and for his own 1937 dance symphony at the Hollywood Bowl, Ito arranged for the classical conductor Konoe Hidemaro (and brother to then prime minister Konoe Fumimaro) to join the production. Ito's increasing engagement with the Japanese community seemed mirrored in his domestic life; in 1936 he was divorced from Hazel Wright and married Ozawa Tsuyako, a Japanese woman originally from Sapporo, Hokkaido. During this decade, Ito took three trips to Japan: in 1931, 1939–40, and 1940–41. In 1934 he also toured with his company to Mexico City.

When Japan bombed Pearl Harbor, Ito's vibrant life in California was interrupted; in the nighttime hours following the bombing, the FBI raided his Hollywood home and arrested him. Donald went to live with some relatives of Hazel Wright, while Jerry went to New York, where he was looked after by Ito's brother Yūji and his wife Teiko. Ito was interned as an "enemy alien," and spent the next two years in a series of Department of Justice Camps: Fort Missoula, MN, Fort Sill, OK, Camp Livingston, LA, and finally Santa Fe, NM, where he was reunited with Tsuyako, who had been incarcerated at Heart Mountain, WY. The two requested repatriation, and in September 1943, they sailed to Japan, with a stop in Goa as part of a prisoner exchange, arriving in Yokohama in November 1943.

Ito spent the remaining years of the war working on behalf of the Japanese imperial project and war effort. With the support of friends and high-ranking officials he founded an institute for performing arts across the "Co-Prosperity Sphere": the Greater East Asia Stage Arts Research Institute. While this effort was, with the exception of one production, entirely unrealized, in his planning documents, Ito outlined an immense organization facilitating theater and dance performance across Asia and cultivating cultural exchange. This plan culminated with his proposal for a mass history pageant to celebrate the Philippines's "independence" from US dominion via the benevolence of Japanese imperialism.

On August 15, 1945, Japan surrendered. As the US-led Allied Occupation moved in, Ito was well positioned to mediate between the occupiers and occupied. He soon began working at the Ernie Pyle Theatre (the requisitioned Tokyo Takarazuka theater), which was the primary entertainment venue for Allied service personnel and billed as the "Radio City Music Hall of the East." There he directed, choreographed, and produced numerous shows, including *Fantasy Japonica* (1946), *The Mikado* (1946), *Tabasco* (1947), and *Rhap-*

sody in Blue (1947). He also helped rebuild theater for Japanese audiences, working on productions outside the Ernie Pyle, such as *Tokyo Carmen* with Hattori Ryōichi and Kasagi Shizuko (1947). During this period, Ito reopened his dance studio and began training a new generation of modern dancers. In 1946, he was also reunited with Gerald, who was serving in the US Navy. As the Occupation wound down, Ito turned his focus to training fashion models, choreographing ice-skating spectaculars, and organizing beauty pageants— all activities in which he could offer dance as a foundation for these high-resourced spheres of cultural production. In 1960, Ito was selected to produce the torch relay and opening ceremonies for the 1964 Tokyo Olympics—the first to be held in Asia. But these plans never materialized, due to his death on November 6, 1961.

Fantasy as Methodology

Beyond the biographical sketch I just offered, more comprehensive accounts can be found in English in Mary-Jean Cowell's forthcoming book, and in Japanese in Fujita Fujio's biography. And, as noted earlier, there has been a proliferation of scholarship about Ito across a variety of disciplines. This growing body of literature provides a wealth of information about and interpretations of Ito that work in similar ways as this book's cover photograph. In this image, taken by Toyo Miyatake, Ito stands in the spotlight, an object of attention. The spotlight is theatrical; Ito is someone who made his life through performance. But the spotlight is also constraining; it holds Ito in its range, and especially given his street clothes, offers a reminder that Ito frequently performed under surveillance. Behind Ito, his shadow looms, distinctly him, but merging with the background into a kind of obscurity. No matter the spotlights we shine on Ito, he remains elusive.

This elusiveness is overdetermined. It is a commonplace that dance, Ito's primary artistic medium, is fundamentally ephemeral.[18] On a concrete level, this means that although we have photographs of his dances, and some of his choreographies have been passed down as inherited repertoire in the bodies of his students and their students, many of his dances remain impossible to reproduce. In any case, none of these are *Ito* dancing. Even during his life, the apparent inaccessibility of dance worked in tandem with orientalist paradigms of inscrutability; for some of his contemporaries, Ito appeared as a cipher for mutually reinforcing notions of both dance and "the Orient" as states of metaphorical escape.

Introduction 15

Ito's elusiveness is also an effect of his apparent adaptability. He had a remarkable ability to make himself into what others seemed to want, whether as the projected screen for Euro-American spectators' orientalist desires, or as a propaganda producer for the Japanese imperial government. This hustler's instinct was accompanied by a sort of willful utopian blindness; his articulated intentions are consistently about producing beauty, self-understanding, and world peace. Ito's opportunism and romanticism have made him a difficult historical subject, seemingly aligned with all the "wrong" things—orientalism, totalitarianism—but with so much idealism that it is tempting to ask: did he know what he was doing?

What I'm getting at is this: there is a problem with Ito's archival traces, and this problem is not the tension between archive and repertoire, or a paucity of documentation, or even censorship or self-censorship (though he was subject to both). Unlike those of many marginalized figures, and in seeming contrast to the ephemerality of his dances, Ito's archives are quite robust. Across repositories in the US and Japan, there is an abundant trail of Ito's material traces: scrapbooks, letters, personal notebooks, reviews, rehearsal schedules, choreographic notations, scripts and scenarios, budget sheets, business plans, and numerous photographs. In addition, Ito wrote numerous magazine and newspaper articles. Seemingly most useful of all are Ito's four book-length memoirs. And yet, these books are filled with fabricated anecdotes, profiles of other famous artists, and descriptions of American and Japanese customs. The pages deflect more than they reveal. Ito's elusiveness is due not to lack of archive but, rather, to an abundance of material that does not reveal what it seems to. *This* is the challenge that Ito exemplifies—a concern that has been overshadowed in the necessary and timely discourses within the humanities that have, over the last several decades, taken up the violence of the archive and its silences. What, alternatively, is to be done with abundance mistaken as fact, that is actually fantasy? This book seeks a critical engagement with that.

If these documents cannot always, or cannot necessarily, be taken as direct documentation of Ito's life, what, then, are they? And more importantly, what do they do? For whom? To what ends? This book posits that they can themselves be taken as performances, and as part of Ito's lifelong performance of self. "Performance," as both a concept and a discipline, is vast, and has been assigned varying definitions. The one I'll use here is the gloss that Ju Yon Kim offers on Erving Goffman's approach: performance is "an individual asking an audience to believe in her or his presentation."[19] While, as Kim notes, Goffman's model seems to involve an assumption of intentionality, I do not suggest that all of Ito's performances were calculated, or even deliberate. But they do all involve a solicitation of a spectator, as a partner in the production of desire. Many of Ito's presentations of self were embodied—in his formal, onstage appearances, in his public persona, and even in the most mundane moments of daily life. But Ito's presentations of self also extend to his many writings, published and unpublished, in which he projects a vision of himself toward a set of imagined spectators—imagined, or fantasized, even when they are "real."

In line with this, and following performance studies scholar Shane Vogel's discussion of Lena Horne's autobiography, I read Ito's books and other writings not "as document[s] of performance history . . . [but] as instance[s] of performance theory."[20] Ito's memoirs, precisely in their fabrications, utopian political statements, and cultural essentialisms, point us to the performance strategies by which he constructed a fantasy of himself as a cosmopolitan, as a modernist artist, and as a cultural mediator—a fantasy that both he and many others invested in. Vogel continues, "I do not necessarily assume that she [Horne] is only writing out of self-interest or self-promotion, but that she offers in her performances some insight into sexual and racial subject formations in modern American culture."[21] Ito was assuredly writing out of self-interest and self-promotion, an activity at which he excelled. But in precisely this vein, Ito's writings reveal what it means for a Japanese male dancer living and performing across Europe, the US, and Japan in the early and mid-twentieth century, to promote himself, and what such promotion required. Ito, then, was always performing—which is not to suggest that there was some true, essential Ito "behind" the performance, nor to suggest that Ito was some kind of empty person, "nothing but a performance." Ito's performances, inevitable and self-sustaining, were his ties to the world around him; they were the fantasies that allowed him to feel that he belonged. In parallel, the archival abundance of Ito's material traces, with all their misdirection, fabrication, incompleteness, and unrealizability, is what allows me to pursue, to reconstruct, to imagine, Ito's fantasies.

Ito's performances, and the fantasies they encoded, are not, as the title of this book suggests, only his; they are also mine, and many others'. To write about Ito's fantasies, and the fantasies he elicited in others, I must also engage in fantasy. And so, I propose fantasy as both a scholarly methodology suited to constructing a history of a career that is impossible to reconstruct, and as a conceptual tool that animates the problems of fiction within abundance—the navigation of uncertainty as a manifestation of desire.

Introduction   17

Take Ito's Olympics plans. The sketch with which I began details a performance that never took place. It is, nevertheless, one that I can provisionally reconstruct from Ito's writings, from newspaper articles, and from my knowledge of his working method and other choreographic endeavors. Here we are in the well-established realm of performance reconstruction as a methodology of history writing. By "reconstruction" I do not mean the physical reenactment of Ito's dances—although I am indebted to the dancers and scholars who have created these reperformances. Rather, I follow dance scholar Susan Manning, who, working as both traditional historian and literary critic, "construct[s] Wigman's dances as structures for the interaction of performer and spectator."[22] The methodology of performance reconstruction, developed in theater, dance, and performance studies, is a way to piece together, through material archival traces, what a performance might have looked like. But performances are not only a matter of lines recited, choreography carried out, costumes worn, and staging realized. Performances are also about the frisson between performers and the audience, and the erotic circuits of energy that animate performances, and reverberate beyond the time of the performance itself. That is, performances can be fantasies, and it is these fantasies that I seek to reconstruct.

A fantasy reconstruction of Ito's Olympics plans, then, involves not only a sketch of what he wanted the torch relay and opening ceremonies to look like, but also imagines what desires those plans encoded. As Ito traveled along with the procession, did he perhaps instruct each athlete to pass the torch with bodily motions borrowed from his own dance method positions, thereby choreographing a broad absorption of his technique into numerous nondancer bodies, and even, through the newsreels shown of the events, out into the population at large? Dance, then, and his own method in particular, could be integrated into daily movement at the scale of the entire globe, an expansiveness that would finally match the scope of Ito's ambitions. Perhaps Ito would meet with heads of state, and local business at each stop, using his charisma to negotiate sticky moments, as municipalities jostled for recognition. Here is Ito the mediator, the cosmopolitan, whose lifetime of living in translation allows him to perform as an artistic diplomatic. These are, as Laplanche and Pontalis have it, some of the desires that Ito's Olympic fantasy offered a setting for. These are the desires, the fantasies of self, with which Ito could construct a sense of solidity in the world.

Fantasy, as a methodology, offers a possible rubric for how to decide what to include in an account of someone's life, and how to narrate that life as a field of possibilities rather than interpretive conclusions. As I've indicated, fantasy insists that we consider both fabrications and unrealized projects as significant pieces of evidence in assembling a story of Ito's careers. It thus offers a possible methodological response to the problem that Pannill Camp has argued the "performance nonevent" poses to theater history; it offers a way of delineating the "constituents of a possible world."[23] Fantasy as a methodology opens up the scope of what counts as part of Ito's oeuvre and alters how we draw connections between his various activities. Fantasy is a way of taking Ito seriously, despite the nearly inconceivable and absurd commitments he had to utopic political programs and a cosmopolitan persona. And fantasy is a tool of imaginative reconstruction, one that both lives within and enlivens the fragments and ephemera of his careers, while embracing the partial, provisional, and personal nature of this rendering.

In the racialized, imperial-nationalistic circumstances of Ito's career, there are ethical implications to reconstruction, certainly as an embodied pursuit, but also in the engagement of Ito's archive. I seek to follow VK Preston's process of writing "speculative and critical reimaginings that reveal [repetition's] fissures and exclusions and set the past askew."[24] Likewise, my use of fantasy has much in common with recent articulations of "fabulation," especially in my disinterest in "setting the record straight" for someone such as Ito, who was constantly enjoined to be both legible and inscrutable; as well as in my attention to fabrication, gossip, and utopian scheming as activities of great consequence. Fabulation, particularly in Tavia Nyong'o's speculative approach, understands Black performance and art as an inventive rearrangement of the false, producing, as he puts it, "a sense of the incompossible, mingling what was with what might have been."[25] It is to address, then, the problems of Ito's archive—of the ephemerality of performance, of global racial hierarchies, and of the instability and unapproachability of the past—that I pursue fantasy as a methodology. This is an approach that owes much to Amy Stanley's *Stranger in the Shogun's City*, in which her extensive archival research has enabled her not to assert a singular historical interpretation, but rather to provide the grounds for imagining a field of possibilities for her protagonist Tsuneno's feelings, thoughts, and experiences, as well as for the conclusions we can draw from this mode of historiography.[26] Fantasy is a way of delineating the possibilities of someone's life.

In performance, watching and being watched are continuous activities, carried out by the formal performers and the audience alike. It is this feeling, of watching and being watched, of sensing, of hearing, of kinesthetically

Introduction   19

engaging, that my approach seeks to inhabit, to trace, and to imagine. Fantasy, as a methodology, invites us to imagine what movement does, what a body elicits in others, so that we can enter into the heady oscillation of seeing, sensing, and performing that structures the circulation of desire. Within this book, the circulation of desire is historical and specific: the global exchange of different forms of embodied orientalism, the celebration of cosmopolitanism and the bodily ambiguity that such avowals of itineracy seemed to allow, the hope that political belonging might be achieved through choreographic assimilation, and more.

But across time and place, fantasy is also categorically about failure. Where performance studies and related fields have invested in performativity as a kind of promise of performance's value,[27] fantasy does not promise an altering of our world, or of possibilities for being. Instead, fantasy as a methodology traces the flights of imagination that launch people, and that may even sustain them across a career, but that also involve disappointed desire, and the abortion of flight. This is one of the ways in which it differs from fabulation; while fabulation operates in the subjunctive, fantasy does not transport us to a different temporality. Instead, fantasy aims at the indicative, and it is there that it falters, shatters, and fails.

In the stead of Ito's unrealized projects, misdirected utopias, and insufficient performances of self, there are traces and there is persistence. Indeed, to attend to the complexity of Ito's fantasies is to attend to his *persistence*, and the persistence of his traces, far beyond his concrete biography, and at times to stand in direct contention with its seeming concreteness. Attending to the fantasies of Ito Michio (his, mine, and others') means sifting up some of the traces of his work, illuminating threads of performance genealogies that are with us today, when we watch the Olympic ceremonies, or eat lunch in Los Angeles's Little Tokyo neighborhood, or shop in a Japanese department store. These fantasies, and the modes of embodiment through which Ito pursued them, continue to percolate and persist, whispering reminders that we are all living amid the traces of the world in which Ito Michio's careers unfolded.

Cosmopolitanism, Orientalism, Empire

As I have elaborated, fantasy is a way of narrating an individual's life and the desires that shape it. And fantasy mediates the individual and the collective. But fantasy also operates on multiple scales; some fantasies are, in and of themselves, collective, involving vast numbers of people. I understand cosmopolitanism and orientalism as two such large-scale fantasies, that were central to Ito's performance of self. And both of these were inextricably bound up in what was perhaps the overarching political structure of Ito's life: empire.

By way of demonstrating my fantasy methodology, and of delineating the forces of cosmopolitanism, orientalism, and empire in Ito's life, let's start with two photographs. The first shows Ito, standing in three-quarters rotation, face front, arms resting in front of him with his hands meeting at his middle. It is the position of formal portraiture, and it matches his outfit—a men's suit from the Empire period. In what looks to be a light gray or blue wool tailcoat, with large silk cuffs, a voluminously tied lace cravat, and a lace handkerchief, Ito here poses as a European aristocrat.[28] This image is not how many people expect to see him. The most commonly reproduced photographs show Ito in some kind of Japanese dress, or in his more typical dance outfits of tunics, loose pants cinched at the ankle, or flowing robes. Such images confirm what seem to be the most obvious, stable facts about Ito—he was Japanese; he was a modern dancer. This image tells us something else.

For one, it tells us that Ito loved to dress up. Part of the appeal of a performance career for him was, assuredly, the pleasure of costume—thick materials, ornate accessories, the way one's comportment transforms under the contours of a particular dress, the way costume induces a kind of bodily fantasizing, paving the way for the acts of imagination that follow. But this image also tells us some particular things about the fantasies Ito was drawn to embody. Because, while this costume references a particular geography (Europe), it is also a historic mélange: the large-cuff sleeves, the oversized cufflink, the clawhammer tailcoat all point to different time periods of male fashion. This referential hodgepodge is characteristic of the genre of "oriental dance"; to see it in this presentation of "European-ness" underlines Ito's agnostic approach to staging history. This costume then, stands for a general vision of cultivated elegance, of debonair worldliness, and of high social class in a political world order in which Europe was ascendant. It represents an abstract idea of aristocratic cosmopolitanism.

As far as I can tell, Ito did not actually dance in this costume. The photograph is by Ito's friend, the photographer Toyo Miyatake, and was probably taken in 1937 in Los Angeles, as part of the publicity and events surrounding Ito's staging of *Blue Danube* at the Hollywood Bowl. In performance, the *Blue Danube* dancers wore costumes of the same overall design as this one, though in satin rather than Ito's wool. I wonder, did Ito wear this outfit not only for

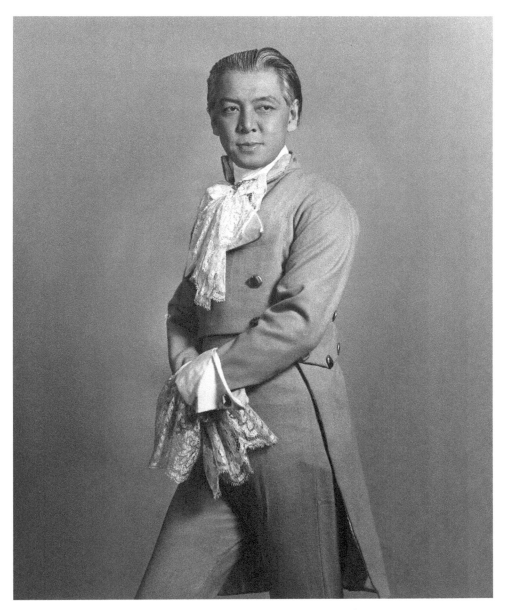

Fig. 1. Ito Michio in *Blue Danube* costume. Photo by Toyo Miyatake, 1937. Toyo Miyatake Dance Collection, courtesy of Alan Miyatake.

studio photographs, but also at the Hollywood Bowl, perhaps as he introduced the program, or as he greeted patrons and fellow artists, presenting himself as the maestro of the fantasy world they were about to see? Perhaps dressing as a European aristocrat allowed Ito to embody the role of cultural mediator that he so frequently enjoyed playing. So too, in the ease and confidence with which he wears these clothes, perhaps Ito is asserting his fundamental compatibility with European (and American) values, at a time when Japan was yet again being framed as unequivocally foreign, and inscrutable to Western mores. That is, if viewers then, as now, felt a moment of surprise at seeing Ito in this costume, then perhaps what Ito wanted to assert was his fundamental belonging in this fantasy, and his access to the European history that this costume signifies. This was a sense of access that began with his own early education at the Jaques-Dalcroze Institute in Hellerau, Germany, or even before, at the point when he decided to leave his classmates who were busy carrying out experiments in Japanese modern theater and instead, to travel to Germany for opera training. The fantasy that this photograph depicts, then, is a condensation of all these longings, crystallized in a moment of costume performance.

In the second photograph, Ito wears a different costume, and seemingly registers a different set of fantasies. His legs are in a wide, turned-out stance, bent at the knees; he is barefoot. His right hand rests on his right hip, arm akimbo, while his left arm flips the position, rising up from the elbow, with the palm stretched out to face the ceiling. He is bare-chested, with a length of fabric that sinews around his right arm, behind his neck and under his left armpit, rising with his left arm so that the rest of the fabric rests in his left palm. He wears dark, billowy pants gathered at the ankles. Another length of fabric is wrapped around and tied at his waist, with the ends hanging down in front. On his head he wears a *gelung* headpiece found in Balinese *wayang wong*.[29]

This photograph tells us something else about Ito's fantasies—as well as the ones projected on him by his spectators, patrons, and collaborators. The photograph might correlate to *Javanese Temple Dance* (1928). Like the *Blue Danube* costume, this one contains a jumble of referents and artistic license: while the headpiece resembles that worn by male *alus*-type characters in *wayang wong*, and the fabrics are Javanese-style dance scarves, the use of two scarves, and the wrapping of the upper one around the arm, undermines its functionality. The pantaloons, meanwhile, seem derived from Indian dance. This photograph can be taken to represent Ito's prolific involvement in the subgenre of "oriental dance," which, alongside "interpretive dance" made up

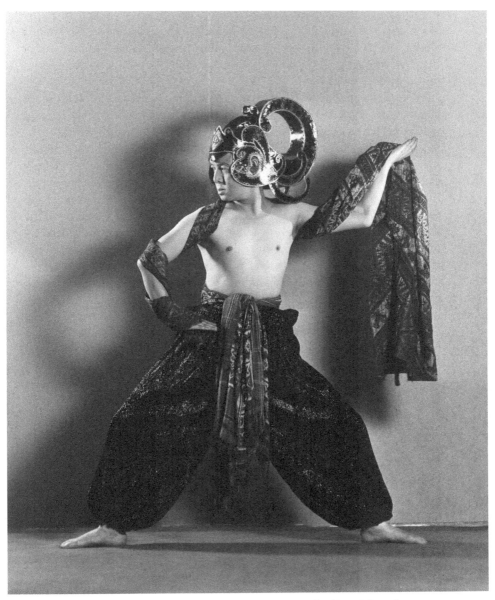

Fig. 2. Ito Michio in Javanese dance. Photo by Toyo Miyatake, Toyo Miyatake Dance Collection, courtesy of Alan Miyatake.

the set of concert dance-making practices in the US that were known, in the 1910s, '20s and '30s as "the art of the dance." In the 1940s, these two strands would become known as "ethnic dance" and "modern dance"—though today the term "modern dance" is also used as an umbrella to describe this entire range of dance practices.

Ito's participation in the genre of "oriental dance" reveals a complex set of negotiations. "Oriental dance" was predominantly executed by white women (and some white men) who, as Yutian Wong writes, identified "with Orientalist imagery in an effort to articulate new models for middle-class femininity."[30] But dancers who today would be identified as, or themselves identify as, Asian were expected to perform their own cultural knowledge within this genre, and to offer their own bodies as authenticating examples for the genre at large. Further, many dancers, including Ito, did not specialize in the dance of a particular region or tradition, but rather, performed a wide array of danced referents, putatively embodying a diversity of Asian countries and traditions, all subsumed under the fantasy of "the Orient." In this mélange, the fact that Ito was Japanese precipitated a slippage wrought by white Western racialization: he was not only Japanese; he was also "oriental." What we see in this photograph is exactly this generalizing abstraction; Ito was not only expected to perform Japanese on European and US stages, but was imagined to have a particular capacity to embody any and all "oriental" traditions, and to be taken as a representative of the fantasy of the Orient at large.

But if this photo is suggestive of the ways in which Ito was abjected into US orientalism, it also shows, like the *Blue Danube* photograph, Ito's own enjoyment of costume, his love of theatricality, and most pertinent, how stage orientalism provided particularly enticing opportunities to pursue these pleasures. Ito's fascination with stage orientalism began early, in Japan, in June 1912 (if not before), when he performed in a production of Welkmeister's *Siddhartha* at the Imperial Theatre. The production boasted sumptuous costumes and opulent scenery that transported spectators to the scene of Buddhism's founding in India.[31] It was, for Ito, a dazzling and enticing introduction to stage orientalism, the theatrical evocation of an exotic racial fantasy.

This photograph offers a glimpse of some of Ito's ongoing desires that circulated through his engagement with orientalism. Perhaps, as he shifted his body into this pose's angles, he found pleasure, or relief, in exploring an "exotic" that he did not feel was reducible to his own culture, his own Japaneseness. Perhaps the heavy headpiece made him more conscious of all his body's movement, and in that consciousness, he found a renewed sense of

Introduction   25

dancerly precision that was useful to his practice at large. Perhaps he enjoyed drawing the audience's fascinated glances to his body, but with a layer of remove, a layer of protection provided by the "oriental" screen. Stage orientalism, with its sumptuous costumes, extravagant scenery, and specified movement vocabularies, seems to have allowed Ito access to a world of fantasy.

The fantasies I have just read into these photographs are important not only because they might offer insights into Ito. Ito's fantasies, and Ito more generally, are important because he gives us a way to understand broader patterns of cultural formation, and the stories and desires that upheld these structures. Take cosmopolitanism, for instance. What I just sketched above was a range of fantasies about cosmopolitanism, about being cosmopolitan, that appear specific to Ito. But cosmopolitanism was, in fact, a very relevant, and precisely defined, concept for Japan as a whole. As both John Namjun Kim and Naoki Sakai have traced, cosmopolitanism became a key term for many of imperial Japan's philosophers, particularly those belonging to the Kyoto School and the imperial think tank, the *Shōwa Kenkyūkai*.[32] For these philosophers, such as Miki Kiyoshi and Tanabe Hajime, Japan's cosmopolitanism manifested in the ongoing creation of a unified East Asia under Japanese rule. Sakai details one instance of this imperializing cosmopolitanism in a 1943 speech by Tanabe, delivered to an audience of volunteer soldier students about to leave for battle. In Tanabe's attempt to incite patriotic spirit, he formulated the Japanese nation-state as a universal entity; it could contain vast diversity, and make all that diversity "Japanese." As Sakai notes, the audience certainly included students from the colonies, who were interpellated as belonging to the nation just as much as their Japanese peers. Japanese imperialism thus proceeded not only through extraordinary violence, but also through a credo of universalism and free will—a norm of imperial cosmopolitanism. When Ito styled himself as a cosmopolitan, then, it was not only a sign of his desire to be included in Euro-American elite culture, or only of his own relatively elite position, both in Japan and then among other Japanese immigrants in the US, or only a sign of his longing to be accepted as a modernist artist. It was also a posture that put him directly in relation to Japan's own avowed ideologies, its own imperial designs, its own desire to be seen as equal to the Western powers.

If cosmopolitanism was thus a fantasy that was at once deeply personal and also intimately related to the geopolitical ambitions of the country of Ito's birth, orientalism offers an amplified version of this tension. For if Ito frequently experienced orientalism as a structure used to demean, exoticize, and abstract him while he attempted to live and work in Europe and the US, orientalism was also a paradigm that had developed a specifically Japanese variant, known as *tōyō*. As Stefan Tanaka has explained, *tōyō* was a discourse and historiographic endeavor to produce for Japan its own "orient"—a discursive entity that included the rest of Asia, but also an earlier, premodern Japan.[33] This paradigm allowed Japan to claim itself as both part of Asia, but also as developmentally apart from it, and thus, its natural leader. One central contention of this book is that when Ito is only portrayed as the object of white orientalism, we miss the fact that long before he arrived in Europe, Ito was well versed in orientalism from the position of a subject of imperial Japan. Likewise, when Ito participated in the genre of "oriental dance," he did so not only as an abjected Asian male dancer working in the US, but also as a subject of imperial Japan. We should, then, understand his "oriental dances" as, at least in part, enacting Japan's own imperial epistemology and fantasy of cosmopolitan assimilation through the paradigm of *tōyō*.

Japanese imperialism was central to Ito's attachments to the fantasies of cosmopolitanism and orientalism; it was a force that took shape in the decades before his birth, and that, along with the United States's own imperial inclinations, structured Ito's life. In 1868, Japan performatively became a nation-state, as the Meiji Restoration returned the emperor to the seat of governmental power in Edo-turned-Tokyo. A year later, Japan embarked upon its imperial project by incorporating Ezo, the northern land of the Ainu, as Hokkaido. The southern Ryūkyū islands soon became Okinawa; in 1895 Japan colonized Taiwan, and by 1910 had annexed Korea by winning the Russo-Japanese war. This victory also resulted in possession of the Karafuto (South Sakalin) and the Kwantung Leased Territory, which provided control of the Southern Manchuria railway lines, and thus a base for the founding of Manchukuo. These territorial expansions were Japan's clear-eyed response to Western imperialism, seen both in the threats by which Commodore Perry had "opened" Japan in 1853, and in China's own disastrous experience. Japan's leaders concluded that in order to protect its sovereignty and be recognized by Western nations as an equal, it must transform into an imperial power itself.

These early conquests involved uneasy incorporations of new populations into Japan. For instance, although the Ainu were defined as Japanese in 1872, they were marked in family registries as "former native" and were excluded from the military until the 1890s. Korea and Taiwan, meanwhile, were subject to the *kōminka* movement—the formal administrative effort to transform colonized peoples into imperial subjects, an effort crucial to the mobilization

Introduction 27

of soldiers and laborers for the war, but one that was dogged by the fear that these people could not, or would not truly become loyal Japanese.[34] From the start, the question of what, or who, could be considered "Japanese" vexed the project of expansion.

Alongside its agenda of territorial expansion, Japan encouraged its citizens to strike out across the globe, seeking their fortunes and acting as unofficial (legally unrecognized) imperial outposts.[35] Other governments, especially the US, responded with anxiety and racial animosity. This could be seen in the proclaimed necessity of the US's annexation of the Hawaiian Islands, as well as in the many exclusionary laws aimed at stemming the "Yellow Peril." Such laws were first aimed at Chinese laborers, but when Congress sought to restrict Japanese entry, it had to negotiate more carefully, given Japan's rising geopolitical power. The resulting 1907-08 "Gentlemen's Agreements" restricted the immigration of Japanese laborers but allowed entry to the wives and children of already settled Japanese, and to an economic class of migrants (students, merchants, tourists, agriculturalist) who had enough money and educational status that they would not become physical laborers in the US.

It was under the terms of the Gentlemen's Agreements that Ito first arrived in the US, and then was able lawfully to travel outside the US and to return to it in 1931, 1934, 1940, and 1941. Indeed, Ito's entry to the US—from the capitals of Europe rather than from Japan, and as an artist rather than a laborer—marks his passage as an exception to the standard narratives of Asian migration to the US, in which working-class migrants arrived as contracted laborers, indentured to farms on the West Coast. And yet, Ito's story is not so exceptional. Several thousand Japanese, including students, artists, merchants, and businessmen, entered under the same terms.[36]

Once Ito settled in the US, he was increasingly subject to the anti-Asian laws that proliferated during his time there. For instance, when Hazel Wright married Ito in 1923, the Cable Act of 1922 meant that she lost her standing and rights as a US citizen. Likewise, the 1922 Ozawa supreme court case confirmed that Japanese could not be considered white, and therefore, Ito could not hope to gain citizenship. The Immigration Act of 1924 (Johnson-Reed), meanwhile, closed the remaining immigration loopholes provided by the Gentlemen's Agreements. Throughout this period, California was a driver of anti-Asian policy. By the time Ito arrived in Los Angeles, in 1929, his first-generation peers had lost the possibility of owning land, or even of entering into lending or cropping agreements; likewise, they had seen any possibility of legal protection or naturalization dismantled.

At the same time that Ito navigated anti-Asian laws while living in the US, he also remained aware of—and in some respects, a beneficiary of—Japan's growing imperial project. In September 1931, Japan launched a full-scale invasion of Manchuria, and established the puppet state of Manchukuo shortly after. In July 1937, the Second Sino-Japanese War officially began after the Marco Polo Bridge Incident, with the Japanese army spreading through inner Mongolia down to Shanghai. In 1938, Japan announced the "New Order in East Asia," and in 1940, as Japan began to press into South and Southeast Asia, it declared the creation of the Greater East Asia Co-Prosperity Sphere, a fantasy of an Asia unified economically and culturally under Japanese leadership. At the peak of its territorial control, Japan claimed Korea, Taiwan, Manchuria, much of China, Hong Kong, Vietnam, Cambodia, Laos, British New Guinea, the Philippines, Malaya, and Brunei as part of its empire, expansion that was carried out simultaneously through extraordinary violence and various forms of cultural suasion.

Empire, then, and its cultural fantasies of cosmopolitanism and orientalism, determined many of the opportunities as well as the experiences of racialization and dislocation that structured Ito's life. While Japanese and US imperialism exerted the greatest force in structuring Ito's life, Britain and Germany's imperial projects also bore upon Ito—whether as partial models for Japan's nation-state building which Ito experienced in his youth, or in the foundation of the Jaques-Dalcroze Institute, and again in the interruptions caused by World War I and Japan's alliance with Germany in World War II. Empire was, in many ways, the fantasy (though immensely real) setting within which Ito had to play out his desires, and to perform himself into history.

On Disciplines, Diacritics, Terminology, and Translation

The problem begins with his name. Should I write Ito or Itō? And should I write Ito Michio, or Michio Ito? This is not simply a choice about transliteration (for much of his life, English texts used "Itow"); it is instead a choice about disciplinary alignment, about how I ultimately see and understand my subject, even as I aim to maintain his elusiveness. The correct pronunciation of his name is with a long o, rendered as Itō in accordance with the Revised Hepburn system of transliteration that is standard. And in Japanese, last names are given first. These two points would indicate that I ought to render his name Itō Michio, in closest accordance with the Japanese.

Introduction 29

And yet, in the subtle signals that shape the boundaries of disciplines and tell potential readers whether they should be interested in a given topic, "Itō Michio" suggests not only that he was Japanese, but that this is a study intended only, or primarily, for readers invested in Japanese studies. It suggests to readers that my subject is someone who properly "belongs" to Japan. The question of national belonging, and of which national histories claim him, is one that percolates throughout this book, and haunted him in life as well. Indeed, in the Japanese press, his name was often rendered in katakana, the Japanese syllabary used for foreign loan words and for visual emphasis—a sign that, even in Japan, Ito stood out. Likewise, his friends, such as Yamada Kōsaku, wrote of him in Japanese with his given name first—another way of marking him as part of a larger world. Taking these cues and considerations, in this book, I render his name Ito Michio (no diacritics, but with Japanese name order).

The question of Ito's name is emblematic of the larger question of this book's disciplinary straddling of Asian studies and Asian American studies, and my position that it is necessary to intertwine these fields to approach the historical and theoretical insights that a study of Ito can offer. The necessity of bringing these fields together is not just, as Takashi Fujitani writes, "that the civil and military leaders of the United States and Japan were much more cognizant of such global connections and comparabilities than are most conventional historians, and acted accordingly."[37] It is also because, like Ito, many, many people found themselves subjected not only to one of these nation-state empires, but to both, especially during the war and its aftermath.[38] Not only did Ito experience, and position himself in relation to, both these empires, he believed them to be deeply alike, and fundamentally enmeshed, and this belief was central to his unrelenting willful utopianism, and what frequently appears to be an overt political blindness. So too, as I have sketched above, was Ito's navigation of orientalism deeply imbricated in both American and Japanese politics. This point pertains to a related, though frequently disavowed, phenomenon, of the relationship between white orientalist and Asian American literature, as Josephine Park has explored.[39]

This book, then, draws from and intertwines the disciplines of both Asian and Asian American studies, even as it acknowledges the historic conditions surrounding each discipline's distinct formation, and the ongoing usefulness of their separate positions.[40] In doing so, and with attention to the needs of Ito's story, this book situates itself within the emerging field of Global Asias. In her 2021 presidential address to the Association for Asian Studies, Christine Yano advocates for a Global Asias paradigm by tracing the international and artistic itineraries of the hit song, "Ue o muite arukō" (known around the world as "Sukiyaki"). As Yano's analysis demonstrates, Global Asias is both a thematic and an interpretive approach that is not only about how peoples, objects, performances circulate, but about the oddities, improvisations, and unresolved contradictions of that circulation. Global Asias is a way of thinking about the desires for legibility, for economic success, and for political efficacy that *move* people. As Yano writes: "Global Asias takes mobility as a given and asks that we look at the meanings, privileges, and conflicts given to movement itself."[41] Yano's words get at the crux of why the field of Global Asias holds utility for this book. But in turn, I want to offer Ito's example as a reminder that "mobility" and "movement" are not only metaphors, or simply ways of describing relocation. They are the words that literally describe Ito's dancing—the work by which he was able to travel across the globe. Ito's dances themselves contain and produce the "meanings, privileges, and conflicts" that Yano cites. We can see this in the tension between Ito's German-derived method and his audience's expectations for Japanese-derived gestures; and we can see this in the sense of aesthetic supremacy granted to much of Ito's work because of its association with Japan. Most crucially, the body itself, in motion, is a site for these things. In the juxtaposition of head and torso, each twisting in opposite directions; in the stillness of feet while the arms dart wildly; in the body moving sometimes with the music and sometimes against it, dance was not simply the vehicle for Ito's global circulation; it was, itself, constitutive of it.

If Ito, in motion, across the globe and on the stage, is paradigmatic of a broader phenomenon of the contingencies and contradictions of global circulation, then the language that I must use to narrate his story—and, indeed, the language used in his own time—is also a site of shifting meanings and historical change. I highlight here a few of the terms that are crucial to this study, but whose usage requires some explanation.

Tōyō (the East/the Orient) is a term that has particular importance because I use it to try to make sense of how Ito negotiated Western orientalism, not simply as an abjectifying and objectifying ideology that he was subjected to, but as the English translation of a concept with which he was already quite familiar. It is with this key parallelism in mind that I use the terms "the Orient" and "oriental" in this book. But a few more words are in order: "The Orient" is a fantasy. It is a fantasy, tied to a putative geography, in service of an ideology of global hierarchies and Western, white dominance.

Introduction 31

"Oriental" is not simply the adjectival form, but a grammatical application that assigns particular things, and particular people, to that fantasy.

The words "the Orient" and "oriental" were the dominant terms in use during the time Ito lived in Europe and the US; they are the terms that we find in writings about him, as well as in his own usage. However, when I use them in this study, it is not to correspond to contemporaneous usage; rather, it is to continually foreground the fantasy aspect of this term, and, crucially, Ito's deep attraction to the concept it represents, as a "future orientated" longing[42]—a longing that cannot be disentangled from his longing for *tōyō*, the Japanese counterpart of this fantasy. When I am not aiming to highlight the theatrical, libidinal fantasy formation that these terms register, I use "Asia"/"Asian."

Between *tōyō* and "the Orient" sat Japan—or so it claimed. Ito helps to problematize what gets called "Japanese," and why. In common usage, "Japanese," as an adjective describing cultural products, indicates that something is "from" Japan, derived from Japanese cultural traditions, or is created by someone who is Japanese. Implicitly in contrast to "Japanese" is "japoniste" (or the term with more commercial connotations, "japonaiserie"). "Japoniste" has been used to describe the artistic products made by artists and artisans in Europe and the US (and sometimes, elsewhere) that are inspired by Japan, but not, so the distinction goes, made by people who are Japanese. But, as Arata Isozaki has argued, the question of "Japan-ness," both in Japan and abroad, is inextricably bound up with Japan's awareness of itself in relation to an international audience.[43] In this study, therefore, I often refer to Ito's artistic projects as "japoniste." I do so for two primary reasons: (1) to flag that Ito's Japan-engaged choreographies worked to produce Japan as a fantasy, in ways that were similar to the works of white Euro-American artists, and were also part of a much larger phenomenon within Japan of selling "Japan" abroad; and (2) to continually move away from the notion that there is some authentic "Japanese" essence—an idea that was very much in vogue at the time, but that also remains quite powerful today.

The complicated, questionable nature of Ito's relationship to these identificatory labels reminds us of the unstable nature of all of these terms, what Kandice Chuh has highlighted as their "internal contradiction."[44] As Chuh observes of the term "Asian American": "'Asian American,' because it is a term *in difference from itself*—at once making a claim of achieved subjectivity and referring to the impossibility of that achievement—deconstructs itself, is itself deconstruction."[45] As Chuh highlights, "Asian American" was the term that community

32 FANTASIES OF ITO MICHIO

members explicitly claimed to replace "Oriental." A generation earlier, however, Ito had embraced "Oriental" as a way to claim his own subjectivity. As I have suggested, Ito is elusive, hard to pin down. But what his complicated relationship to all these terms illuminates is that subjectivity, at large, is hard to pin down, and though it frequently appears to reside under one identificatory label or another, in the end, it exceeds (and eludes) them all. [46]

Following Japanese language convention, when referring to Japanese people, I generally write the last name first, except for individuals who are broadly well-known in English via a First Name/Last Name order. I use macrons to indicate Japanese long vowels, except for place names and very common Japanese words that have either been absorbed into English without diacritical marks, or under a different spelling (e.g., Tokyo and noh, rather than Tōkyō and nō). Likewise, I use macrons for Japanese names of individuals who predominantly lived in Japan (but drop them for someone like Toyo Miyatake, whose name is given in English order, and without macrons). I give the kanji for Japanese names, productions, and other significant concepts in the index, alongside the romaji transliteration by which they appear in the main text. All translations are my own, unless otherwise indicated. However, an immense thanks is due to Kushida Kiyomi, Asako Katsura, and Andrew Leong, whose suggestions, edits, and general support have been so valuable to me.

The Pageant of Chapters

Ito transformed himself in relationship to each place he resided, with a responsiveness to local conditions that enabled him to nearly always perform some version of what his audiences desired. The term of his assimilation to each place, however, was always his exceptionalism (artistic, racial, national), and thus he was also always performing for himself, constituting himself in accordance with his own desires. Place was an organizing category of Ito's life, and so it is of this book; each chapter covers one locale, and proceeds more or less according to the chronology of his movement from one place to another. An exception is chapter 5, which covers the same period as chapter 4, but in focusing on Ito's trips abroad, pulls out additional thematics and employs different methodologies.

Chapter 1 addresses Ito's two years in Germany to consider how both the fabricated and the "real" can serve as a kind of fantasy. I propose that the stories Ito told about this period are documents of the desires Ito held

Introduction 33

for himself—to be recognized as a modernist artist, a cosmopolitan, and as a Japanese subject connected to other Asian people. Alongside these narratives, Ito's actual experience at the Jaques Dalcroze Institute for Eurythmics in Hellerau, Germany, was a kind of realized fantasy. At Hellerau, Ito learned the eurythmic technique that formed the basis of his dance method; I discuss its influence, both choreographically and ideologically, and offer a description of Ito's technique. The Dalcroze Institute is also where Ito learned to "perform Japanese" as a strategy of simultaneous singularity and representativeness. In his first months at the school, Ito experienced an isolation that I call "racial arrhythmia," a sense of being out of time and place that I liken to the "arrhythmia" that the school's method was supposed to resolve in its students, and, theoretically, in all of German society. Ito found that the resolution to his racial arrhythmia was to join the school's international community as one of its constitutive elements. This performance of Japaneseness, as the predicate of difference, but also inclusion, helped establish his mode of cosmopolitanism thereafter.

Chapter 2 contends that the quality of compressed, internalized energy that is a hallmark of Ito's choreography emerged from his engagement with two artistic movements during his time in London (1914–1916): the Japanese dance poem movement, and London-based vorticism. Ito's relationship to the dance poem movement, begun by his two close friends, Yamada Kōsaku and Ishii Baku, has been almost entirely overlooked. I argue that Ito understood many of his experiments in England, and his own developing aesthetic, as part of Japan's developing modern dance movement, even as he remained abroad. I then highlight Ito's relationship with Ezra Pound, to suggest that Ito sought to assert dance as the foremost vorticist medium (and thus, himself as a key theorist and practitioner of vorticism). In the chapter's last section, two photographs taken by Alvin Langdon Coburn—one of Ito in a female-type noh kimono, and the other in his Hawk's costume for *At the Hawk's Well*—serve as provocations to fantasize about how Ito created a space for his own desires, and constructed a persona that reflected them, even as he was always a compelling object of desire for those around him.

In New York, the site of chapter 3, Ito choreographed the bulk of his solo repertoire, developed his teaching practice, and established himself as a general promoter of modern dance. I understand Ito's activities in the late teens and 1920s through the framework of the japoniste collection, an interpretive lens in which desire—the collection's motivating affect—emerges as a key analytic. In New York, Ito engaged with Japanese performance forms, other

Japanese artists, and even the small local Japanese immigrant community in ways that should be understood as "japoniste"—creative engagements that drew power from the widespread notion of Japan's aesthetic universalism. This framework gave Ito's work an artistic sheen even when he worked in other genres or the commercial theater (such as his 1922 Broadway revue, *Pinwheel Revel*). As a corollary to his japoniste activities, Ito was interpellated into the genre of "oriental dance," which, I argue, both was a site of abjection and, in its resonances with Japan's own orientalist paradigm of *tōyō*, also affirmed his position as an imperial subject. Ito's embrace of both japoniste and orientalist dances entailed a slippage that later in his career reappeared as a commitment to the ideology of Pan-Asianism. I close with a consideration of the desire of the fetish; a photograph by Nickolas Muray and Ito's own narrative of his relationship with the dancer Vaslav Nijinsky prompt a reading of Ito as the desired object who collects desires in turn.

When Ito moved in 1929 to Los Angeles, he entered a region intent on growing its cultural reputation—and one that had a substantial Japanese population. Working with Nisei (second-generation) dancers, Ito gave special lessons and included them in his large-scale dance symphonies. These activities were part of Ito's involvement in the broader community arts movement, whereby he asserted dance, and local Japanese, as significant to the formation of local political community. If Ito's efforts at danced integration cohered with goals held by both local white progressives and some of the Issei elite, it is harder to know what these opportunities meant for his young dancers, who were captured in a photograph by Toyo Miyatake. I wonder about the possibilities that Ito's dances might have held for these Nisei, for whom the promises of citizenship and belonging were to dissolve within the decade. Likewise, Ito's own example complicated the idea of integration; the concept of *kokutai*, or national body, suggests how both American and Japanese assimilative projects hinged on absorbing foreign-marked Others—who could then appear to threaten the nation, as Ito and his students would be charged with only a few years later.

Chapter 5 examines the four trips out of the US that Ito took during his time in California: to Japan in 1931, to Mexico in 1934, again to Japan from November 1939 to the summer of 1940, and once more over the winter of 1940–41. By focusing on Ito's reception in each place, I consider how Ito's audiences interpellated him as a figure for their own fantasies of national embodiment. Employing Eiichiro Azuma's concept of Japan's borderless empire, I argue that across these trips, Ito suggested that Japan's imperial expansion could be a corporeal phenomenon, accomplished through his cos-

Introduction 35

mopolitan career and choreographic embodiment of other racial-national forms. In each site, Ito's masculinity became a site for discursive contestation, as reviewers saw in him an embodiment of what a nation such as Japan could achieve—or conversely, how it might be threatened from within.

Chapter 6 takes Ito's wartime writings as the basis for considering his turn to the ideology of Pan-Asianism—and as an opportunity to entangle the disciplines of Asian American and Asian studies, toward the field of Global Asias. I maintain that moving between Ito's experience of internment *and* his participation in Japan's imperial effort requires an integrated historiography. I offer an account of Ito's FBI file and the purported reasons for his internment, and a discussion of his wartime notebooks' brief glimpses into his life in the internment camps. After repatriation, Ito spent the war's final two years under the desperate conditions of Japan's total war mobilization. Under these circumstances, Ito drew up—and submitted to government officials—plans for a massive Pan-Asian performance organization, the Greater East Asia Stage Arts Research Institute, among which are proposals for a mass festival pageant to be staged in the Philippines. I read these documents as evidence of Ito's persistent fantasy of an artistic cosmopolitanism. These documents also occasion a demonstration of the methodology of fantasy: the Philippines festival pageant never took place; but its unrealized status allows us to recognize unacknowledged themes that were central to his career (such as the pageant), and to reconsider what counts in his choreographic oeuvre.

Chapter 7 covers the Allied Occupation of Japan and Ito's postwar activities to show how Ito remade his own career by offering dance as a practice by which war-weary Japanese could remake themselves in this tumultuous period. Ito's work of corporeal rejuvenation was particularly aimed at Japanese young women—at the major entertainment venue for Allied troops, the Ernie Pyle Theatre, in Japanese women's magazines, and in courses offered for aspiring models. The tension inherent in the Allied Occupation lies in the tantalizing, but always somewhat illusory promises of democracy, subjecthood, and freedom that the Americans appeared to offer, and that so many Japanese, in many different ways, pursued. That these are yet another set of fantasies makes clear the peculiar form of performance that Ito had to teach his students: in the Occupation, he, and they, not only sought to remake themselves, but had to do so *as a performance*, for Occupation authorities and the world at large. Thus Ito's lessons during this period all involve instruction in self-consciousness, as a performance strategy that does not resist or subvert the gaze of others, but responsively produces oneself as part of—but never completely coterminous with, others' desires.

CHAPTER ONE

Japanese Exemplarity and Exceptionalism

Germany, 1912–1914

Michio is inseparable from his dreams.

So writes the composer Yamada Kōsaku in his foreword to *A Classroom for Beauty* (Utsukushiku naru kyōshitsu, 1956), one of Ito's postwar autobiographies.[1] Yamada was both a friend and mentor (*sempai*) to Ito. He was the central figure of Ito's first six months in Europe, keeping an eye on him in Berlin, introducing him to other artists, and ultimately leading him to the Jaques-Dalcroze Institute in Hellerau. So it's a bit curious that Yamada doesn't appear at all in Ito's recollections of his time in Germany, not even in the book for which Ito asked his friend to write the foreword. In Ito's narrative, he instead goes to Paris, and then to Egypt, befriending famous French modernists and an inspiring Egyptian teacher. And yet, Yamada doesn't seem offended by this erasure. Like so many of Ito's students and friends, and the scholars who have engaged his life, Yamada is captivated, a willing audience for his charismatic friend and the stories he told.

Michio and his dreams—his fantasies, as I call them—are key to understanding his career. We need Ito's fantasies to understand not just the concrete things that happened, but to understand the desires and engagements that allowed him to fashion a sustained sense of self, and to withstand the ruptures and dislocations of his career. In this chapter, I attend to his experience at the Jaques-Dalcroze Institute for Eurythmics in Hellerau, Germany. The Jaques-Dalcroze Institute was the formative site of Ito's choreographic training and exposure to the ideology of modern dance. It was also where he learned to "perform Japanese"—to present himself as an embodied instantiation of what European (and later, US) audiences already esteemed about Japan. Before we get to Hellerau, though, I want to spend time with some of Ito's stories, the ones that he claimed filled the period before he arrived at the Institute, because these anecdotes reveal Ito's fundamental desire to

Japanese Exemplarity and Exceptionalism

cast himself as a cosmopolitan artist. In these narratives, Ito figures himself as the protagonist of a *voyage imaginaire*, constructing, through this orientalist literary itinerary, a sense of himself as not just Japanese, but "Oriental," and as not simply a student of modernism, but as a self-making artist. In his memoirs, by the time he arrives at Hellerau, he has begun to understand the singular path he will need to take in order to make a name for himself.

At the Jaques-Dalcroze Institute, Ito recognized the necessity of a performance of Japaneseness—a performance that was, certainly, responsive to the orientalist expectations projected on him, but that also reflected his own desires. And in this performance, Ito began to perfect an oscillation between Japanese as exemplary and Japanese as exceptional. Because he came *from* Japan, Ito was understood as representative of it—as well as of "the Orient" at large. This exemplarity is what enabled him to integrate into Hellerau's international community. At the same time, his ability even to arrive at Hellerau, to move freely and expansively (across the globe or the stage), was a sign of his exceptionalism, and in this, his Japaneseness also served as the sign of his fundamental uniqueness. Hovering between these two significations, Ito cultivated "Japaneseness" as a fantasy by which he might be known.

Ito's narration of this period, both in his wholly invented anecdotes and in his recounted stories, should be taken less as records of his experience in Europe, than as traces of his own fantasy of what his time there meant. In this we might follow Shane Vogel, building on Thomas Postlewait, who proposes that we read performer autobiographies such as Ito's as "instances of performance theory" rather than as "document[s] of performance history."[2] In their imaginative flights of fancy and wry commentary, Ito's memoirs offer insights into how he wanted to be read; they theorize how he might be understood. His memoirs also present a performance within a performance: in these writings he recounts stories of his earlier performances as a cosmopolitan Japanese artist; but the very narrative act carried out in this writing is another kind of performance, and the virtuosity of this second, narrative performance must be recognized as the accrued prowess that he built up through those earlier, more youthful performances—whether "real" or "imagined."

Voyages of the Imagination

Ito's ship docked in Marseille on December 23, 1912. According to his postwar memoirs, here's what happened next:

"I deliberately set my eyes on Paris. There, I found dazzling brilliance, but with my youthful understanding, I could make no response."[3] Immediately upon his arrival, Ito forms friendships with a catalog of notable modernists. He spends hours with Auguste Rodin, Claude Debussy, and Anatole France, listening to them debate the meaning of art. In these conversations, he depicts himself as uncomprehending, his French too poor to grasp their debates. But "having gained the opportunity, I continued my visits, yearning for the key to explain my quiet anguish."[4] He explains that he is innately drawn to the same questions as the artists whom he claims as his peers: "What is art? What is beauty?"[5] In Ito's account, a shared aesthetic impulse, more powerful than linguistic barriers, asserts the connection of artistic kinship and marks Ito as present in the history of modernism.

But he is not satisfied by these theoretical discussions. Isolated by linguistic barriers and yearning for a more direct impulse, Ito spends days wandering the halls of the Louvre. He is drawn again and again to the Egyptian Room:

> Even at the time I could not have clearly explained what in this room, what of Ancient Egypt grabbed me in this way. But I had the sense that here, truly, the enigma of art was hidden.
>
> Spread across unrestrained picture scrolls were [images of] the first of mankind to establish the city-state, with a religion of nature worship as its underlying basis. I felt in every point it was the inverse of Paris's maelstrom of modern sensation.[6]

Egyptian art and artifacts, calling to Ito from an ancient world, seem to hold the answers that hours of debate could not penetrate. Ito invokes a sense of directness, of naturalness, of artistic freedom that he opposes to the confinement of Paris's swirling urban modernity. But the museum is not enough, for it is, itself, a dampened, restrained version of what Ito seeks. And so, yearning for the immediacy of personal, physical encounter, he goes to Egypt.

The dusty road leading from Alexandria to Cairo is filled with camels and donkeys carrying luggage, weary under the blazing sun. Ito wanders along with the crowd and makes his way to an oasis.[7] Under the shade of a tree, he discovers an old man teaching a group of rapt children about astronomy:

> Then, suddenly, this old man whom I had by chance come face to face with there in the middle of the road, he determined the course of my life.

Japanese Exemplarity and Exceptionalism

> The old man was called Abdellah Hassan. After meeting him, I stayed in Egypt for half a year, educated by the man's fluent French. Whenever he was struck with an idea, regardless of time and place, he would speak about the stars and the universe, discussing philosophy and art. He was also well-versed in modern literature, and explained his theories with numerous [literary] examples. . . . Abdellah Hassan was a person whom I could never forget, because he opened my eyes to art.[8]

Another version of the story, recited in a lecture Ito gave at Tokyo Christian Women's University in 1955, provides more details about this unexpected and consequential education:

> When the old man discovered that I was a student with an interest in the performing arts and dance, he began to draw examples from Maeterlinck, for he was the man of the moment. . . . [Hassan] was the one who gave me the desire to become a dancer. The performing arts are expressed by human movement, and what counts is balance. The old man told me, "A fifty-fifty balance is ordinary and tedious. The ratio of the center to the periphery must always be in flux. If one hundred is perfection, balance can be achieved at 70:30, 40:60, 99:1. Our mistake is that we always place ourselves in the center. This is why we can't keep our balance. When you stand teetering at the edge of something you can remain balanced. . . ." His point was that we must catch the center of a movement. From a technical point of view, no matter how freely we perform, we never fall if we find our center.[9]

Under the old man's tutelage, Ito gains the knowledge he has sought—an enigmatic but lyrical statement of the body in balance. This wisdom, of course, is both choreographic and philosophical: the body finds its balance by holding itself in tension, by perching on the precipice of a fall; so too, an individual who locates himself on the edge, rather than at the center of a social world, will maintain his perch, and his suspension.

After six months, having run out of the funds supplied by his father, Ito returns to Berlin, and with his brother-in-law's support, goes to Leipzig to study with a woman named Margaret Lehmann,[10] and thence, to Hellerau. But for Ito, the sojourn in Egypt points the way for his artistic career: "The problems that, in Paris, had made me fall into such agony, I had at last gained an understanding of here [in Egypt.]"[11]

Ito began to tell these stories while in New York, but it is in Tokyo, during the period of the Allied Occupation, that he writes them in detail, and has them published, in Japanese, for a Japanese audience. These are performances, then—as all autobiography is[12]—that produce for his readers an "Ito" specifically drawn as a cosmopolitan figure. As will be further discussed in chapter 7, in the aftermath of war, imperialism, and a pervasive ideology of national loyalty and sacrifice, Ito understood that his postwar Japanese readers were eager—if anxious and ill-equipped—to re-engage with the world outside Japan and to position themselves as ready for a new kind of internationalism. Ito's performance of cosmopolitanism in his memoirs was particularly geared to meet this moment, but it was also an identity he embraced, and aspired to, from the early moments of his career.

The fantasies that Ito offers as the early stories from his time in Europe are crucial, then, precisely because as fantasies, they tell us how Ito most wanted to be seen, and what being cosmopolitan meant to him. The very fact that Ito expands his geographic experience to include Paris and Alexandria coheres with a basic precept of cosmopolitanism: the ability to travel anywhere in the world and to be warmly received. Moreover, his particular choice of Paris rather than Berlin places him at the perceived center of artistic innovation and modernism. Ito surrounds himself with recognized luminaries—but they are not the figures of early twentieth-century Parisian modernism, such as Gertrude Stein, Pablo Picasso, and Henri Matisse, who were Ito's contemporaries and who were all in Paris at this time. Instead, Ito places himself among Anatole France, Auguste Rodin, and Claude Debussy, artists of the prior generation, whose importance to the development of modernism was, in effect, already acknowledged, and whose reputations, therefore, had already begun to be recast as conservative. In situating his education among these older modernists (all of whom died within a decade of when these conversations supposedly took place), Ito positions himself, both geographically and relationally, as their heir. Moreover, in this rather atypical slip, where he aligns himself with the "wrong" generation, he also composes an unintentional reproduction of the discourse of "oriental" belatedness, to which I will return.

While Ito duly places himself in Paris, he also asserts that Paris cannot hold the answers to his artistic quest; only Egypt—that is, the Orient—can provide the education he seeks. Ito's trip to Egypt, then, is a fantasy in two senses: it is fabricated, and it narratologically executes the fantasy genre of the "oriental" travelogue—modes that are, in this case, inextricable from each other. By the time of Ito's supposed trip, and then his setting it down in writing decades later, the genre of the "oriental" travelogue was well estab-

Japanese Exemplarity and Exceptionalism

lished in both European and Japanese literary practice. As Susanna Fessler and Joshua Fogel have explained, the Japanese travelogue (*kikōbun*) differs from the European genre in that while the latter is usually a kind of adventure story, and a record of encounters with the unknown and alien, the former prioritizes travel to the same spots as those who came before.[13] The Japanese travelogue thus installs the writer within a poetic lineage of the *utamakura* (famous spot), where she can see and experience what she has already read about, and, in subsequently writing about it, feel herself to be part of the location's tradition of poetic inspiration. Ito's narrative conjoins these two forms. Like the *kikōbun*, his account feels familiar because it reproduces the classic details of the orientalist scene: the dusty road, the oasis, the ancient sage. Indeed, the very contrast that Egypt offers—immediacy of understanding rather than hours of unresolved discussion in Paris—was a common orientalist trope, especially connected to contemporary theories of the hieroglyph.[14] But at the same time, Ito's narrative follows the European model, in that this is a solitary voyage of (self-)discovery, where he accesses knowledge and insight unavailable to others. Crucial to Ito's reworking of these genres is the fantasy status of "the Orient" itself. The *utamakura* in his text come not from actual geographic sites, but rather from his familiarity with the florid descriptions of literary fiction or the sensual scenes laid out in oil paint. These are details that are familiar because of the repeated allure of the Orient, as a setting for uninhibited exploration and self-invention. We might even say that Ito's invented account could take place only in the Orient, itself an imagined geography.

Ito's trip to Egypt, then, demonstrates his total fluency with the tropes of orientalism. But, while embracing generic conventions, Ito also suggests that *his* experience of Egypt is specifically Japanese, that is (and this is an intentional slippage), "Oriental." We see this when Ito understands Abdellah Hassan's French, while he failed to comprehend that of Debussy and Rodin. Successful communication is thereby rendered less a matter of shared linguistic knowledge, than of affinity. We see this again when they discuss Maeterlinck, the Belgian dramatist whom Ito had studied in Japan. Hassan's teaching is not detached from Europe, but instead, European art appears to serve as a shared reference point for two "Orientals" who can then plumb greater depths of knowledge than might be available in Europe. The "East-East" contours of this fantasy are crucial. As Joshua Fogel writes of Japanese literary accounts of travel to China, "Whereas Western travelers would have assumed they would find an alien culture and people in China, perhaps impenetrable to the Western mind—'inscrutable'—Japanese travelers presumed an uncomplicated capacity to comprehend."[15] Japan's relationship with China, of course, stretched back centuries, and, as Fogel notes, "understanding China," whether in a positive or negative valence, was crucial to Japan's conception of itself. Egypt, by contrast, was far less familiar, and almost paradigmatic as a site of orientalist projection. But we see in Ito's narrative the positioning that Fogel observes in Japanese travelogues to China—a presumption of access and comprehension, and an insistence on a shared identity (whether essential or interpellated) that became key to Ito's construction of his own Japanese persona.

If Ito's trip to Egypt embraces the narrative conventions of the "oriental" travelogue, in which the fantasy of the Orient serves as a projection screen for a particular construction of the self, this trip was also a fantasy in the more mundane sense of the word. The genre of the imaginary voyage, or *voyage imaginaire*, had a close relationship with the fantasy epistemology of the Orient. Lisa Lowe has traced how the literary *voyage imaginaire* cast the Orient as always, fundamentally, elsewhere, but in that elsewhere, it also always stood as the eternally tantalizing site of colonial desire.[16] We cannot dismiss the colonialist aspects in Ito's own desire for an "oriental" encounter. As I traced in the introduction and will further explore in chapter 3, Ito was fascinated by the theatricality of Western stage orientalism, and was also steeped in Japan's own discourse of imperial orientalism, *tōyō*. Ito's imagined ability to travel to Egypt, to receive a warm welcome, and to enjoy deep understanding with Hassan, then, are all marks of the assumption of *access*—bodily and otherwise—that underlies colonialist orientalism. Indeed, as Rana Kabbani shows, the colonialist thrust of the orientalist imaginary voyage is found not only in the act of fantasizing the voyage, but in the act of writing it down: "The onlooker is admitted into the Orient by visual seduction [. . .] and armed with language—*he* narrates the encounter in a reflective, post-facto narrative; *he* creates the Orient. [. . .] The Orient, then, [. . .] is the seraglio of the imagination disclosing itself."[17]

Ito's Orient, like everyone else's, is a reflection of his own imagination and desires, even if his fantasy does not have the seraglio's sexual overtones that were so typical of the genre. Or does it? It's worth observing that Ito's *voyage imaginaire* to Egypt is also where he erases the presence of his friend, Yamada Kōsaku. Yamada was the friend and mentor who acclimated Ito to Germany, acquainted him with other artists there, made sure Ito focused on his studies, and in fact introduced him to the Jaques-Dalcroze Institute—which is to say, Yamada was the key to Ito's artistic education and awakening. This is a curi-

Japanese Exemplarity and Exceptionalism 43

ous surrogation, then, at once suggesting a repressive closeting, as well as, at the very least, a performative insistence on ipseity. Hassan, an untraceable and generic—but importantly, "oriental"—figure, allows Ito to emerge as the unique, but also exemplary, Japanese artist, who can take the wisdom of the Orient and manifest it through his own artistic genius and Western modernist forms.

Written, as this anecdote is, many decades later, it is also interesting that Ito does not include a scene of himself learning any traditional Egyptian dance forms. Such ethnographic training "from the locals" was, after all, a primary source of authentication and publicity touted by early modern dancers (most especially Ruth St. Denis) to authenticate their "oriental dance" repertoires. Given that Ito had developed a substantial "oriental dance" repertoire, and indeed, so many of his later large-scale productions and proposals were grounded in this kind of "folk research," his disinterest in writing a scene of imagined choreographic transmission here is notable. The Orient, it seems, is not a site of technical training, but rather, one of personal development, self-making, and deep, artistic insight. For Ito, then, the Orient is a place where he imagines inter-Asian affiliation and understanding, but it is also the place where he stands alone, and alone becomes the representative of Asia to Europe and the US.

Ito embellished and proliferated the narratives of his travels to Paris and to Egypt. These accounts appear in *America and Japan* (1946), the lecture "Reminiscences" (*Omoide wo kataru*) (1955), and *A Classroom for Beauty* (1956). But in this last publication, which contains the most comprehensive account of his experiences in Paris and Egypt, Ito titles that chapter "Fantasy of Egypt" (*egyputo he no gensō*), a title printed at the bottom of every single page of that section. Within the text, Ito makes no mention of the fabricated status of his account. Instead, the story is rich in detail, and, as he does with all his other reminiscences throughout the book, he draws meaningful lessons from the experience, and attributes his particular artistic perspective to his encounters. In some ways, then, the fact of fantasy is marginal to the story Ito is trying to tell, even as it is boldly announced, on every page and in the table of contents. This is an apt figuration for how we might understand the role of fantasy in Ito's life. Fantasy offered Ito the pleasure of producing a vision of himself that had room for his own desires; it was a way of making up for his own sense of absence, even as it was also a way of gestating projects, and his own sense of self, into being. And fantasy, proclaimed at the beginning and around the edge of the page, is also an apt way to describe my approach to this book's reconstruction and accounting of Ito's career. Amid substantial archival evidence and a narrative that might, at times, seem nearly complete, I highlight how much I still do not know, and linger on these absences as fields of interpretive possibilities. Fantasy is what we, as readers, spectators, historians, and theorists, must do to catch glimpses of Ito. To call this work fantasy is not to dismiss its capacity to reveal something akin to truth; nor is it to dismiss the pleasure of a good story.

Ito's Method and Dalcrozian Foundations

If Ito's first six months in Europe occasioned postwar narrative flights of fantasy, the Jaques-Dalcroze Institute at Hellerau *was* the fantasy. It was a space of artistic training and creativity, a space of modernist invention to quell the ills of modernity. It was a place where the body was celebrated as the foundational source of rhythm, of musicality, of movement, and of expressive freedom. It was a site where national identity interwove with international projects, so that cosmopolitanism as both an ideal and a sort of lived reality permeated the halls. The Jaques-Dalcroze Institute at Hellerau was the fantasy, and for one magical year, Ito belonged.

The Dalcroze eurythmic method served as the basis for Ito's choreography throughout his career and for the development of his own dance technique.[18] The most significant echoes can be seen in his two series of poses that resemble Jaques-Dalcroze's sequence of twenty poses, and in Ito's use of embodiment exercises in which the body beats out multiple rhythms at once. The parallels between eurythmics and Ito's technique are not limited to the formal, however, for at Hellerau, Ito also absorbed the ideologies that underlay the method, and these also became central to his own artistic philosophy.

The Swiss composer Émile Jaques-Dalcroze originally developed the eurythmic method at the turn of the century as a technique for music students. Rather than experiencing music as an external, intellectual phenomenon, Jaques-Dalcroze developed a series of physical exercises that would enable students to internalize the music, perceiving it in and through their body. As Julia Walker has recently highlighted, Jaques-Dalcroze developed his method drawing on his education at the Paris Conservatoire in the 1880s, his work playing improvisatory piano at the famed Chat Noir cabaret in Montmartre, and most crucially, from a year spent in Algiers in 1886–1887—a sojourn that perhaps inspired Ito's own "voyage" to Egypt.[19] Working as an assistant conductor and chorus master at the Théâtre des Nouveautés, Jaques-Dalcroze was in Algiers as part of France's colonial apparatus. While his job was to entertain the bureaucrats with Western music, as Walker traces, Jaques-Dalcroze had many opportunities to encounter Arab music, with its rhythmic variations, expansive scale, and the philosophical principal of a cosmological musical unity. This principal, wherein the body's expression of the music was understood as a manifestation of a co-extensive spiritual unity, can be seen in a similar set of beliefs grounding Jaques-Dalcroze's method and his Institute. Differently articulated, a similar idea would be foundational to Ito's own artistic ethos.

At the Jaques-Dalcroze Institute, students learned not only a technique of musical embodiment, but also a conception of the body as an organic whole. Central to the method's premise was the idea that eurythmic training would enable students to have perfect control over their bodies; with their minds precisely attuned to each limb, students could approach their creative work as self-possessed individuals. Students enrolled at the Institute took classes in rhythmic gymnastics, solfège, and improvisation, and additional ones in dance, gymnastics, and anatomy. They were encouraged to develop different ways for their body to express music, as Selma Odom explains:

> He [Jaques-Dalcroze] would play, and after listening carefully, the students would immediately repeat what they heard in movement, matching their steps to the duration and sequence of notes they perceived. Sometimes they would "echo" the pattern, moving in silence, immediately following the example played, or they would move in canon, making one pattern while listening to the music for the next one. Often exercises involved singing as well as listening and moving, so that patterns and whole phrases might be stepped together, the students becoming the source of both sound and movement.[20]

The increasingly complex exercises produced in the students greater bodily control and—it was argued—internal harmonization.

While Emile Jacques-Dalcroze had originally envisioned his method as a music education system, the technique, combined with its principle of corporeal restoration, was quickly embraced as an approach to dancing-making that drew students from across Europe and beyond. In the method, the exercises in rhythm were structured by a series of twenty positions. These positions gave the bodily shapes that students could move through as they explored and built their rhythmic capabilities. By moving through these positions in varied orders, tempos, and dynamics, students could interpret the music and improvise to it in unlimited ways. These twenty poses, like musical scales or a corporeal alphabet, were the building blocks with which students endeavored to embody the music, and ultimately, to choreograph original dances.

The Dalcrozian method formed the foundation for Ito's own dance technique. Recalling the Jaques-Dalcroze series of twenty poses, Ito's method relied on a sequence of ten arm poses, which could be performed in either an A or B mode, for a total of twenty positions. For example, in the B sequence, (1) the arms first raise overhead, slightly bent at the elbow; (2) then float down to the sides of the body; (3) next the palms are lifted to hip height; and (4) then up to the heart, with the backs of the fingers nearly touching; (5) next the palms flip forward and push the arms slightly open and forward; (6) then with a slight pull back the arms fully straighten in front of the body at shoulder height; (7) then they return to the chest, crossing at the wrists; (8) then the arms open a bit and the hands rest, nearly horizontal, in front of the mouth; (9) next the palms flip open and pull out to either side of the head; (10) then the elbows push forward and the forearms form parallel lines in front of the face; the arms return to the raised position overhead, and then again to rest at the body's sides.[21] Ito at times called these modes "masculine" and "feminine," with the B/feminine positions having a softer feel. However, these categories were not indicative of performer or character; all students had to master both, and exercises and choreography freely moved between the two. The poses could be ordered in any number of combinations, and transitioning from one position to the next created a fluid, complex choreography. As Mary-Jean Cowell comments, "While individual positions have a two-dimensional design quality, the path of the feet changes direction as the torso twists. Consequently, both the basic gestures and the entire sequence achieve more three dimensionality, the figure interacting with the surrounding space."[22]

Just as important as the positions themselves was the technique's breathwork and the concept of the "one-arm lead." In most of Ito's dances, rather than the body going through a sequence of the postures symmetrically, one arm (or side of the body) leads, moving through the positions; the other arm follows later, or carries out a different, supporting sequence. Dana Tai Soon Burgess, who takes Ito as a kind of historic mentor, and who learned the method from a mix of Ito's Japanese and Japanese American students, explains: "So much is about how to breathe life into the form. There is a natural rise and a fall, and a generosity in the way the body brings in energy and

Japanese Exemplarity and Exceptionalism

sends it away. [. . .] The one-arm lead keeps the dances fresh because it takes you seamlessly through the entire piece. If you know the imagery intention of the dance and where to breathe in the choreography, then you know how the postures are linked together."[23] Two photographs show this concept in motion: one, by Arnold Gente, taken in 1921, shows Ito in a field dancing. His left arm, stretched forward and overhead, leads his body, while his right arm is also raised, but bent at the elbow behind his head, which helps sharpen the overall shape of the body in motion. The second is of Sarah Halzack, a dancer in Dana Tai Soon Burgess's company, performing *Ave Maria*, which was Ito's examination piece at the Dalcroze Institute and so registers a particularly close connection between Ito's technique and the Dalcroze method. Halzack is in a low lunge, left leg forward, and her torso tilts forward to form a descending line with her back leg. Her left arm is raised, slightly bent at the elbow to arch over her head with the palm facing up. Here, it is her right arm that leads, as it stretches out and gently downward, pulling the body forward. The taut balance of Halzack's limbs create planar juxtapositions of the body in space. The one-arm lead takes the dancer through the dance, so that rather than the choreography feeling like a sequence of frozen positions, it is a dynamic flow of breath and motion.

As in his Dalcrozian training, Ito's students trained by moving through the poses in rhythmic across-the-floor exercises. A masterclass in the Ito method, taught by Satoru Shimazaki in 1980 and recorded on film, demonstrates the approach:[24] students traverse back and forth across the studio, walking in time to the music, while their arms move through a sequence of the basic arm positions. In the next round, the arms move in canon, with the right arm one or two positions ahead of the left. The legs then follow another sequence, with lunges, transfers between plié and relevé, and half-turns, while the arms continue their paths through the air. As dancer and choreographer Pauline Koner explained in an interview in 1975, "He developed a whole context technically of arm shapes and arm movements, and he was a very fine musician, and transferred it to multiple rhythms in the legs and the arms. . . . He had ten positions with variations and [. . .] doing them in ways where you didn't do both arms together but they were rather like a canon, one would follow another so the variations were infinite that he could achieve in that way."[25] Having his students move back and forth across the floor, Ito required them to attend to the basic activity of walking as key to any form of rhythmic expression. From this foundation, additional movements could be understood as complications or embellishments of rhythm.

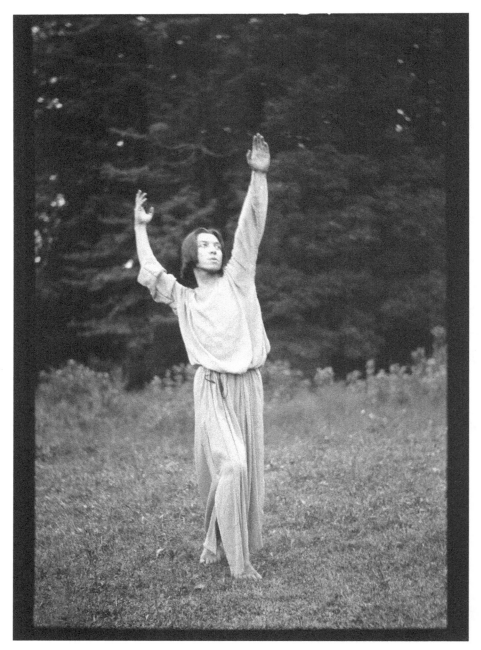

Fig. 3. Ito Michio by Arnold Gente, 1921, courtesy Library of Congress, Prints and Photographs Division.

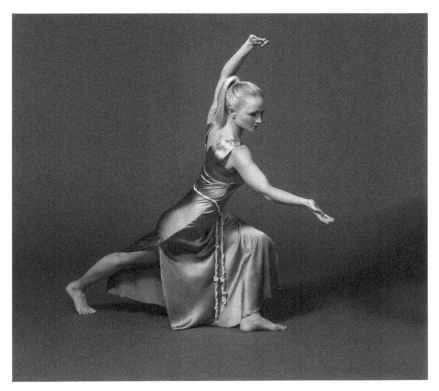

Fig. 4. Sarah Halzack performs *Ave Maria* (Itō, 1914). Photo by Jeff Watts, courtesy of Dana Tai Soon Burgess Dance Company.

The foundational practice of walking was a part of Ito's technique from the beginning. Beatrice Seckler, who studied with Ito in New York in the early 1920s, recalled, "And I remember one thing that was difficult. You walked very straight with one foot in front of the other and not turned out at all. And the balance was interesting. You had to get your balance."[26] Carrie Preston, informed by conversation with Ito's student Ryūtani Kyoko (and her student, Komine Kumiko) in Japan, suggests that this mode of walking was also influenced by Ito's brief teenage training in *nihon buyō*. In Ryūtani's postwar study with Ito, she identified his walking with *suriashi*, a technique of moving across the floor with a smooth sliding of the feet and the torso kept level that is common to many Japanese movement practices.[27] By the time Ito arrived at Hellerau, his body was certainly already habituated to particular Japanese corporeal practices, such as *suriashi*. The general fascination with Japan that he encountered in Germany and then England must have encouraged him to embrace these bodily habits, rather than attempting to erase them, as often happens when students learn a new movement form.

Working with a body stamped with early Japanese dance experiences and habits of bodily comportment, Ito developed his take on the Dalcroze method by foregrounding a series of stationary poses that were then recombined in sequences that required dancers to carry different rhythms in different parts of their bodies. Unlike other Dalcroze students, such as Mary Wigman, whose approach to dance moved away from what she had learned at Hellerau, Ito remained devoted to his education there. Most notable, in fact, was his persistent belief in the importance of music in dance. While many modern dancers (spearheaded by Wigman) soon renounced musical accompaniment, preferring to present dance as a self-sufficient artistic medium, for Ito, music was a necessity. As he commented in 1927, "When I dance, the music does not accompany me—we become as one. Sometimes the instrument has the melody, sometimes I have it, and sometimes the melodies are intertwined."[28] Across his career, music allowed Ito to realize the body's expressive capabilities; in his choreography and teaching, rhythmic harmony remained a central ideal in his dancing, a way of conducting his own body through space.

Like most of the Institute's students, Ito was drawn by the school's modernist reputation and the artistic possibilities it offered. The Jaques-Dalcroze Institute's founding, however, was a result of more industrial-national concerns. The period of imperial expansion following Germany's unification in 1871 required both economic-industrial growth and an increased sense of national cohesiveness. But industrialization, though necessary for the nation's prosperity and empire-building, also seemed to threaten its health. Where the rural, farm-laboring body was seen as healthy and vigorous, the urban, factory-laboring body, denied sunlight, nutrition, and wholesome, free-moving activity, was weak and degenerate. Thus emerged the "Life Reform Movement," a wide-ranging set of practices and efforts, including land reform, housing reform, *Körperkultur*, and the applied arts movement, all aiming to heal the ills and alienation of modernized urban living. As Didem Ekici writes, "The ultimate aim was to restore harmony to modern society in all its aspects. This would be achieved through the aestheticization of society, from the body to the built environment, as a *Gesamtkunstwerk*."[29] Across Germany many came to believe that the individual, replete with a sense of organic wholeness and health, would not only best serve the nation's industrial, cultural, and military needs, but

Japanese Exemplarity and Exceptionalism 51

would also represent, and give life to, a healthy, vigorous, and beautiful nation. We will encounter this idea again, when I turn in chapter 4 to *kokutai*, Japan's notion of the national body politic.

In this context, Jaques-Dalcroze's method rose to prominence as a life-reform solution for the problems of modernity. In particular, eurythmics seemed to resolve a specific part of the bigger problem, as articulated by the economist Karl Bücher in his widely read book *Arbeit und Rhytmus: arrhythmia*, or the disintegration of man's natural rhythms due to industrialization, urbanization, and the unrelenting sense of constant acceleration in modern life.[30] If man's arrhythmia could be resolved, the worker would no longer be alienated from his own body; his productivity, his health, and his sense of connection to community and nation would be repaired. Bücher's writing had wide influence on contemporary German thought, and in particular, on Wolf Dohrn, a leader of the German *Werkbund* (a reform organization dedicated to integrating arts and industry) and a financier of the industrialist Karl Schmidt's plan to found the garden city of Hellerau to provide holistic housing for the workers in his furniture factory. In October 1909, Wolf Dohrn saw Jaques-Dalcroze give a lecture-demonstration. Dohrn recognized in Jaques-Dalcroze's method a solution for this problem of arrhythmia and alienation. The following day, Dohrn and Schmidt invited Jaques-Dalcroze to move to Hellerau and to build his institute for rhythmic education there. By the spring of 1910, plans were underway to construct the theater hall, designed by Adolphe Appia, that would house Jaques-Dalcroze's institute, and by the fall of 1911, the school had opened.

The Jaques-Dalcroze Institute was thus not only where Ito gained the foundations for his choreographic technique. It was also where Ito gained his belief in art as a force for social harmonization and cosmopolitanism. This belief might seem contradictory to the Institute's founding justification as a site for producing more vigorous national-imperial subjects. But, as Julia Walker observes, "the political objective of the modern nation-state at the turn of the twentieth century may have been the creation of a common culture forged out of different languages, ethnicities, beliefs, and customs, but it did not necessarily require the homogeneity of an ethno-nationalist ideal that would underwrite the violence of the twentieth century."[31] The practice of eurythmics, which taught individual bodies to give expression to multiple, simultaneous rhythms through different body parts, and then systematized how those bodies could be orchestrated into a unified whole, offered a formal technique for the actual practice—and political imagining—of producing "multi-ethnic and multi-cultural harmony."[32] For Ito, as for many at the Institute, cosmopolitanism was an obvious corollary of the method's underlying principals. Moreover, for Ito, that the Dalcroze method's fundamental solution to society's ills was rhythmic movement—dance—was a belief that served as the bedrock of his own abiding belief in dance as a force of social transformation.

Belatedness and Becoming a Japanese Cosmopolitan

If Ito's time at Hellerau provided both the choreographic and the ideological foundation for the rest of his career, it was nevertheless an experience marked by a sense of missing the moment. Indeed, his time at the school (August 1913–August 1914) was characterized by an accumulating number of near-misses with the luminary figures and events of modern dance's origins. The extraordinary teacher Susan Perrottet, whom students adored, had already defected to Rudolf von Laban's colony in the summer of 1912. The star pupil Mary Wigman, who had been offered the opportunity to open a Dalcroze school in Berlin starting in the fall of 1913, instead also followed Laban to Monte Verita. The 1913 School Festival, with its production of Hector Berlioz's score revision of Christoph Gluck's *Orpheus and Eurydice*, which drew spectators from across Europe and the United States, and was immediately spoken of as a pilgrimage event that recalled Wagner's Bayreuth, was not to be repeated the following year. In February 1914, Wolf Dohrn died in a skiing accident at the age of thirty-six; plans for a 1914 School Festival were dropped as the Institute mourned. In any case, Jaques-Dalcroze had agreed to oversee an immense pageant performance celebrating Geneva's history for the Fête de Juin, held there in July of 1914, which prevented his involvement in another festival at Hellerau. Ito had missed his chance to appear in one of the school's legendary festivals.[33] While in Geneva, Jaques-Dalcroze signed the "Geneva Protest," a document that condemned Germany's shelling of the cathedral at Reims. His contract at the Institute, which would have run to 1920, was canceled. But by then, students had already begun to leave in droves, as World War I terminated the school's happy pastorale of international collaboration. Ito's anecdotes about his time at Hellerau, then, are marked by nostalgia, but also by an insistence on his thereness; they are narratives intent on claiming his place within this legendary site of modernism, in the face of a sense that he came too late.

Japanese Exemplarity and Exceptionalism

The idea that Ito came too late, however, is discursively overdetermined. Coming from Japan, from the stagnant "Orient," Ito had, in one sense, no chance to be "on time," to be present for the history of modernity as it unfolded. We might recognize this as what Homi Bhabha has termed the "time lag of modernity."[34] Or, as Lisa Lowe puts it, "the *colonial division of humanity*, or *colonial difference* within the present, is not a fixed binary distinction; it operates precisely through various modes of spatial differentiation and temporal development."[35] Tropes of "oriental" stagnation, and even degeneration, made the colonial paradigm of belatedness particularly sticky, such that Japan also employed it to describe its own colonies—not yet modern, because not yet "Japanese."[36]

If Jaques-Dalcroze's method aimed to resolve an arrhythmia that was caused by the speed of modernity, then we might recognize Ito's sense of belatedness at the Institute as a kind of racial arrhythmia. "Racial arrhythmia" names the sense of being out of step, and even out of time, not only with a putatively European and white modernity, but also with the notion of a "natural" bodily rhythm, where that "natural" has been established as the domain of an unmarked body. As Harry Harootunian has argued, in a similar vein as Bhabha, Japan's program of modernization-as-Westernization bound the country within a script of "time-lag," in which modernity is an essentially Western temporality. Nations such as Japan were thus caught in an impossible game of catchup, in which the equivalence of "not quite modern" and "not quite white" perpetually barred them from entry into modern time.[37] Suspended in its own almost-modern time signature, Japan was thus out of tempo with the West. The artists, intellectuals, and many other Japanese who, like Ito, traveled to Europe to study and observe were, in effect, trying to sidestep this supposed chronological variance, plunging into the temporality of European modernity in order to return to Japan with something more up-to-the-minute than Japan's own modernity. We can thus think of racial arrhythmia as a constitutive shadow of the arrhythmia identified by Karl Bücher, an unmistakable product of the colonialism that powered Europe's modernity. And this sense of racial arrhythmia drives a desire not simply to be in time, but, for Ito, to be at the center, to be so fully a part of modernism's unfolding that it could not fully materialize without him.

Racial arrhythmia manifested in Ito as an intense loneliness, which he spent the first few months trying to hide. As he recalled, "In my youthfulness, I mixed with peers from other foreign countries, merrily playing piano, dancing, playing tennis; nevertheless, I was prone to homesickness, overwhelmed by the feelings of loneliness that welled up. But I wanted to become a good dancer, and so, solely pursuing that which was my heart's desire, I didn't particularly care that I had not made close friends."[38] The bravado woven into this anecdote, written more than three decades later, enunciates Ito's sense of isolation but also his determination to perform the part of happy student. Only he knows how out of sync he feels with the rest of the school.

In its sense of suspension and internalization of racialization, what I am characterizing as Ito's racial arrhythmia might also be recognized as Anne Cheng's racial melancholia. But unlike melancholia, which, Cheng shows us, cannot be resolved (though it may offer "transformative potentials for political imagination" through surviving grief),[39] arrhythmia is supposed to be curable; indeed, that is the entire point of the Dalcroze method. As Jaques-Dalcroze wrote, "Arrhythmy can be radically cured only when the general functions of the human organism have been completely regulated, when constant regularity has been set up in its various manifestations, and when there has been normally developed the instinct of muscular and nervous harmonisations."[40]

The racial arrhythmia of colonial modernity cannot simply be resolved through physical training, however. (Though, as we will see, Ito masters the corporeal techniques of control central to the method, and quickly finds himself styled a "genius.") Instead, as a belatedness of development and sociopolitical difference, in Ito's narrative racial arrhythmia is remedied by cosmopolitanism, by a bringing of different national and racial representatives into international harmonization. In his memoirs, the event that brings Ito into synchrony with the Dalcroze community is Christmas—a holiday that is all about time: calendrically, as a common and set date; individually, in the experience of waiting and the affect of anticipation; and communally, in the observation of its rituals of celebration.

A few days prior, Ito tells us in his narrative of the holiday, he had gone into the town of Dresden. Packed in with the crowds of Christmas shoppers, he had purchased a green tobacco case, a necktie pin with a coral stone at its head, and a little crimson box of Japanese-made lacquerware, though he had no one to exchange gifts with. Sitting alone in his small room on Christmas Eve, amid a few flickering candles, Ito tries to keep himself occupied by carefully unwrapping and then rewrapping the small presents. "When I had finished re-wrapping the presents once again, like a child without anyone to play with, I was enveloped in loneliness."[41] Ito's memory illustrates his isolation through meaningless activity; instead of wrapping presents *for* some-

Japanese Exemplarity and Exceptionalism

one, or unwrapping a gift he has received, he goes through the motions of gift-exchange alone. Time here loops, rather than progressing, signaling that Ito's isolation has left him outside of time. Meanwhile, the gifts themselves—clearly meant for him, but also representative of him (the Japanese-made lacquerware)—reiterate his arrhythmia as both temporal and geographic. They are items he might have bought *in* Japan, as souvenirs for others, but instead he has bought them in Dresden, for himself, so that rather than signifying the curiosity of the foreign object (as they might for other German shoppers), they represent Ito's displacement.

Just at that moment, there is an insistent knocking at his window, and Ito sees several faces, pressed against the glass, stifling laughter. On opening the window, Ito is pelted with paper snowflakes, as cries of "Merry Christmas" echo around him. The group invites him to join their celebrations, and he recognizes one of the men—Kristiansky from Poland, who thrusts himself through the window to press a gift into Ito's hand, before darting off to catch up with the others, singing as they walk down the snowy road. Ito's unexpected joy increases as, soon after, the bells of a horse-drawn sleigh draw near, with the voices of seven or eight young women bouncing around. This time, he recognizes one of the female Russian students, as the group invites him to come caroling with them. The feelings of unbearable loneliness evaporate as Ito senses the camaraderie shared by these students, drawn from across the world.

> On this night of blessings, I dare say, they purposefully turned their sleigh towards my boarding house, out of thoughtfulness for that certainly lonely Japanese youth. And it was not just those young women. After the sounds of the bells of the horse-drawn sleigh had grown distant in the snowy village, then from a female classmate from Norway, from some men from France, from a group from America, one after another, I received words of celebration and presents. . . . As I wrote in the pages of my notebook, that year, that Christmas, for the first time, the light of my life abroad burned brightly.[42]

As in all of Ito's writings, his sense of dramatic timing and pathos renders this account a perfect model of the genre of Christmas stories, as holiday joy rescues him from miserable loneliness. On that night, the rituals of Christmas bring Ito into rhythm with the school's community.

Ito's narrative of the Christmas episode as the occasion of his inclusion in Hellerau's community is also notable for the way in which his integration is structured as a blossoming of internationalism. Poland, Russia, Norway, France, America; one after another, different nationalities represented at the school make an appearance. Each one does so because someone has thought of the "lonely Japanese youth" and invited him to join their celebration and their community. The episode thus becomes an experience where Ito moves from national and racial isolation to a euphoric experience of community, which he portrays—with groups dashing through the snow amid the peals of sleigh bells and the sonority of different languages—as an idyllic utopia of internationalism. But, as Ito's narrative makes clear, joining the Hellerau community does not erase the fact of his racial and national difference. On the contrary, Ito's inclusion is predicated on the logic of internationalism, in which nationality must remain distinct. Indeed, a curious detail of the story is that Ito receives gifts, Christmas greetings, and caroling visitations, but does not give anything in return. Instead, he stands at the window, as these tokens of Christmas are bestowed on him by one group of students after another, as if they are a series of tributaries to the "lonely Japanese youth." Here, Ito not only finds a way to resolve his racial arrhythmia, he begins to recognize Japaneseness as a performance strategy with which he could enter the international community and position himself as a singular figure within it.

Indeed, Ito soon discovered that being Japanese was not only the characteristic that enabled him to integrate into the Hellerau community; it was also the thing that made him unique, and exceptionally artistic. In one episode recounted in his book *America*, Ito recalled the headmaster giving him piano sheet music to learn, as all students at the institute were required to study an instrument. Recognizing the piece as a Mozart sonata he had studied in Japan, he went out to play tennis. When the headmaster found him on the tennis courts, Ito was dragged to the music room to demonstrate his ability.

> Because I had more or less practiced the piece [in Japan], I was able to play it without looking at the score. The headmaster was considerably surprised. I let pass the chance to say to him, "In truth, I played this when I was in Japan." . . . The following day, when it was the end of the headmaster's morning lecture, he said, "We have in our school a prodigy. That is the Japanese Ito." And saying this, he invited me to the platform. . . . There was nothing for it, so in a daze, I played the tune. And at that moment, I again missed the chance to say, "When I was in Japan, I played this song, that's why." From then on it was hard. For three years I could not escape having to play the role of a prodigy, which was a huge trouble. To be a genius is really a disagreeable thing.[43]

Japanese Exemplarity and Exceptionalism 57

The passage laughingly dismisses the appellation of prodigy, even as it demonstrates the youthful Ito's virtuosity, if not at piano, then at performance. But it also records Ito's interpellation as Japanese, his nationality becoming part of his identity and an explanation of his genius. Indeed, Ito frames this story by explaining that he was taken to be a representative of Japan, and therefore, felt compelled to excel in all his activities.

If at Hellerau, Ito learned a performance of Japanese exceptionalism, he was also cognizant of the interpellation of his person as more broadly representative of "the Orient" at large. At times, he experienced this racialized generalization as an obstacle preventing him from expressing himself as an individual:

> I alone was Japanese, the only Oriental person. Therefore, everything I did appeared a curiosity; a Japanese person speaks in such a manner, an Oriental person does things in this way, as if I were the representative for all Japanese and all Oriental people. [I wanted to say:] "Since I was born in Japan, it is well and good that I am called a Japanese person, but it is entirely wrong to believe that my thoughts are those of a Japanese person, or an Oriental person." But without such an explanation, I could not say anything.[44]

We see here the frustration and impossibility of being taken as racially representative, and the bewildering loss of self entailed in assimilating himself to this epistemology. But there is also a striking slipperiness of identity here. In each iteration, "Japanese" slides into "Oriental," collapsing the distinction between nationality, ethnicity, and race. Responding to his classmates' sweeping categorization, Ito, in turn, began to understand himself as not just Japanese, but also as "Oriental," a broad performance that continued to inform his career. In time, the embrace of "the Orient" as a site of identity would re-inflect Ito's understanding of himself as Japanese, an overlap intertwined with the plot of geopolitical history.

I want to take us ahead, for a moment, to see the effects of Ito's newfound awareness of the meanings generated by his Japaneseness. A photograph taken in London, by Alvin Langdon Coburn, shows Ito wrapped in a kimono and looking up at a huge mask mounted on the wall—probably a *namahage* of folk ritual practice. The bulging whites of the demon's eyes are mimicked by Ito, whose own eyes are opened wide and spun all the way to the side to focus on the mask. Ito's wry smile, the suspension of his hand, and his mouth open in speech, suggest that as much as he is engaging the demon, he is also

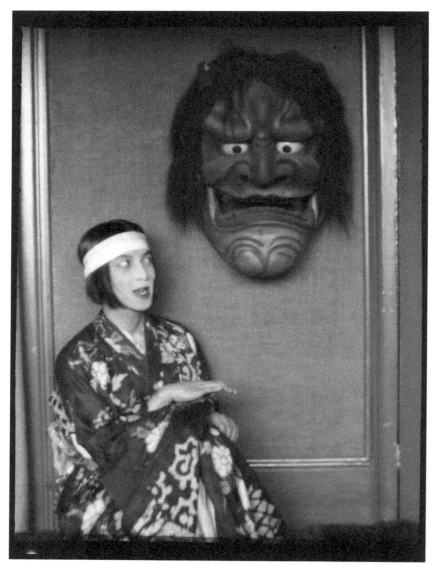

Fig. 5. "Dancer Michio Ito" (Ito with *namahage* mask). Photo by Alvin Langdon Coburn, ca. 1916, courtesy of the George Eastman Museum.

Japanese Exemplarity and Exceptionalism

engaging the camera, the photographer, and whomever else is in the room. Indeed, it seems as if his eyes, rolled all the way sideways to catch the demon, will in a moment flip back forward to look straight at the camera, catching it in the same game. We see here an example of what Robin Bernstein has taught us to recognize as a scriptive thing—"an item of material culture that prompts meaningful bodily behaviors."[45] The demon invites Ito to mirror it, to pose with it, to interact with it like another character in a play. (In another photograph Ito presses his face up against the demon's cheek, with his arm circled under its chin in a sort of hug, as if it were a cute oversized stuffed animal.) The mask draws Ito into a set of activities and poses, but these gestures are for the camera, and others who may be in the room.

The demon, I would argue, is here scripting Ito's performance of Japaneseness. In its clear, larger-than-life referentiality of folk craft and traditional practice, it prompts Ito's own exaggerated response. Japaneseness, here, cannot escape an association with Japan's traditional arts, but also allows for wry commentary on these traditions. The close relationality of Ito and the demon also suggests Japaneseness as a quality produced through a proximity with objects.[46] And, through the mask's theatricality, and the theatricality it thus induces in Ito, it also fundamentally suggests Japaneseness—ontologically—as a performance.

Ito's performance of Japaneseness here is also a carefully modulated response to the confluence of associations that he senses are the desires of this photograph's offstage observers. It is thus that we see, in his body turned out to the camera, and in his wry smile, that he is very much aware of the performance taking place. Ito is aware that this posing constitutes not just a performance of a role, but a performance that will be read as self. Michelle Carriger calls this "awareishness": "a sort of theatricality—a conscious choice of playing one's self on at least two levels: the personal and the public."[47] For Carriger, rather than being a consolidation of identity, the self-consciousness of awareishness holds open a space between "essence and expression." I will further suggest that we understand this particular kind of performance as fantasy because it is structured by the circuitries of desire, where spectator and performer each project and respond to the performance unfolding. Indeed, the desire for Japaneseness as a performed set of meanings permeates this photograph, but it would also overflow it, becoming an ongoing and reverberating practice of fantasy engagement.

At Hellerau, then, Ito learned to construct a performance of himself as Japanese—where Japaneseness was both a sign of his artistic talent and utter exceptionality, but also the identity of which he was taken as exemplary, and indeed, as a sort of diplomatic cultural representative. Ito's embrace of Japaneseness was, ultimately, tied to his understanding of the mission to renovate society held by the Jaques-Dalcroze Institute and the broader *Lebensreform* movement. At the Institute, the most public manifestations of the school's program of reform were the school festivals held each summer, and the "plastic music representations" that were staged as each festival's centerpiece.[48] These performances, most notably the 1913 staging of Gluck's *Orpheus*, were intended as demonstrations of the school's work: each student, performing, stood as an individual instantiation of the Dalcrozian principles of expressive bodily control and internal harmony. The dancers all performing together, and moving in concert with each other in precisely balanced group formations, represented a society filled with rhythmicized, beautiful bodies. Just as their bodies on stage vivified an ideal relationship between individual and society, so too did the very process of making the pageant offer a scale model of social renovation, as one individual choreographed the mass of dancers, who in turn, represented the far greater masses of society. This scaling, between exceptionality and exemplarity, was precisely the function that Ito recognized his Japaneseness could effect. Always singular, but also always representative, Ito could play the role of artistic international mediator, and in that role, pursue the utopic vision of sweeping social renovation that had become his abiding dream.

• • •

The international utopia of the Jaques-Dalcroze Institute was rapidly dismantled at the outbreak of World War I. As their nations were one by one drawn into the war, the school's students left Hellerau. Yet Ito held out, "By no means had I decided [to leave]. I had barely just mastered the fundamentals of dance training, and after all, the hope that the international situation might yet become peaceful had not yet entirely vanished, so I kept praying."[49] But with an inescapable feeling of tension in the town of Hellerau, and with entreaties from his friends, who warned that Ito might find himself trapped, he finally agreed to leave. Traveling with other Japanese, including the actor Soganoya Gorō, the writer Ikuta Kizan, and the Marquis Maeda Toshinari, Ito left Berlin on August 14, 1914, a week before Japan declared war on Germany. Two days later, Ito arrived in London.

Like the exchange of glances in the photograph that marks Ito as both playing a role and playing himself (and that complicates the distinction

Japanese Exemplarity and Exceptionalism

between the two), Ito's memoirs offer a doubled temporality—the remembered past and the postwar present—in which Ito performs, in his narratives, a version of himself performing in the past. Both cases—the recounted past and the recounting present—are fueled by a desire to make himself matter. At Hellerau, Ito's initial sense of isolation and being out of place becomes the story of how he integrated into the student community there. Read from the moment of Japan emerging from fifteen years of war, the narrative also takes on aspects of a fable, teaching his readers a strategy for recovering a sense of international belonging after its wartime isolation. Might Ito's point of integration at Hellerau—his performance of an exceptional Japaneseness—serve as a tactic for Japan's rapprochement with the world at large? I don't want to read this parallel too hard (though commentators on *nihonjinron* [the theory of Japanese uniqueness] and the 1980s economic boom argue exactly this idea of exceptional Japaneseness). I think it is enough to say that Ito desired that his own experiences stand as a sort of model for Japanese postwar international re-engagement, if only because such a view would also secure his own significance back in the nation of his birth.

The fantasies that Ito wrote into his first six months in Europe would reappear in London, where he began to make a name for himself as a dancer. This professionalization built on the performance of Japaneseness he had begun to construct in Hellerau, but it also, in crucial ways, relied on the slippage between Japan and Orient, and between his own "oriental" desires and those he recognized in the eyes of his spectators. Just as we might say that in his memoirs, Ito turned his friend Yamada into the Egyptian sage Hassan, so too, in London, did Ito himself transform into the Egyptian-styled hawk of the dance-drama *At the Hawk's Well*. In these transformations, whole people become the figurative vessels of desire—for singularity, for artistic expression, and for the capacity to self-mythologize.

CHAPTER TWO

Modernist Mythologizing

London, 1914–1916

Pizzicati is Ito's most iconic dance. Set to Léo Delibes's "Pizzicato" from the ballet *Sylvia*, it is brief, barely a minute or two. A spotlight, set low at the front of the stage, beams up on Ito, casting an immense shadow on the white backdrop behind. Throughout the dance, Ito's feet, planted in a turned-out second position with knees slightly bent, do not move. Only his arms, thrusting and slashing through the air, oscillate around his body, in time with the music. On the backdrop, the magnified shadow dances as well, the swift plunges and swinging of the arms dominating the stage. Many commentators, reading the frequently reproduced Toyo Miyatake photograph of the dance, characterize it as menacing, or as an intimation of the violence soon to befall the world and upend Ito's life.[1] But set to Delibes's bouncing, flitting music, the dance seems to stage an ebullient game of chase, as figure and shadow compete to keep up with each other, and we lose track of which leads and which follows.

To understand this dance, and the desires Ito tried to express through it, I want to look to a sketch of the choreography in motion. In the drawing, Ito imagines a sort of Vitruvian man whose being is defined by movement, as opposed to a classical stasis. The limbs radiate out, turbine-like, while the figure's torso holds center. Dramatizing the tension between the silent, rooted torso, and the striking, whirling limbs, Ito offers up the human body as a subject of poetry and of self-realization.

Ito's *Pizzicati* drawing resembles other dance drawings from the same period. As Arabella Stanger argues in her reading of choreographic renderings done by Rudolf von Laban and Oscar Schlemmer, these are "living diagrams" that, like the *Lebensreform* and Bauhaus movements from which they emerged, "imagined new types of body and living space as the basis for a repaired social future."[2] As was discussed in chapter 1, Ito was significantly shaped by the discourse of the natural body and the experiments of the *Leb-*

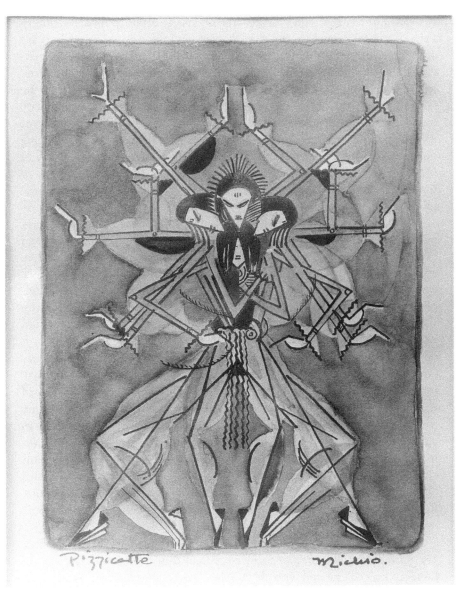

Fig. 6. Drawing of Pizzicati by Ito Michio. Toyo Miyatake Dance Collection, courtesy of Alan Miyatake.

ensreform movement, and thus his drawing has a certain familial relation to Laban's and Schlemmer's. But both Laban's and Schlemmer's drawings are abstracted: they are A dancer, or we might say, THE dancer, where the renderings represent the generalized, idealized figure of the universal dancer. Ito's drawing, by contrast, is of himself. The hair flopping down over the face, the rendering of the eyes which we see in many of his other publicity drawings, and the costume indicated with squiggly lines and ruffled sleeves are all particularized, personalized details. For Ito, dance, and the dancing human, are always universal, but also pointedly particular. Where many of his modern dance peers started with an abstraction or depersonalization of the dancer, Ito started with himself, and understood dance as a fundamental mode of self-making.

This drawing helps us understand not only *Pizzicati*, but Ito's choreography more generally. In Ito's dancing, energy gets pulled in, rather than expelled outward. This trait, I suspect, blossomed during his time in London, and it notably differs from much modern dance. For instance, Isadora Duncan's "motor in the soul" originates in the solar plexus and propels the dancer's expressivity out into space; so too, Ito's dancing diverges from Rudolf von Laban's pendulous movement scales and his sketches of the human body, in which limbs stretch out to the farthest reaches of the kinesphere; likewise, it deviates from Martha Graham's pioneer woman in *Frontier*, who projects her energy out into the land.[3] Ito's dancing is markedly grounded and internal; rarely projecting himself into the space through leaps or spins, he instead concentrates energy within himself.[4] While we might connect this quality to movement practices in both noh and butoh, Ito's treatment of energy in dance should not be reduced to some essentialism about Japanese movement. For Ito, this quality can be traced to the particular influences on his choreographic development, and perhaps as an embodied expression of his desire to be at the center of artistic worlds. Pulling in the space around him, Ito also pulled in desires—the myriad fantasies that spectators project upon, or cast him as—and braided these desires with his own.

I take Ito's desire to be at the center as the core thematic of this chapter. The period covered here has received a great deal of attention because, in London, Ito collaborated with W. B. Yeats and Ezra Pound (and a coterie of other modernists) to work on the dance drama *At the Hawk's Well*. I postpone discussion of that production to the end of the chapter, however, to focus on two other major influences on Ito's development as an artist: the Japanese dance poem movement (*buyōshi undo*) and vorticism. The dance poem

Modernist Mythologizing

movement—Japan's first modern dance movement—was formulated by two of Ito's good friends, Yamada Kōsaku and Ishii Baku, at exactly the time Ito was working with Yeats and Pound. The dance poem movement centered the body as a medium that could express things beyond the capability of words. I argue not only that Ito drew from his friends' work, but that he desired to participate actively in the development of this program, even from afar. Turning to Ezra Pound's vorticism, I delineate how Ito's choreographic style responds to this avant-garde program; at the same time, precisely because of vorticism's claims for expressive immediacy, I argue that Ito understood dance as the paradigmatic vorticist medium.

Ito's desire to place dance—and thus himself—at the center of artistic modernism is the key to reassessing his London period. While he has often been portrayed, first by his collaborators and then by some scholars, as a sort of hapless, if providential, muse, we should recognize these characterizations as the traces of his performances—if not entirely intentional, then certainly not un-self-aware. London was where Ito fully learned to perform himself in responsive attention to the desires that circulated around him—those of his spectators, his collaborators, and also his own. With such a framework, I re-approach *At the Hawk's Well* not necessarily to identify and assert Ito's agency in the project, but to explore how he at times held himself as a sort of cipher—especially with respect to his constant interpellation as Japanese. I propose his embodiment of the Hawk as Egyptian as an instance of this slipping out from the expectations of representation held by those around him, and as a way Ito made room for the indulgence of his own fantasies.

This ability, to occupy the center but hold himself as a sort of blank screen for the projection of myriad desires (others' and his own) was crucial to the work of self-mythologizing. In this, he received help from his notable collaborators, who all understood that part of modernist art-making was the attendant work of modernist myth-making. Thus, the Irish poet W. B. Yeats would famously write of Ito, "I see him as the tragic image that has stirred my imagination. There, where no studied lighting, no stage-picture made an artificial world, he was able, as he rose from the floor, where he had been sitting cross-legged, or as he threw out an arm, to recede from us into some more powerful life."[5] The poet here gives tribute to Ito's persistent, haunting corporeal power, and at the same time, marks how Ito has become a poetic figure of Yeats's own creative force. Ito's collaboration with Yeats and Ezra Pound has been taken as almost accidental, and certainly not as deliberately occasioned by Ito himself. But I think that you do not become the spectral embodiment of artistic expression for Yeats (not to mention Pound) by accident. I think that the power attributed to Ito's dancing presence, and indeed, the power that both poets began to recognize in dance, was very much the result of Ito's intentional efforts to cast himself as central to their literary experiments.

Ito's finely attuned responsiveness to the tremors of desire in performance made him an apt subject for modernist myth-making. Yeats, Pound, and Yamada were all, in their own ways, crucial to this myth-making, but so, of course, was Ito. And so, it should come as no surprise that *Pizzicati*, too, comes with a story:

Once, Ito visited the famous Russian ballerina Anna Pavlova, who "danced exquisitely Delibes' Pizzicati on her toes." She then asked Ito to return the favor, but having brought none of his own music, he asked the pianist to play the same tune. "Planting his feet firmly on the floor he danced the entire dance using only his arms and hands."[6] As with all his stories, Ito's mythologizing of the origin of his most famous dance was a characteristic modernist gesture. In referencing his friendship with Pavlova, a dancer who, despite her devotion to classical methods and even repertoire, was lionized for her "modern spirit," Ito also positioned himself as an inner member of the avant-garde. And in rejecting the constricting and explicitly female tradition of balletic point, Ito declared his allegiance to modern dance's explorations of the human body in space. As with the other tales from his European period, this act of self-invention through narrative registers the question of what performances make up a person (or persona). *Pizzicati*'s whirling figure, pulling space and the spectator's gaze into himself, was perhaps the very method of Ito's own compulsive, striving self-mythologizing. With arms and legs occupying everywhere all at once, Ito pressed himself into the memories of others, and in doing so, held himself still—a striking feat for someone who was to become known for his movement, in dance and across the globe.

Developing the Dance Poem

Ito's solo dances are often called "dance poems." The term seems casually appropriate for his choreography, and as Helen Caldwell explains in her early biography of Ito, people use the phrase because "that is what he called them."[7] The descriptive aptness of the term has meant that its precise historic reference has been overlooked—and with that omission has gone the story of Ito's relationship to Japan's early modern dance movement, a relationship that

Modernist Mythologizing 67

developed alongside his more well-known collaboration with London's literary modernists. Ito's use of the term "dance poem" staked a claim of belonging in Japan's modern dance history, even as he remained geographically distanced from it.

The dance poem movement (*buyōshi undo*) was Japan's earliest modern dance movement, and it was launched by Ito's good friends, Yamada Kōsaku and Ishii Baku. Born in Tokyo in 1886, Yamada (also rendered as Kôsçak Yamada) graduated from the prestigious Tokyo Music School, and with this intensive training in Western orchestral music, went to Berlin to study at the Hochschule für Musik from 1909 to 1913. In Germany, in addition to his musical studies, Yamada immersed himself in the avant-garde art scene, drawn especially to the work of expressionist artists.[8] He also became interested in the experiments of the dance reform movement, going to see performances by Vaslav Nijinsky, Anna Pavlova, and Isadora Duncan, three dancers whose work and modernist reputations especially inspired him. Curious about the principles of free movement and natural rhythm that had become important to theories of musical education, in 1912 he visited the Jaques-Dalcroze school at Hellerau, accompanied by the artist-musician Saitō Kazō. Yamada's time in Hellerau was brief—a few days at most. Nevertheless, the Dalcroze eurythmic method deeply informed Yamada's own work as a composer and music educator; on returning to Japan, he introduced Dalcrozian methods broadly, both to other music professionals and as a general education method.[9] We will encounter Yamada again in chapter 3, when he next crossed paths with Ito during a US concert tour from 1917 to 1919, and the two collaborated on several recitals. (And we will see him a third time, in chapter 6, after Ito repatriated to Japan during the war.) Yamada and Ito continued to work together at various points throughout their careers as the composer gained a reputation as one of the leaders of the development of *yōgaku* (Western-style music) in Japan.[10]

The other major figure in the dance poem movement is Ishii Baku (given name: Ishii Tadazumi; first stage name: Ishii Rinrō [1886–1962]), who is considered the father of modern dance in Japan. He began his training at the Imperial Theater, in the same group as Ito studying opera and *nihon buyō*. His early interest in dance led him to work under Giovanni Vittorio Rosi, the Italian ballet master brought in to lead the dance section of the opera department at the Imperial Theater. In 1915, Ishii began working with Yamada, newly returned from Europe, and Osanai Kaoru (who had similarly made a trip to Europe, stopping by Dalcroze in April 1913); the three formed a group called the New Theater (Shingekijō). Yamada trained Ishii in Dalcrozian methods, and together they began to develop the dance poem movement. This collaboration continued through 1922, during which time Ishii was also active in the Asakusa Opera movement.[11] Ishii then went on his own performance tour abroad to Europe, from 1922 to 1924, where he saw performances by Mary Wigman and Harald Kreutzberg, and to the United States, where Ito helped arrange his first recital in New York. On returning to Japan, Ishii continued his choreographic work. He also founded what is considered to be the first modern dance school in Japan, educating generations of dancers who subsequently spread modern dance not only in Japan, but elsewhere in Asia.

For Yamada and Ishii (and for Ito), "dance poem" named a belief in dance as a distinct art form (and in this it was similar to claims simultaneously being made by European artists). The key to the movement was the use of the poem as a sort of formal analogy: a dance poem is a dance that is *like* a poem. That is, the dance expresses an idea, or an image, which is never explicit, but is revealed, obliquely yet with force, through the accumulation of mood, rhythm, and physical expression. A dance poem does what a poem does, but through movement. As Ishii explained, "Our art of the dance must be poetry achieved through movement of the body."[12] The dance poem concept was thus distinct from casual usage of the term as a synonym for "dance-drama," or for dancing accompanied by the recitation of poetry.

Yamada explicitly attributed the genesis of the dance poem to his observations at the Dalcroze Institute. His emphasis on rhythm as the source of artistic expression is present in all his writings on the dance poem:

> When a rhythm is expressed through sound, that is music; and when it is represented through movement, it is called dance. So, I believe, it is by this mediator, rhythm, that true dance must be expressed as a single whole of music and movement. From this premise, I have arrived at the creation of a field of research called "buyōshi," which, for the first time, makes a perfect art form through the harmonization of music and dance.[13]

For Yamada, the power of rhythm, expressed through music *and* dance together, offered the purest articulation of the image, or impulse at the heart of a dance poem. As Nohara Yasuko has traced, in addition to the Dalcrozian exaltation of rhythm, Yamada's theorization of the movement incorporated shadings of German expressionism and mysticism borrowed from the composer Scriabin.[14] The pieces that Yamada and Ishii developed were fre-

Modernist Mythologizing

quently preoccupied with the deranged, the marginal, and the supernatural, representing, as expressionist art often did, the human condition through moments of anguish.

Yamada and Ishii's dance poem experiments were first presented on June 2, 1916—exactly two months after the first *At the Hawk's Well* performance—at the Imperial Theater, under the aegis of the Shingekijō. The program consisted of two dramas, Yoshi Isamu's *Asakusa Kannondō*, performed by Ubukata Kenichirō, Tanaka Eizō, and Miyabe Shizuko, and Strindberg's *Thunder*, translated by Mori Ogai. There were also two dance pieces, Yamada's *A Page from a Diary* (Nikki no ippen), performed by Ishii, and *A Tale* (Monogatari), performed by Ishii and Otobane Kaneko. A second program, given June 26–28 at the Hongo-za, featured Rabindranath Tagore's *Chitra*, again translated by Mori Ogai; Nagata Hideo's *Starvation* (Kikatsu); and Yamada's *Bright and Dark* (Meian), performed by Ishii Baku and Komori Toshi to a poem by Ochiai Namio. As these mixed programs show, the dance poem presentations were part of a larger movement of artists in Japan experimenting with performance forms, with material from international modernism, and with dance's relationship to text.

The piece *A Page from a Diary* represented, literally, a page from Yamada's diary—September 20 of the previous year. Rather than a depiction of the day's events, however, it was "a record of his feeling on that day."[15] In his article "Dance-Poem and Dance-Drama," published a few months after the Imperial Theatre performance, Yamada asserted "the world of sound and movement is not the world that is manifested in words. More than words, sound and movement have an intimate connection to us."[16] To portray the "feeling of the day"—that which could not be expressed in words—through dance, was to allow dance its own particular power of communication. The music composed for *A Page from a Diary* was later performed under other titles, such as "Poem," "He and She," and "Oto no Nagare," while the original title was applied to newer works developed out of the same creative process—different days, with different spirits to express.[17]

Yamada and Ishii experimented with multiple approaches to their new form; their writings and performances reflect options they tried out, as well as, later on, their differing aesthetic preferences. For instance, while the premise of the dance poem was an analogy between the two artistic media, they also experimented with more literal pairings of dance and poetic recitation, a format that echoed the work of Isadora Duncan, whom Yamada had seen dance in Germany.[18] Similarly, some pieces were still narrative-based, such as *Bright and Dark*, which dramatized the shifting fortunes of two Buddhist priests. Across their experiments, both artists emphasized that they were interested not in the "the imitation of various forms of real life," but rather, in giving expression to "something that gets filtered out, passing through the head to the chest."[19] They sought an expression that escaped the "head's" verbal realm, to be shaped instead by the logic of the body itself. Not surprisingly, as a composer, Yamada maintained a belief that the dance poem should be composed with and accompanied in performance by music. By contrast, Ishii, especially after his own tour to Europe, where he saw Mary Wigman perform without music, began to abandon musical accompaniment. Perhaps recognizing that Yamada, already a famous composer, could exert greater authority over the movement's articulated purpose, after Ishii returned from Europe he largely stopped using the "dance poem" designation, simply calling his pieces "dances" (*buyō*).

The official dance poem movement fared badly in Japan. Only twenty-seven people came to the first performance, in the grand hall of the Imperial Theatre. The experiments were seen as yet another foreign import, at a time when calls were being made to develop domestic forms of modern art. One reviewer dismissed the genre by writing, "Like being made to eat the West's fermented tofu, this makes no sense."[20] (By which, it is assumed, he meant "cheese.") Another critic panned the performance without even bothering to attend, apparently basing his evaluation on the opinions of a few spectators he knew.[21] Ishii's 1922 tour through Europe, however, was very well received; because the movement developed out of European dance trends, audiences there were more receptive to the form. Despite (or perhaps because of) the lukewarm reception in Japan, the dance poem experiments are considered to mark the beginning of Japanese modern dance. Recognizing Ito's role in the movement therefore means not simply acknowledging the transnational foundations of the dance poem, as it was shaped by Yamada's and Ishii's trips to Europe, it also requires us to think about nation-based movements as actively shaped by individuals residing outside that nation.

With the exception of a brief reference to Ito by dance scholar Funeyama Takashi, Ito's commitment to the dance poem as a form of artistic theory and practice has gone unnoticed.[22] And there are a range of possibilities for how Ito came to use the term. Coeval or even coincidental development of the term is entirely possible. "Dance" and "poem," after all, are two common words, and the notion of a communion between dance and poetry was a prevalent theme in early modernist artistic circles.[23] Ito also might have adopted the

Modernist Mythologizing 71

term later, once in New York and again collaborating with Yamada. Indeed, Ito performed there in a version of *A Page from a Diary* and *Blue Flame*, and Yamada later wrote that the New York experiments "further strengthened my belief in the harmony between music and dance."[24] But as I suggested in chapter 1, Yamada and Ito were very close. As Yamada wrote in his foreword to *A Classroom for Beauty*, "It is a relationship where we call each other 'Michio' and 'Yama-chan'"—"chan" being a Japanese address of close friendship and endearment.[25] The options I imagine as most likely are that right after Yamada began to conceive of the idea, following his own visit to Hellerau, he shared it with his eager, enterprising friend, or perhaps Yamada shared his ideas with Ito by letter, after the older musician had returned to Japan. The clearest indication that Ito knew about the dance poem movement while he was in London comes from Ezra Pound, who organized a recital in October 1915 in which Ito danced to Pound's "Sword-Dance and Spear-Dance" translations. Pound, writing in the literary magazine *Future*, calls these pieces "dance poems."[26] Although many scholars have attributed this naming to Pound himself, it just as likely came from Ito intentionally naming his work.

Ito's *Fox Dance* (1915) serves as an example of how he might have involved himself in the dance poem experiments while in London. A description of this dance was published the following year, by the New York critic H. T. Parker:

> His dance of the fox, his one distinctively Japanese number, disclosed him bare-footed, in the mask aforesaid and in the dress of his country. Beginning in writhings like to the motion of an excited animal it rose to a frenzy of such movement, for the fox of the legend was the Pierrot of beasts, moonstruck into a delirium of the dance until ecstatic death stayed him. There was no questioning the vividness of Mr. Ito's dancing or of the imagination behind it, or yet again of his rare command of singularly rhythmical movement in which head, limbs and body all answer to a mutual beat.[27]

Parker's description offers a vivid sense of Ito's experimentation, as he moves between the semimimetic/diegetic and the abstract. A studio photograph taken by Alvin Langdon Coburn likewise helps us to imagine how the dance poem informed Ito's early choreography. Ito, wearing the mask created for him by Edmund Dulac, bends forward at the waist, one leg raised up behind him in a low *attitude*, while his supporting leg is bent in a *demi-plié*, foot in *demi-relevé*. His arms stretch forward like a cat's, his hands curled like lightly clawed paws. This is a difficult position to hold; movement is imminent; the fox is running. As with Parker's description, there is an obvious mimeticism here, but it is in service not of realistic imitation, but of some unspeakable essence of Fox. It is an expression, perhaps, of what a fox's spirit might be. Indeed, Ito said as much in an interview he gave to the *New York Tribune* in August 1917: "My fox dance is furtive and independent and cunning and staccato. I studied a fox and his ways with a biscuit long before I practised my fox dance. Then I went to a great hill in Hampstead and I made my soul into the soul of a fox, and so I evolved my fox dance."[28] To make his soul "into the soul of a fox" is to understand dance—and the practice of dance-making—as transformative. Ito's articulation of his artistic intentions here parallels Yamada's statements on the power of movement and sound to express something about the world beyond the indicative capacities of language. This is dance as a conduit of impressions, and an aestheticization of perception, or as Ishii put it, "poetry achieved through movement of the body."[29] Such a characterization, as we will see, paralleled what Ito recognized as dance's role in Pound's vorticist program.

Ito's investment in the dance poem movement illuminates a few things. First, it identifies an important intertext for Ito's choreographic approach; not only Dalcroze and London modernism, but ongoing experiments in *Japanese modernism*, were crucial to Ito's development as an artist. Second, the dance poem requires us to think of Ito as a multiply-located figure, participating in multiple modernisms at once, and tying his reputation to those movements. If it is unsurprising that Ito continued to use *At the Hawk's Well*, and his relationship with the famous London modernists, as a sort of calling card to confirm his modernist distinction each time he moved, then it should also be unsurprising that he continued to use the term "dance poem" for the rest of his career—even as he let its historic signification go unexplained. Always hustling and attentive to the ways he could make himself legible, and indeed desirable, to his many audiences, the dance poem became, perhaps, the constitutive shadow of his choreographic practice, unacknowledged in words, but present nonetheless in his bodily approach to artistic dance.

The Japanese Dancing Body as a Medium of Poetry

Because W. B. Yeats's play established Ito in modernist history, and because Ito returned to it throughout his career, we readily connect him with Ito. But

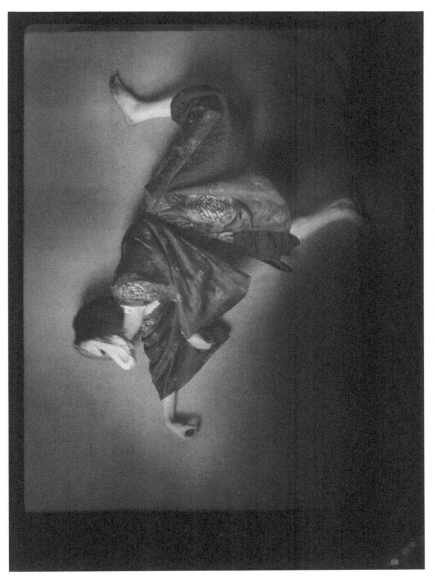

Fig. 7. "Michio Itō performing his *Fox Dance*." Photo by Alvin Langdon Coburn, ca. 1916, courtesy of the George Eastman Museum.

I suspect that Ezra Pound was in certain respects more influential than Yeats, because of the amused affection that Ito and Pound seem to have had for each other, and, not least, for a shared talent in self-promotion and effective self-placement. In particular, Pound's vorticism should be recognized as a significant influence on Ito's continuing development as a dance-maker (far more so, perhaps, than either noh or *At the Hawk's Well*). But more than simply acting as a receptive protégé, Ito aimed, I suggest, to assert dance as the paradigmatic vorticist form, and choreographed himself as its very embodiment.

Ito's appearance on the Anglophone modernist scene intersected with important shifts in both Yeats's and Pound's poetic practice, wherein Japanese poetics appeared as the solution to their literary blockages. At the beginning of the century, Yeats had aimed to overturn European trends toward naturalism with the development of a nonnaturalistic theatrical style, rooted in Irish myth. The aim here was not simply stylistic, but anticolonial: Yeats joined John Millington Synge and Lady Gregory in founding the Abbey Theatre in 1904 as Ireland's national theater, with the ambition that the theater could provide the basis for a strong, independent, historically grounded national identity. But, following the 1907 riots surrounding Synge's *The Playboy of the Western World*, Yeats became disillusioned with commercial theater that could be disrupted by "the mob"—not the working class or peasants, but portions of the middle class who censured artistic expression on religious and moral grounds. He turned, instead, to what Elizabeth Cullingford calls an "aristocratic populism" and a search for a private and poetic theater.[30] Pound, meanwhile, having arrived unknown in London in 1908, quickly made a name for himself as a provocative avant-garde poet and editor. In the summer of 1914, Pound renounced his original poetic program, imagism, in response to the American poet Amy Lowell's announcement of her own planned imagist anthology. Proclaiming that vorticism was what he had meant all along, Pound refined his artistic program to make a claim for poetry as a form expressing vigor and movement.

For both poets, Japan offered literary models that appeared to point the way out of the artistic impasses they faced. This turn to the East was part of a much longer engagement with "the Orient" as a source of formal rejuvenation. For Yeats, there was a long-running investment in various orientalisms, seen in his interest in Indian literature and his relationship with Rabindranath Tagore, his fascination with Arabian art, Chinese history, and Japanese aristocratic traditions. These interests were all tied to his commitment to the project of Irish nationalism; in each "oriental" permutation, he believed he

Modernist Mythologizing 75

had found a parallel with which to reconstruct an ancient Celtic sensibility.[31] Pound, meanwhile, has long been recognized as invested in China/"China," as seen in some of his most important works, such as *Cathay* and *The Cantos*.[32] A more recent wave of scholarship has reasserted the significance of Japan to Pound's poetics, well beyond his famous interest in the haiku.[33]

Ito's arrival in London came as a providential coincidence for both poets. London was the first place Ito had to make his way on his own—Yamada Kōsaku was back in Japan, and he no longer had the same familial support as in Germany. But he quickly established himself in a circle of Japanese and European artists by frequenting the Café Royal, a bohemian haunt popular with Japanese expatriates, where one could speak French and German freely—a boon to Ito, whose English was limited. When he received a letter from his father urging him to come home, Ito responded that he was not ready to leave Europe, but could manage on his own. His father sent a final hundred pounds sterling for a return ticket, which Ito promptly spent. His friend the painter Augustus John introduced him to the conveniences of a pawnshop, which allowed Ito to live for some time, until November 1914, when he had pawned nearly all he owned. In a now-famous episode, he pawned his last necktie, and with the few coins he earned, bought a loaf of bread to make "bread soup" and put the remaining change in the gasometer. Shivering in his room from hunger and cold, his misery was interrupted by the painter Richard Nelson dropping by to bring Ito to dance at a party at the house of Lady Ottoline Morrell. Despite his protestations, Ito soon found himself at the mansion, and though dizzy with hunger, when Lady Morrell showed him a closet full of sumptuous "oriental" costumes he could wear for his dancing, he agreed to perform. To accompaniment by the chamber orchestra of Sir Henry Wood of the London Philharmonic playing Chopin, Ito performed the dance he had choreographed for his Dalcroze examination.

The following day, he received an invitation from Lady Cunard to perform that evening. He again performed the Chopin piece, repeating it twice more as an encore, as it was the only work he had choreographed at that point. Regardless, the high-society audience was taken with him. On the basis of these impromptu appearances, Ito earned a two-week booking at the London Coliseum, running May 10 to 23, 1915. His program offered four pieces: *Dance of the Green Pine, A Seated Movement, Japanese Lady with Umbrella and Fan,* and *A Fox Dance by Moonlight*. As Ito later commented, "I was promoted as a Japanese dancer, and needed to evoke a Japanese atmosphere. For this purpose, I created dances like *Sho-jo* or Fox."[34] The sense of compulsion to perform Japanese was something Ito was already aware of from his year at Hellerau. With Ito's first public appearance, he also developed his showman's instinct, as well as a growing appreciation of how Japan—both "real" and imagined, could provide a fertile source of artistic inspiration.

Pound, meanwhile, was in search of someone who could demonstrate noh to him. In November 1913, Mary Fenollosa, widow of the recently deceased art historian and curator of Japanese art, Ernest Fenollosa, had sent to Pound the first batch of her husband's papers, charging the young poet with the task of polishing and publishing them. He and Yeats spent that winter at Stone Cottage in Sussex, working over Fenollosa's noh manuscripts. By this time, Pound was steeped in local discourses about Japanese aesthetics, and had become enamored of Japanese poetics: "In a Station of the Metro" had been published in April 1913, and his June essay "How I Began" delineated how Japanese poetic models had illuminated his way to that poem's structure.[35] But, as David Ewick demonstrates, noh was to have a far greater and long-lasting influence on Pound, in terms of his approach to poetic structure, emotional evocation, and the idea of "unity of image."[36] Pound spent the first Stone Cottage winter working on his "noh translations." These plays were the result of several layers of translation: Hirata Kiichi, a scholar of English literature at the Higher Normal School in Tokyo, had been a colleague of Fenollosa's, and had produced literal translations of noh plays for Fenollosa to read prior to seeing them performed.[37] Fenollosa, working off of Hirata's translations and marginal notes, began to compose literary translations of the plays, but died before he could finish. Pound then stepped in to complete the project, stamping on these plays his own artistic choices, which involved numerous instances of misunderstanding, mistranslation, and creative interpretation.

Around the time of Ito's Coliseum performances, Ezra Pound sought him out at the Café Royal to request a demonstration of noh.[38] Ito recruited two friends, the painter Kume Tamijurō (1893–1923) and his *senpai*, the writer Kōri Torahiko (1890–1924), to demonstrate noh to Pound and Yeats (and probably Edmund Dulac) in June 1915. This was the first of several demonstrations offered by Ito and his friends. Both Kume and Kōri were better versed in noh than Ito; Kume had even trained as a child in the Kanze noh family. For this demonstration, the two sang *noh utai* while Ito danced—which Kōri later described as an "imitation of *noh*" and a "strange dance."[39] Here, as Carrie Preston has argued, although Yeats and Pound may have assumed that Ito offered an unmediated and reliable window into noh, his performance was much more complicated; Ito can simultaneously be recognized at this demon-

Modernist Mythologizing

stration as himself a student of noh, but also as an adaptive performer who had already been "disciplined by movement techniques" common to many repertoires of traditional Japanese performance and pedagogical technique.[40]

This demonstration is another of the mythologized moments of Ito's London period. In his memoir *A Classroom for Beauty*, Ito recounted that when Pound requested that he teach him about noh chanting and dance, Ito responded, "My uncle is a noh enthusiast; when I was a child he often made me wear hakama to go see it, but on the whole, my impression is that noh is pretty boring. By no means should I become your assistant."[41] Though this exchange has become a mainstay of literature on *At the Hawk's Well*, its source is Ito's own postwar narratives. This is not to suggest that the conversation did not take place, but rather to highlight that this anecdote is also a precisely honed performance. While the story has been taken as evidence of Ito's ignorance of noh (true enough), given that it comes from Ito himself, I take it more as a self-aware, purposive illustration of himself as modernist hustler: if the poets wanted noh, noh is what he would give them. Moreover, as is true throughout his memoirs, Ito's anecdotes are written for a postwar, Japanese readership. His own turn to noh, as motivated by Yeats's and Pound's interest in the form, offered a lesson for Ito's fellow Japanese: the turn to Japanese traditional arts—which emphasized a vision of Japan as supremely aesthetic, and as long predating its period of fascist totalitarianism and empire—could serve as a ticket to international engagement and appreciation for them, as it had done for him, thirty years earlier.

While noh was a foundational form for Pound's poetic production, I do not believe the same to be true for Ito. Although Ito restaged *At the Hawk's Well* on several occasions, he did not really experiment with noh as a form. It was not a productive spur, in the way that, for example, the mass pageant was to be. But Ito did embrace, and continued to use as the basis for his own choreography, Pound's concept of vorticism, as informed by his notion of Japanese aesthetics.

Pound had, a year earlier, articulated why noh was so illuminating for his concept of vorticism: "I am often asked whether there can be a long imagiste or vorticist poem. The Japanese, who evolved the hokku, evolved also the Noh plays. In the best 'Noh' the whole play may consist of one image. I mean it is gathered about one image. Its unity consists in one image, enforced by movement and music. I see nothing against a long vorticist poem."[42] What noh unlocked for Pound was a way to deal with scale and temporal duration. Instead of plot, or development, there was Image, of such crystalline force

78 FANTASIES OF ITO MICHIO

and layered significance, that the play could be experienced as an accordion, stretched out in its literary expression, but compressed around its rendering of the Image.

We see how this concept was vivified—and what it might have meant for Ito—in the program of poems and dances Pound and Ito put together in the fall of 1915. "Sword-Dance and Spear-Dance" was presented in a small theater studio in Kensington on October 28 and November 2 and 9. The program consisted of five of Pound's translations of classical poems written in Chinese by Japanese poets.[43] These were recited by Utchiyama Masami, with Ito dancing, and a Mr. Minami accompanying on a flute. After Ito's departure to the United States, Pound published notes from the performances along with his translations in the December 1916 issue of *The Future*. As Carrie Preston has traced, at least one or two of these pieces probably resurfaced later in Ito's repertoire as *Sword Dance, Kenbu*, and *Warrior*.[44]

As Pound was quick to point out, these poems were not related to noh:

> Among the finest things Michio Itow showed us, very different from the delicate women's dances and fox-dance, the finer movements of which were lost and almost invisible on the Coliseum stage; different equally from the splendid and stately dances of the Japanese classical plays which need so much knowledge of Japanese history and literature before they can be fully comprehended, were the sword and spear dances which were seen by only a few people when he performed almost privately in a Kensington studio-theater.
>
> Each dance was in itself a drama in miniature, having within the few lines of its text not only the crux of a play but almost the form and structure of full drama, Mr. Minami accompanying on a weird oriental flute and Mr. Utchiyama's voice booming ominous from behind the curtain. Itow himself, now rigid in some position of action impending, now in a jagged whirl of motions, slashing with the sword-blade, sweeping the air with the long samurai halberd.[45]

Pound here draws an important generic distinction: Ito's solo compositions (the "delicate women's dances and fox-dance") as well as noh are both challenging genres to comprehend, the former because of its delicacy and the latter because of its rich allusiveness. Though he does not say it explicitly, Pound suggests by this comparison that the sword dances are graspable—intellectually, emotionally, and artistically. Indeed, though he has just contrasted these pieces to noh, his description in the second paragraph, of dance

Modernist Mythologizing

communicating the plays' "crux," "form," and "structure," suggests that he saw in the choreography exactly what he so valued about noh: the communication of a totality through a condensed Image.

The Image, for Pound, could not be a static one. The distinction Pound drew between imagism and vorticism was movement—a distinction that Ewick, Andrew Houwen, and others have traced to the poet's understanding of noh.[46] Thus we have Pound's characterization, at the beginning of his introduction to the sword- and spear- dances, of Ito: "Itow himself, now in a jagged whirl of motions, slashing with the sword-blade, sweeping the air with the long samurai halberd." Pound's very description of Ito's dancing *moves*, following the choreographic shapes and the gestures that call up one scene and then another, the account evoking the energy unleashed in the dance. Ito does not simply carry out jagged, slashing movements, he *becomes* the "jagged whirl of motions"—his body both a representation of vorticism, and its instantiation.

I do not believe this was coincidence on Ito's part. Rather, Ito's choreography of *Pizzicati*, either during or on the heels of his collaboration with Yeats and Pound, suggests that he was explicitly thinking about vorticism as a choreographic mode. We see this best by returning to Ito's sketch of the dance, which we might take not only as a kind of choreographic blueprint, but as a fantasy of what Ito envisioned dance could do. We might, most obviously, read this drawing as collapsing temporal duration into a single visual representation. Thus, the various positions of the limbs indicate different positions that Ito's body moves through, one after another. But we might also read the drawing as an indication of Ito's choreographic desire—not a record of its actual choreography, but rather a record of the overall impression he intended the dance to impart. This interpretation—in line with the goals of the dance poem movement—sees that in this dance, Ito is everywhere at once; his limbs do not so much move *through* space, as occupy it all, simultaneously.

If we understand Ito's vision for *Pizzicati* as one in which the body is able to exceed the constraining dimensions of time and space, such that one glance at the dancer shows him in full possession of both, then we can also understand *Pizzicati* as a dance that is about the particular expressive potential of dance itself. Indeed, I'd like to suggest here that Ito aimed, with his Sword-Dance and Spear-Dance, and especially with *Pizzicati*, to out-vorticist Pound, and to assert dance as the preeminent form of vorticist expression. In his "Vorticism" essay, Pound explains that the image underlying his Metro Station poem first imprinted itself in his mind as "splotches of colour":

> That is to say, my experience in Paris should have gone into paint. If instead of colour I had perceived sound or planes in relation, I should have expressed it in music or in sculpture. Colour was, in that instance, the "primary pigment"; I mean that it was the first adequate equation that came into consciousness. The Vorticist uses the "primary pigment." Vorticism is art before it has spread itself into flaccidity, into elaboration and secondary application.[47]

Here, Pound argues that any given powerful experience will impress itself on a subject through some particular sensation—color, sound, dimensionality—and that the artist should, in fact, employ that qualia's artistic corollary in translating that experience into art. I think Ito thought differently. Ito, though skilled at drawing, and an accomplished baritone, believed that dance was the "primary" pigment par excellence. This was a belief he imbibed at Hellerau, and it was to become one of the fundamental principles guiding his career. For Ito, dance was primary because it was, fundamentally, the intentional aestheticization of impulses registered within the body. Without the use of any outside tools—pen, brush, musical instrument—the body was its own expressive medium, capable of summoning into itself the Image, and then expressing itself *as* the Image, or, as Pound would put it, as a "radiant node or cluster; it is what I can, and must perforce, call a VORTEX, from which, and through which, and into which, ideas are constantly rushing."[48] Ito did not think of dance as a tool to create a poetic vortex, but rather, as the medium through which he himself could become the vortex.

Ito's embrace of vorticism evinces the complicated nuances of his own shifting relationship to Japan, and how he saw other artists relating to it. To be sure, that Pound had found his inspiration for vorticism in Japanese aesthetics must have been appealing, and perhaps, personally validating. Moreover, as Christopher Bush and Diego Pellecchia have both suggested, Pound's attraction to noh was not only stylistic or generic; noh contained "geopolitical" or "ethical" value for the poet.[49] As Bush argues, in Pound's vorticist program, the (moving, frequently extended) Image was not a "solipsistic moment, but rather a condensation of collective aesthetic experiences and traditions."[50] For Pound, noh expressed a more general, indeed, civilizational history, and crystallized a public's collective participation in that history. Noh thus served as a stylistic model, and also as a model of "selective inclusion" in the manner of epic—that is, a literary form that allows a community to see itself in its texts.[51] As Bush demonstrates, noh's capacity in this regard was particularly significant because of Pound's understanding, following Fenollosa in *The Chinese*

Modernist Mythologizing

Written Character as Medium of Poetry, of Japan as the nation and culture that could best absorb and selectively merge Asia and Europe "in a new composite type worthy of becoming a model for the world."[52] Ito may or may not have read Fenollosa/Pound's *The Chinese Written Character*, which Pound was, with more and more irritation, trying to get published at exactly the time of his collaboration with Ito.[53] At the very least, it seems likely that Ito would have encountered some of this essay's ideas through Pound. Moreover, he assuredly would have heard about Pound's conversations and correspondence with the poet Yone Noguchi, who had been in London from October 1913 to April 1914, visiting Stone Cottage that winter, and giving lectures on haiku at Oxford University.[54] As Sato Hiroaki traces, Noguchi by that time had already become "a full-fledged 'advertiser of Japanism'"[55] (Noguchi's own phrase), a loose ideology emphasizing Japan's uniqueness and valorizing its traditional culture and "spirituality" in contrast to Western "materiality" (capitalism) and individuality. I suspect, then, that Ito paid particular attention to Pound's pronouncements about Japan, precisely because the poet envisioned Japan as bearing an historic and artistic particularity that held universal (that is, global) significance, and this was, for Ito, an alluring and gratifying vision. Where, for Pound, noh was the art that condensed this collective tradition into an exemplary and revelatory form, Ito confidently envisioned himself as that condensation, and that selective repository. That is, Ito's energy-absorbing, vorticist fantasy upheld his own dancing body as representing, and mediating, a world-historical alignment of civilizations.

As others have remarked, there is a striking parallelism in that both Pound and Ito were imprisoned by the US during World War II and its aftermath. Particularly significant in this parallelism is the correspondence of Ito's and Pound's stated intentions in appearing to work against the US. In a 1936 letter to the Japanese modernist poet and artist Kitasono Katue, Pound wrote that there were "two things I should do before I die, and they are contriving a better understanding between the U.S.A. and Japan, and between Italy and Japan."[56] Ito, meanwhile, stated in his internment trial that his recent (suspect) activities in Japan had been for the purpose of "cementing friendly relations between the United States and Japan."[57] As Pellecchia has traced, Pound imagined that noh, if shared widely with the American public, would convince the US to turn away from war with Japan—a proposition he shared in personal letters and in public radio addresses from Rome.[58] Ito, as I have suggested and will continue to elaborate, believed that dance could serve as the basis for both cross-cultural appreciation and a training of bodies toward peace rather than war—and he explicitly and repeatedly brought this idea to high-ranking officials in Japan and the US. Both artists, then, insisted on the idea that art was the key to resolving international conflict—especially between Japan and the US—and that art could thus serve as the foundation for a new vision of a universal world culture. Moreover, both artists did not simply imagine art as the key to world peace; they fantasized themselves as its mediators. This, perhaps, is the shared vision of the vorticist, and the basis of Ito and Pound's compatibility—an insistence that art could be both world-making and self-making, and that these might be one and the same.

Whose Desire Is This?

If, in London, Ito developed a vision of dance—and himself—as central to the aesthetic-political expressive projects of artistic modernism, then we should expect this same deliberateness in his participation in his best-known work of the period, *At the Hawk's Well*. And so, I want to consider how Ito understood his role in this collaboration, and what desires, artistic and otherwise, he pursued, either for himself or as a knowing, willing circuit for others. To do so, I turn to two photographs of Ito taken by Alvin Langdon Coburn. In both photographs, what interests me are Ito's costumes. The first is a studio photograph of Ito in a female-gendered noh kimono. The second is a photograph of Ito, in his Hawk costume, in a garden (probably belonging to Lady Ottoline Morrell). These photographs, and the costumes Ito wears in them, tell us a great deal about how he understood desire—both that of his spectators, and his own—as a force that structures performance. Both photographs also register Ito's engagement with Japan—as the place where he grew up and to which, as a citizen, he still belonged, but also as a complex fantasy that he was as enthralled by, as were his collaborators and spectators. Rather than understanding Ito's engagement of japonisme as a matter of acquiescence, abjection, or self-orientalizing, I suggest that Ito's embrace of "Japan" as a mode of performance allowed him to set himself at the center of any number of overlapping and mutually constituting desires.

In the first of these photographs, Ito stands close to a wall, wrapping himself in the long sleeves of a women's kimono, with one hand hovering delicately below his chin. His head is encircled with a white band, and his eyes are downcast to the right, glancing out of the frame of the photograph. On the wall to his left is a hanging scroll *ukiyo-e*, "Tori-oi street singers for New

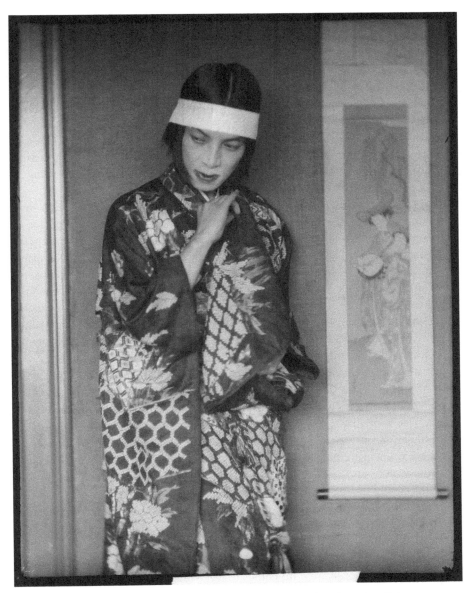

Fig. 8. "Dancer Michio Ito" (Ito with *ukiyo-e*). Photo by Alvin Langdon Coburn, ca. 1916, courtesy of the George Eastman Museum.

Year celebration," by Isoda Koryūsai.[59] The *ukiyo-e* depicts two women, one holding a *shamisen* and the other a *kokyū* (both stringed instruments). They are *tori-oi*, literally "bird chasers"—street performers of the *hinin* (outcaste) class, who especially walked the streets of Edo and Kyoto around New Years, knocking on the doors of houses to sing for money. The *tori-oi*, who wore the finest cotton kimono allowed to their class, were thought of as highly charming and even, with their wide-brimmed hats, beguiling; at the same time, they were ultimately considered beggars, and as is so frequently the case with female performers, as disreputable women.[60] Ito looks away from these beautiful street singers, but nonetheless mirrors them, at once embodying and parodying this clipping of Japanese theatrical and print culture.

This is a photograph of crisscrossing looks. And so, I want to begin by asking, who else is in Coburn's studio? For whom does Ito enact this performance, which lies comfortably on his body, and yet, because of the accompanying picture scroll, so obviously also sits as citation? The American Coburn was part of the *At the Hawk's Well* production group, and he was also part of a broader circle of modernist artists for whom Japan held a particular allure—as both a source of artistic renewal, and as a screen for homosexual desire. As Christopher Reed explains, Japan served as a culture "distant in time or place to forge identities that resist the pejorative terms of their own culture by imagining allegiance elsewhere."[61] Japan's image as a land of pure artistry *and* as having a historical tradition of male-male intimacy offered a site for fantasies of aesthetic, queer expression. Grace Lavery observes of this period, "Aesthetic investments in Japan metastasized into libidinal ones, and vice versa; 'Japanese young man' became a euphemism for an effeminate aesthete; Japan was imaginatively transformed into a space of sexually dissident utopian longing."[62] These longings structured the intertwined social, professional, and personal possibilities for a number of young Japanese men moving through Europe and the US, such as Ito's more senior acquaintance, the poet Yone Noguchi.[63] Ito's presence in this scene, then, inevitably coalesced overlapping desires for the exotic and the erotic. I imagine that this studio session perhaps involved other spectators, others of the artistic circle invested in Japan and curious about this young Japanese dancer.

I also want to ask how Ito comes to wear this kimono, which is that of a female noh character? I don't think the kimono belongs to Ito, since he was famously penniless in London. So I could say that someone (Coburn? another of their circle?) possesses a feminine kimono and has offered it to Ito. The camera's gaze records the material traces of a culture of Japanophilia, as well

Modernist Mythologizing

as, perhaps, desires for Ito in particular. But these have become inextricable. The desire for Japan represented by the purchase and possession of this garment is given an outlet when it is offered to Ito, the beautiful Japanese youth. We see here, then, desire as a continuous substance, where desire for Japan becomes desire for Ito, and the substitutionality of person, place, and thing that is a key feature of Euro-American japonisme again manifests as a capacious kind of longing.[64]

But perhaps Ito himself chose the kimono from a trunk or closet in which there were both male and female Japanese garments. Perhaps he is titillated by this drag, running his hands over the silk and embroidery, luxuriating in the feel of the heavy cloth as he binds it against his torso. Ito's pose is highly self-conscious and theatrical. His hand position, not a coded gesture from any Japanese theatrical repertoire, is generically feminine. Ito, at least, knows that this is a female garment intended for the theater, and he seems to step into the role with pleasure. The kimono was not an item of everyday wear for Ito during childhood. It was rather, a nostalgic garment specifically associated with the theater. In the notebook he kept during his internment, Ito recalled a memory of going to the Kabuki-za with his mother, who, with her hair specially done, wore a black kimono and black crested *haori* (jacket).[65] Her beauty on that day, and her happiness to be so attired and for such an occasion, remained for Ito a cherished impression. Conversely, as his dismissal of noh to Pound revealed, he also found having to dress up in *hakama* (and thus, also kimono) to go see noh with his uncle to be rather tiresome. By the time he had settled into London, however, Ito understood the exotic allure and symbolic appeal that the kimono held for Japanophiles, suggesting aesthetic elegance and rich tradition. What the photograph captures, then, is the complicated development of Ito's own desire for Japan—a "Japan" that is a mix of his own memories and threads of domestic discourse about Japanese "essence" as well as the orientalist projections of his European collaborators and spectators. Ito's "Japan," then, like all projections of a nation, is a fantasy, one that he embraces for the way its attributes can become his, and for the web of meanings and evocations that he can step into, wrapping around himself like the thick panels of the kimono.

Though he looks away from the camera, Ito intentionally and effectively holds its gaze. I sense, in this photograph, Ito's awareness of the spectators in the room, and perhaps his enjoyment of being the object of their attention. There is an erotics here, to be sure, but not one we can or should pin down too pointedly. As J. Keith Vincent writes in a discussion of Mori Ogai's *The*

Wild Goose, "The sexuality being enacted here cannot be localized within a single interiorized consciousness. It is distributed among all three minds in the scene, and that of the reader as well."[66] The erotics present in this photograph, coursing among Ito, the kimono, and *ukiyo-e*, the spectators in the room, and ourselves viewing the photograph, exceed any particular relationship or sexual identity. I might say that it is the theatricality of this moment that serves as an erotic circuit: the acts of dressing up, of arranging the body into a pose, of holding still for the camera's shutter—these are all acts in which consideration of the spectator is central to the circuitry of desire; watching and being watched are sources of pleasure. These are all acts in which desire is not about consummation, but rather the enjoyment of the thick palpability of desire itself.

The kimono Ito wears is richly decorated and looks to be of a fine material. But there is something a little makeshift about this outfit as well. The white band tied around his head is reminiscent of the *kazura obi*, the headband worn by noh actors to hold down their wigs. But the female *kazura obi* that would match this kimono would be highly decorative, embroidered with flowers. White *kazura obi* are, instead, worn by male characters. It is as if Ito has found a white ribbon or strip of cloth to improvise a noh actor's headpiece; he is raiding the costume trunk. But it is also as if he is intentionally playing with the semiotics of noh's gender performance, aware that even if his London spectators do not understand these signs, the overall sense—and allure—of gender ambiguity has been achieved.

It is rumored that in London, Ito had a relationship with the Chilean artist Alvara Guevara.[67] Gossip, especially in queer histories, is a crucial kind of historical evidence. But Ito's actual sexual practices are less relevant here than his awareness of desire as a force structuring the performer's work, both in formal theatrical venues and in the more mundane or domestic spaces of the private salon or photography studio. In London, Ito learned to play with, and to weave together, his spectators' desire for Japan with their desire for him, *as well as* his own desire for Japan, and his desire to be desired. That is, the act of "playing Japanese" that is present in this photograph is not something Ito does "for" others. Rather, this performance enacts his own fantasy, where much of the allure of that fantasy lies in the meanings his audience associates with Japan.

Ito, then, is perhaps not entirely dissimilar from the *tori-oi* he archly mirrors. To say that these female performers were driven to perform their street songs because of economic exigency and a rigid social hierarchy is true. But

Modernist Mythologizing

such a statement does not account for the pleasures of performance, the thrill of being desired, and the joys of strolling the streets, finely dressed and singing. The hard, insecure work of hustling also involves the indulgence of becoming the stuff of fantasy—whether in the floating world of Edo's woodblock prints or of London's studio photographs.

• • •

It's worth a moment of surprise that the kimono Ito wore for Coburn's studio session did not serve as the costume he wore for *At the Hawk's Well*, and it was nothing like it. Instead, for the play he wore an Egyptian-inspired sheath, designed by Edmund Dulac with Ito's input. The tunic, with a slit in the back to allow for free movement, may have borrowed from common attire at Hellerau, while the costume's long wings, which could be stretched out with the support of two hidden rods, may have nodded to kimono sleeves, but more obviously borrowed Loie Fuller's "serpentine" technology to produce fabric in motion. Much has been written about *At the Hawk's Well*'s relationship to Japanese noh—the ways in which it approximated elements from noh (intentionally or not), and the ways in which it failed to do so (again, intentionally or not).[68] The fact that Ito's Hawk is Egyptian, by contrast, is duly noted in all treatments of the play, and then quickly explained by the group's general ardor for all things "Oriental." But for many of the production's collaborators, Egypt held specific attraction. Not least was this true for Yeats himself, who during this period belonged to the occult Golden Dawn secret society and drew some of the play's scripted rituals from the order's rites.[69] As we saw in chapter 1, Ito, too, was drawn to Egypt, as a site of "oriental" discovery and self-invention. These and other fascinations with Egypt condensed in the role of the Hawk, which seems to invoke the god Horus.

At the Hawk's Well draws its source material from one of the legends of the Irish mythic hero Cuchulain, in addition to the noh dramas *Hagoromo* and *Yoro*. The well of the title, guarded by a mysterious Hawk-woman, contains water that promises immortality. An Old Man, who has wasted away his life waiting to drink from the well, warns Cuchulain to leave. As they speak of the well's soporific effect, which causes the Old Man to fall asleep every time the water bubbles up, the Guardian of the Well begins to dance, with mesmerizing, hawklike movements. She lures Cuchulain away, and as the well water rises, the Old Man falls asleep. When Cuchulain rushes back on stage, the waters have receded—both he and the Old Man have missed their chance to drink the immortal water. Cuchulain again charges offstage, to fight the warrior women whom the Guardian Hawk has called into battle, leaving the Old Man in solitude to again await the waters of the well.

Rehearsals began for *At the Hawk's Well* in mid-March 1916. The group involved in the production put Ito at the center of Anglophone modernism's fixation with "oriental" art. In addition to Yeats and Pound, the latter serving as stage manager, also involved were the illustrator Charles Ricketts, known as an expert in *ukiyo-e*; Edmund Dulac, known for his 1907 *Arabian Nights* illustrations, who designed the costumes and composed the score; and the photographer Alvin Langdon Coburn, who took pictures of the cast during a dress rehearsal. The other cast members were the actor, director, and later compiler of Yeats's letters, Allan Wade, as the Old Man, and the Shakespearian actor Henry Ainley as the Young Man. The musicians comprised Dulac on the drum and gong, along with a Mrs. Mann (singing and flute) and a Mr. Foulds (guitar). The group gave two performances, on April 2, 1916, in the drawing room of Lady Maud Cunard, and on April 4, at the home of Lord and Lady Islington.[70] Spectators were a mix of the society and artistic elite, including T. S. Eliot, Edward Marsh (Churchill's secretary), and Queen Alexandra.

Ito's famous Hawk's dance, which induced Yeats to cut more and more lines of poetry as he saw the choreography express his words in embodied form,[71] was described by Ito's student, Helen Caldwell, who saw him teach the part to Lester Horton in 1929:

> The dance performed by the hawklike Guardian, as composed by Michio Ito, was, in fact, a modified Noh dance—tense, continuous movement with subtle variations on its monotony, inducing a trancelike state in both personages and audience—but its increase in tempo was more rapid than in genuine Noh and the arm movement was broad and smoothly dramatic, recalling Egyptian representations of the hawk with spread wings and giving a feeling of a great bird's gliding and wheeling.[72]

Caldwell's description, like many others, frames Ito's performance within the paradigm of noh, and then notes the suggestion of Egypt as a vague set of references established through the costume and choreography. But what if I shift the common weighting of frames here, to focus on Ito's Egyptian Hawk, and to ask what she is doing here, in such a guise, in this modernist "noh" dance drama?

Evidence suggests that it was Edmund Dulac who suggested an Egyptian Hawk. Such a suggestion fit with the artist's general attitude—Ito later described him as "an exceedingly oriental person" (*hijōni tōyōtekina hito*).[73]

Modernist Mythologizing

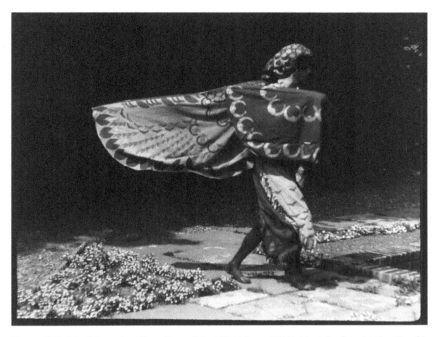

Fig. 9. "Michio Itō as the Guardian of the Well from W. B. Yeats's play *At the Hawk's Well*." Photo by Alvin Langdon Coburn, 1916, courtesy of the George Eastman Museum.

Ito then helped design the costume and worked out the climactic dance in accordance with this inspiration. Coburn's rehearsal photographs give some sense of the dance and of how Ito created a choreographically "Egyptian" Hawk. In this image, there is a striking flatness to Ito's choreography, much as if he were imitating the lines of figures painted in Egyptian tombs. To be sure, we see lots of movement; Ito spins, he flaps his arm-wings, he stomps. But when his torso is directed front, his face is still turned in profile; when his arms stretch out, one in front of the other, they do so across the picture plane, in a horizontal array.

This is, to be clear, Ito's fantasy of Egypt, gleaned from artifacts in the British Museum and his own, desiring imagination. And the fantasy-status of this performance helps open up Ito's role in this famous modernist event: perhaps Ito didn't want to be "Japanese" all the time. Did the Egyptian tomb paintings' famous flatness feel especially resonant with Jaques-Dalcroze's series of positions? The Hawk, then, is Ito's fantasy, and I understand Ito's imaginative transposition of this character as a sign of the magnitude of Ito's ambition, of his desire. Egypt, which he had described in his memoirs as "the cradle of civilization," was mythic enough to be the vessel of Ito's desire for mythic status.

Ito's period in London—his efforts to tie himself to the dance poem movement in Japan, his vigorous embodiment of Pound's vorticism, and his performance as the Hawk—coalesced as the turning point of his career, the moment when he could start to lay claim to a place within the unfolding history of modernism. Just as he was to remain the "tragic image" of Yeats's imagination long after he had departed London for New York, so too would Ito reappear as a poetic apparition in Pound's *Pisan Cantos*[74]:

> So Miscio sat in the dark lacking the gasometer penny
> but then said: "Do you speak German?"
>
> to Asquith in 1914

This is the story that marks Ito's debut, his ascension from hunger and obscurity to a place in London's artistic world. Frequently read as evidence of Pound's racial and political alignments, it is also a canny articulation of Ito's own mythology. The scene describes the dinner held after Ito's performance at Lady Cunard's. Ito found himself seated across from a distinguished-looking gentleman who attempted to engage Ito on the topic of Japanese art. Frustrated at his inability to communicate, Ito asked to speak in German instead, to which the man laughingly agreed, and they amiably conversed the rest of the evening. Ito learned the next day that he had been speaking with the prime minister, H. H. Asquith, in the language of the enemy.

In Pound's poetic recollection, the section turns on the "but" of the second line. When we look closely, however, we see that the moment staged by this "but" is not what we might expect; it is not Lady Morrell's invitation to perform at her salon, nor even the debut moment of his dance itself. Rather, the "but" marks the moment when Ito seizes the chance to navigate his own foreign status, and to make it the basis of his mythic allure. Pound's description here is frequently read as a sign of Ito's linguistic helplessness, if not general naiveté. These lines in fact record a moment of charismatic aplomb, and genial, but certainly intentional, self-realization. When Ito left London for New York in September 1916, he carried with him this sense of having been at the center, and with the confidence that he could, again, draw audiences into his fantasies, and make himself into theirs.

CHAPTER THREE

Japoniste Collections

New York, 1916–1929

Ito's 1927 *Tango*, set to Isaac Albéniz's "Tango in D," begins with a darkly clad figure emerging out of the shadows in a slow walk downstage. He wears the quintessential costume of the Latin dance—black pants, starched white shirt, black bolero, and black cordobés hat, the long brim obscuring the dancer's face. As in *Pizzicati*, a spotlight set low at the front of the stage casts his shadow large against the stage's backdrop. The principal steps of the dance are quickly introduced: simple half box steps with a drag of the following foot; pivot steps ending in low extensions of the leg; lunges back and forth in a plié second position, with a tilting up of the front foot onto its heel; slow, controlled pivot and soutenu turns. Occasionally, he delivers the expected foot stomp; twice, his fingers snap. Rarely moving beyond the area of center stage, the dancer moves back and forth along the diagonal axis, his direction more a function of shifting body weight than literal travel.

The tango was an immensely popular dance for early modern dancers and their audiences.[1] Drawn from Argentina and alternately configured as Spanish, early modern dancers drew on the tango craze of the early 1910s, adapting the form for stage performance. For many male dancers, such as the famous, closeted modern dancer Ted Shawn, it offered a chance to exhibit a highly hetero-masculine persona, as it cast male and female in the dramatic tension of heterosexual pursuit. Embodying the familiar moves of the tango, dancers tended to take on the partnering, and thus narrative, inherent in its movement, even when choreographed as a solo. Ito's *Tango*, however, is coolly restrained. Where other dancers heightened the tango's smoldering sexuality, using its deep lunges and turns to seduce their partner or the audience, Ito's version is a solo that enjoys its self-sufficiency. Brief, subtle rocking of the hips, and an almost imperceptible shimmy, which takes place more in the feet than the torso, is all that evokes the dance's usual sultriness. The

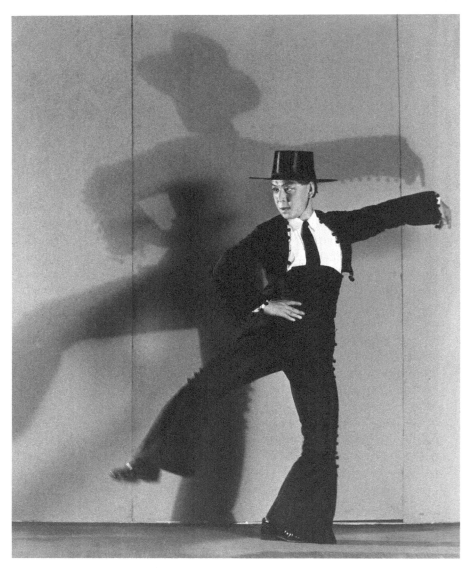

Fig. 10. Ito Michio in *Tango*. Photo by Toyo Miyatake, Toyo Miyatake Dance Collection, courtesy of Alan Miyatake.

Japoniste Collections

dance is melancholy, as if it retraces the memory of a tango, rather than vivifying its usual drama. The shadow cast against the wall reinforces the sense of the dance's solitariness, and even nostalgia. Exemplary of his dance poem approach, discussed in chapter 2, Ito takes up the tango, almost impossibly overdetermined in narrative and character, to meditate on the very idea of the tango and the desires it choreographs.

As restrained as it appears, Ito's *Tango* is an expression of desire. Ito's desires here, I imagine, are many: stepping into the role of male tango dancer, Ito explores the echoes of a seductive masculinity through a particular ethnic type—even as he refuses to enact its stereotyped *machismo* sexuality. This is, on the one hand, a fantasy of mastery, not of the missing female partner, but of the genre of tango and of its weight as a representative cultural form. But this is also the fantasy of being desired, longed for, and accruing power as the object of a desirous gaze. Even as this is a dance about solicitations of longing, it is, as I noted, remarkably self-sufficient. There is, within the dance's small circle of movement, a withholding and a self-preservation, a will to outlast the exhaustion of more fiery expressions. Ito's *Tango* allows, and indeed recognizes, that the audience will read onto Ito's dancing body a variety of interpretations and expectations of race, gender, sexuality, and nationality. And yet, in this piece Ito leaves space for his own desires, for the indulgence of his own imaginative and corporeal fantasies. And in this play, between being a screen for others' expectations, and standing self-sufficient in his own aspirations, Ito collects all these desires and holds them close, in the taut, charismatic, yet understated movements of his dance.

This chapter takes up the question of desire, and the fantasies that desire fuels, by interpreting Ito's repertoire and reception through multiple significations of the "japoniste collection." The aesthetic framework for most of Ito's performance in New York was "japonisme"—a term that broadly refers to the fascination with Japan, and the artistic production flowing from that fascination, notably (but not only) in Europe and the US, from the late nineteenth on through the early twentieth century (if not far longer).[2] Many of Ito's spectators, patrons, and collaborators were engaged in the phenomenon of japonisme, and their appreciation of Ito cannot be disentangled from this particular form of orientalist enthusiasm. I also use the term to describe aspects of Ito's own relationship to Japan—an attitude of aesthetic valorization, innovative use of traditional forms, and self-conscious identification— that he shared with many of his Japanese modernist peers. Recognizing Ito as "japoniste" emphasizes that his own relationship to Japanese aesthetics and creative use of "Japan"/Japan was not necessarily natural, inherent, or authentic, simply because he was Japanese.

Alongside japonisme, the collection provides a useful way to think about Ito's navigation of the structures of imperialism, racialization, and aestheticism that undergirded his time in New York. The collection has been understood by many scholars as a practice of desire—acquisitive, possessive, erotic, fetishistic, and self-defining—but also as a primary mode by which Asia (with and without quotation marks) has come to be produced and known. As Charlotte Eubanks and Jonathan Abel write, "As a construct and product of powerful institutions from empires to nation-states, museums to universities, Asia has long been formulated at the level of the collection."[3] Ito's japoniste collections manifested in his many concert dance and commercial entertainment activities, from his experiments with Japanese performance forms and cultural referents to his participation in the genre known as "oriental dance."

This chapter explores the intertwining of japonisme and orientalism, and the meaning of these politico-aesthetic formations not only to Western hegemony, but also to Japanese imperialism. Japonisme has been predominantly understood as an aesthetic phenomenon underpinned by Western imperialism. But for many Japanese, the fantasy of Japan's aesthetic supremacy was also entwined with Japan's own imperial project, whereby the "universal appeal" of Japanese aesthetics could be seen as the artistic corollary of the political justification for Japan as a world power. Japonisme thus figured in the broader discursive concept of *tōyō*, which, as Stefan Tanaka has delineated, was the historiographic and ideological concept of "Japan's Orient"—the notion of Asia as a counterforce to the West, with Japan as its leader.[4]

As he established himself in New York, Ito found immediate opportunities within the genre of "oriental dance," in which dancers presented pieces that corporeally imagined—and claimed to be from—"the Orient." In "oriental dance" group recitals, such as the presentations of Adolf Bolm's Ballet Intime, Ito appeared as a kind of Japanese curio within larger "oriental" collections. As his choreographic reputation grew, Ito also put together his own "oriental dance" collections, and in this, his status as a subject of imperial Japan is crucial. For Ito's "oriental dance" activities can be understood not only as an expression of Western orientalism, but also of *tōyō*, by which Ito stood as a kind of imperial collector himself.

Both as Japanese collector and as Japanese curio, Ito's participation in "oriental dance" involved presumptions of access and racial structures of objectification. The concept of the fetish, then, with its history of imperial trade,

Japoniste Collections 95

racial objectification, and psychoanalytic sexual desire, is an apt framework for thinking about Ito's performances in New York. I propose that precisely when Ito was framed as an abjected, fetishized object, he could also be seen as an object that itself collects the desires of those around him. Intertwining these desires with his own, Ito pulled in spectators, patrons, and other artists as participants in his alluring performance of self. In this chapter then, Ito appears as both collectible object and object collector.

As newspapers noted, Ito was extraordinarily busy in New York. In addition to my argument about desire and the japoniste collection, this chapter tracks many of Ito's activities in order to provide a full sense of his endeavors, and to lay the groundwork for events and thematics that will emerge in later chapters. Ito's thirteen years in New York, from 1916 to 1929, saw him truly establishing his career as a dancer, and expanding his reach into as many spheres of artistic production as possible. In concert dance, he developed a substantial repertoire that included numerous "interpretive" works, such as *En Bateau* (Debussy, 1919), *Ecclesiastique* (Schumann, 1922), *Caresse Dansée* (Scriabin, 1926), and *Passpied* (Delibes, 1927); as well as a robust array of "oriental dances," such as *Siamese Dance, Chinese Buffoon*, and *Gypsy Dance* (all 1921, accompaniment unknown); *Chinese Spear Dance* (1927) and *Impressions of a Chinese Actor* (1928) (both to musical accompaniment by Maurice-Joseph Ravel); and *Lotus Land* and *Mandarin Ducks* (both 1928, to Cyril Scott pieces). Ito drew not only from "oriental" sources and rising modernist approaches for his repertoire, but also from popular culture. A dance such as *Golliwog's Cakewalk* (1917), set to Debussy's composition of the same name, involved complicated performances of cross-racial identification and appropriation; Ito's experience of racialization in New York was part of a much broader landscape of US racial logic, though the presence of Black racialization only occasionally surfaces in the archive.

Nearly from the start, Ito refused to be confined to concert dance, working in theater (both experimental and commercial), teaching, and working as a dance and arts advocate. Spanning concert dance and theater, he produced a number of Japan-engaged pieces, including noh, *kyōgen*, and *kabuki*-inspired productions such as the 1918 *Tamura* at the Neighborhood Playhouse, dances such as *Te no odori* (unknown, 1917) and *Kappore from Suite Japonaise* (Yamada, 1918), and regular appearances at charity benefits for Tsuda College in Tokyo. In 1919, Ito joined with his former teacher Miura Tamaki, to help stage a pageant representing Japan as part of the World Peace Festival in Washington, DC.[5] Ito also worked in commercial venues providing choreography for large-scale endeavors, such as *The Mikado* at the Royale on Broadway (1927) and the Habima Players' production of *Turandot* at the Manhattan Opera House (1929), and he produced and choreographed his own Broadway revue, *Pinwheel Revel* (1922). He supported himself through an active teaching practice, giving private and group lessons in studios across the city, which eventually supplied him with dancers for his own company. He also became a more general advocate for modern dance, spearheading the creation of a dancer's guild, and drawing up plans for a housing and performance complex for dancers in the city. In 1923, Ito also married one of the dancers in his troupe, Hazel Wright, a union that was the topic of many news stories, as a proxy for the nation's broader anxiety about miscegenation, as I will examine in chapter 4.

Collecting is often thought of as a material practice; collectors collect objects. What might it mean, instead, to collect dances? As such, collecting is not simply a matter of amassing repertoire, though repertoire is, of course, a straightforward answer to this question. Rather, collecting dance can be understood as a practice of possessive self-definition, and as an iterative practice of desire. If, as Susan Stewart has put it, collections are "objects of desire" then Ito in 1920s New York reveals the close relationship between being a curio and being a curator, and how production of self can unfold from the interplay between these two positions.[6]

Japanese Universalism

In 1917, a writer for *Vogue* rhapsodized, "To see him dance is suddenly to seem to see a thousand silken paintings, and wood-carvings, and paper screens, and lacquer lockers, and dwarfed gardens, and falling petals of pink blossoms, jiggled into momentary oscillation and lyric, living ecstasy."[7] This reaction echoed the reception afforded the *shinpa* actress Sadayakko twenty years before, and patterned the reception of innumerable Japanese performers after Ito. White audiences did not simply see Ito as representative of what they perceived as Japan's uniquely artistic culture, they also saw him as a breathing, moving—but no less collectible and consumable—embodiment of Japan's material production.[8]

In the late nineteenth and early twentieth centuries, Japan enjoyed a reputation in the West as a country of extraordinary artistry, a land of dedicated artisans, preindustrial craftsmanship, and an aestheticism that pervaded

Japoniste Collections 97

every person, even in the most mundane activities, as Christopher Bush, Christopher Reed, and Grace Lavery, among others, have shown.[9] This was a reputation that Japan itself carefully devised in its bid to have the unequal treaties of the 1850s and '60s revised. The country's exports, its presence at international expositions, and its negotiations around immigration were all geared toward producing an image of Japan as a civilized nation, equal to the Western powers, through its reputation for artistry. As Bush, in particular, has traced, the effect of this campaign, as well as the ardent fascination with Japan exhibited by artists in Europe and the US, was that Japan was not simply seen as deeply artistic, but rather, as so supremely aesthetic as to represent a sort of universality of artistic expression.

Ito's reception in New York recapitulated all the tropes of this framework. As the *Vogue* article continued, "The dancing of Michio Ito is authentic, because it tallies absolutely with all that we have ever seen exemplified in all the other arts in which the Japanese excel."[10] Ito's reception, as a Japanese, was deemed legible and pleasing because it conformed to the expectations of spectators who felt they were already familiar with a Japan that they encountered through material objects—at home, in restaurants, and on stage—a world of goods whose popularity marked the multiple waves of what was known as the "Japan craze."

Barbara Thornbury and Rosemary Candelario have each drawn attention to a long-running mainstream US cultural paradigm of "Japanese performing artists as purveyors of cultural heritage, an understanding that was then unconsciously transferred to any artist who was seen as 'authentically' Japanese, even if that artist's practices were not actually traditional."[11] As Candelario shows, the American "kabuki discourse" (Thornbury's term) that asserted a fundamental continuity in Japanese culture was so sticky that even butoh and other avant-garde performers such as Eiko & Koma were absorbed into its vision of Japanese timelessness and tradition. While Thornbury and Candelario's studies both analyze artists working after the Asia-Pacific War, the vision of Japan as a realm of aesthetic tradition was already widely accepted by the late nineteenth century, and this vision guided Ito's reception as well. On the one hand, as we will see, Ito and his peers readily performed versions of classical Japanese theater, accommodating white American spectators' interest in Japan's traditional arts. On the other hand, they freely presented programs in which these traditional forms were shown alongside their modern dance experiments. This amalgamation, done with very little framing, may in fact have helped lay the ground for the continued

98   FANTASIES OF ITO MICHIO

notion that Japanese artists all draw from some putatively shared cultural essence, a notion that, as Candelario underlines, still impacts contemporary Japanese artists today.

In this section, I analyze several of Ito's japoniste performance activities to understand how the paradigm of Japanese universal aestheticism offered Ito both a certain artistic imprimatur and the freedom to experiment with modern forms. Within Ito's japoniste activities, I highlight those he created with fellow Japanese artists Yamada Kōsaku and Komori Toshi. Ito's collaboration with Yamada and Komori parallels his noteworthy, if limited, engagement with the local New York community of Japanese immigrants, who were, likewise, interested in what Ito's artistic achievements might signify for more general opportunities for Japanese people in the US. I also consider Ito's teaching practice, in which he framed Japanese aestheticism as a foundation that could allow his students—regardless of background—to express themselves as individual artists.

Ito's early years in New York are rich in japoniste engagement. Midori Takeishi and Carrie Preston have both insightfully analyzed Ito's numerous Japan-related projects in New York, in terms of their modernist, noh, and musical elements, and their reception in the mainstream New York press.[12] Here, I home in on Ito's japoniste activities in 1918, because they are some of his most notable engagements with Japan-sourced material, but also because they foreground a crucial though sometimes overlooked aspect of his work: far from being the singular Japanese artist alone in New York, he frequently collaborated with other visiting Japanese artists, most notably the composer Yamada Kōsaku and the dancer Komori Toshi. Yamada (whom we met in chapters 1 and 2) was already an important composer in Japan; he was also important to Ito, as both a friend and mentor, and as the person who had introduced him to the Jaques-Dalcroze Institute in Hellerau. Komori Toshi (1887–1951), meanwhile, shared Ito's initial performance training in Tokyo, and had collaborated with Yamada and a third friend, Ishii Baku, on the dance poem experiments discussed in chapter 2 (and who briefly visited Ito in New York in 1924). Like Ito, Komori developed a repertoire that moved between interpretive and "oriental" dance; following his stay in New York with Ito, Komori moved to Paris, where he spent the bulk of his career, from 1922 to 1936, and established the Ecole de Danse Orientale in Montmartre.[13]

Ito's 1918 programs were notable for the way they accentuated a contemporary Japanese perspective and intentionality. In February, Ito presented a dance recital, assisted by Komori and Tulle Lindahl (Ito's dance partner from

Japoniste Collections 99

1916 to 1919), in which a majority of the pieces were new. The titles of these pieces were given in romanized Japanese, without a translation—a contrast from his first eighteen months in New York. For music, Ito used original melodies arranged by Lasalle Spier, who also provided live accompaniment. By April 1918, Yamada had arrived in New York, and the three collaborated on a recital that featured a dance portion, a mime play called *The Donkey* written by Ito with music by Spier, and the noh *Tamura*. For the dance and mime play portions, Ito was again assisted by Komori and Lindahl. Komori and Ito each danced a new piece by Yamada, who provided musical accompaniment; Komori performed *Harusame* (Spring Rain) and Ito performed *Nikki no ippen* (A Page from a Diary), the dance poem that Ishii Baku had originated in Tokyo two years earlier. As discussed in chapter 1, Yamada used the title "A Page from a Diary" for more than one musical composition; it is not clear, therefore, whether Ito danced to the same piece as Ishii had, or whether he simply engaged in the same creative process, whereby a page from Yamada's diary was used as the basis for the poetic expression of a feeling of a day. Together, the three forms of performance found in this April program—the noh play, the mime play, and the modern dances—offered a complex gloss on Ito's engagement with Japanese forms. Under the title "Modern and Classic Japanese Pantomimes and Dances,"[14] the group used their spectators' familiarity with, and desire for, Japanese traditional arts as an opening to present their own modernist experimentation.

Another recital in April, at the Greenwich Village Theatre, offered a program primarily featuring new pieces by Yamada. As Takeishi has shown, this recital foregrounded Yamada's experiments in adapting traditional *koto* works to the practices of European modernist composers such as Scriabin.[15] Ito performed his sword dances from London, and both he and Komori (with Lindahl) created new choreography for Yamada's compositions, such as "Petit Poem, Vision of Hope," "Blue Flame, Mystic Ballet," and "Kappore, Suite Japonaise."[16] The three friends thus freely wove material from traditional Japanese instrumentation and folk music with European references and aspects of their training. Unhindered by programmatic loyalty to national forms, their gloss on modernist expression espoused an aesthetic receptiveness and cosmopolitan belief in cultural amalgamation.

Ito, Komori, and Yamada's efforts at modern Japanese expression coalesced in their production of *At the Hawk's Well* at the Greenwich Village Theatre on July 10, 1918. For this production, Ito, Komori, and Lindahl danced the three roles, while Yoshinori Matsuyama, Anne Wynne O'Ryan, Gwendolyn Gower, H. Asheton Tong, and Martin Birnbaum chanted the verse. The music, composed by Yamada, was performed by musicians listed as Ichikawa and Sakan. The art dealer Martin Birnbaum arranged to have sent over the original production's masks and costumes designed by Edmund Dulac. The most evident change in this version of the play was the music: Takeishi has found that while Dulac attempted to approximate traditional noh music in structure and by employing Japanese scales, Yamada composed a "simpler, folk-like style colored with a light Japanese tint" for harp accompaniment. She also notes that Yamada did not compose new music for the Hawk's dance.[17] While Ito's choreography may not have significantly changed, the overall shift in music suggests a subtle alteration in the meaning of Japaneseness signified by the production. Whereas in the London version traditional Japanese instruments and musical composition served to guarantee the production's "Japaneseness," in New York, Yamada felt free to compose for the harp. This version was "Japanese" because of the artists involved in the project, who nevertheless felt free to pursue their own artistic interests under the guise of this modernist noh. Across the spring and summer of 1918, Ito's collaborations with Komori and Yamada bear this sense of artistic self-sufficiency. While they certainly all contended with the expectations of tradition and authenticity held by white US spectators, they seem to have felt no compunction about hewing to their own artistic goals.

Though Ito and his friends primarily performed for a dominantly white and elite audience, they were aware of another set of spectators, whose interest was important even if they never made it to the theaters in which Ito performed. These were the members of the Japanese immigrant community, who took a clear interest in Ito's activities. As Mitziko Sawada has detailed, these immigrants were notably different from many of their West Coast counterparts, in that they usually came from more elite backgrounds and had higher educational and professional status.[18] They were, as Sawada suggests, drawn to the US not necessarily out of economic pressure, but because of the fantasies that New York represented to them: bourgeois success, urban identification, romantic love, American adventure, and national expansion. But life in New York rarely matched these fantasies, as they found that the only jobs open to them were positions in menial labor, as domestic workers, fairground booth operators, and cooks. Ito then might have felt like a peer, in terms of his similar background, but he also stood out because he had managed to retain his elite status on coming to the US—a feat he had accomplished through his work as a dancer, another kind of physical labor, but one

Japoniste Collections

that could parlay Japan's reputation for aesthetic achievement into personal advancement.

Reading through commentary in the newspaper *Nyū Yōku Shinpō*, it is clear that Japanese immigrants in New York found Ito to be a compelling and instructive figure. Readers recognized in Ito the ongoing endeavor to use Japanese art to assert Japanese enlightenment and equality with Western powers—a strategy embraced by both the Japanese government since Meiji, and by leaders in the Japanese immigrant community in the US and elsewhere.[19] For many, Ito's performances were not only examples of Japanese achievement, but being primarily aimed at white audiences, they offered insights into white perceptions of Japan and Japanese art. For example, a feature on Ito's production of *Tamura* interviewed one Helen Rosenthal, described as an "American" (*beijin*), who shared with the paper that even though she could not understand the play and its traditions, she found it exceedingly beautiful.[20] Detailed descriptions of Ito's concerts paralleled the English-language press's reception, but with the Japanese community's distinctive take. For instance, being familiar with actual Japanese noh, the *Nyū Yōku Shinpō* characterized Ito's *Hagoromo*, in January 1923, as "performed in a new style," recognizing in the music and movement the innovations being carried out under the name of noh.[21] Similarly, in a review of *Pinwheel Revel* (to be discussed shortly), the journalist suggested that the contrasts present in the program would "entice the strange tastes of Broadway's kind"—a subtle commentary on how members of the Japanese community might have viewed New York's center of theatrical entertainment.[22] Ito drew notice as far away as California, as one writer observed that Ito was at the center of a "Japan craze" in the theater.[23] Again and again, Ito marked a point of cultural strength that the Japanese-language press in New York hoped might translate into increased respect in the increasingly restrictive and threatening years leading up to the Immigration Act of 1924, with its total foreclosure of Japanese immigration to the US.

It is not only that members of the Japanese immigrant community took an interest in Ito. There is evidence as well of Ito beginning to make ties with the Japanese community in New York, hints of the kind of relationship he would fully develop in Los Angeles. He ran ads for his dancing classes in the *Nyū Yōku Shinpō*, and even placed a casting call for four Japanese girls who had kimono to perform in his 1922 *Pinwheel Revel*—assuring interested readers that they would simply need to stand, silently, on the stage.[24] While the papers frequently encouraged their readers to attend Ito's recitals, I have found no record of their attendance. But the attention directed his way, and

Ito's efforts to involve Japanese individuals in his activities, suggest that in New York, Ito began to work out possibilities for tying his aesthetic performances of Japaneseness to the local population, a relationship that he would fully materialize in Southern California in the next decade.

In New York Ito also laid the groundwork for the development of his teaching practice, which in California and back in Japan after the war was to be one of his lasting legacies. Ito first opened a summer school at Dobbs Ferry in 1918, and then a school at 9 East 59th Street in November 1919. By October 1920, he had moved to a studio at 1400 Broadway. In 1924, he was teaching in a studio at 61 Carnegie Hall, a popular place for teaching dancers, but by early 1925, he had moved to Chatsworth Roof, at 344 West 72nd. In February 1926, John Murray Anderson opened a school with Robert Milton as part of Anderson's new Park Avenue Theatre. There, Ito taught interpretive dance with Martha Graham.

The itinerant nature of his teaching probably reflected both his tendency to become involved in new endeavors and the difficult economics of dance instruction, even when it was an important source of income. Many of Ito's students became members of his troupe, performing with him in New York and joining a US tour in the late '20s. But a distinguishing feature of Ito's teaching, compared to his peers, was his eagerness to set up his students in their own careers. Around 1928, he began presenting his students in individual recitals, offering his experience and name recognition as a way for them to debut as solo artists. The mainstream press took notice of Ito's success as a teacher; as the *Times* observed, "Ito's protégés have a way of distinguishing themselves. Not so long ago Martha Lorber, Angna Enters and several dancers only slightly less well known were members of his ensemble. For that reason it may be interesting to note that the ensemble which will appear with him in his concert at the Golden Theatre this evening is made up of Isa Ellana, Lillian Shapiro, Beatrice Seckler, Sylvia Heller, Mercedes Krug and Marguerite Hirth."[25] Such noting of Ito's students in press coverage was common in New York, and, in the following decade, in Los Angeles; it suggests Ito's real talent in teaching.

Ito taught his students the audience-pleasing "oriental" dances that could be a reliable source of income. But even as he did, he framed his teaching as imparting the very opposite of ethnic type: expressive individuality. An ad for his classes placed in *Vogue* in November 1920 exemplified this stance, explaining, "Everyone has his own feeling and his own expression; dance as you feel and as you want—that is the better dance for you than any other

Japoniste Collections

kind. I will not teach you as others do; I will stand by your side as assistant and advisor and help you make your own dance. I sincerely hope that many dancers of this kind will come into this world and that is why I have started my school."[26] The emphasis on developing a student's individuality as a dancer certainly had roots in the philosophy at Hellerau, which embraced rhythmic movement as a way to restore to each individual their own internal balance and expressiveness. But what is striking is how Ito advertises himself as a catalyst for self-expression and self-realization. That is, individuality here is not something casually arising, but rather something that must be carefully nurtured, with the guidance of an expert such as Ito. Though he advocated an individualized, deracinated approach, the assurance of his method's efficacy was the unspoken imprimatur of Japanese artistry, and Ito's promise that he would, somehow, pass this exceptional aestheticism on to his students.

In some respects, it was, perhaps, the pervasiveness of the fantasy of an artistic Japan that allowed Ito to maneuver and create space for himself as an artist. But, as I will suggest in the next section, sidestepping the japoniste expectations held by his audiences, patrons, and students seems to have involved aligning himself instead with the broader fantasy of the East, or, the Orient. We might thus understand the complicated performance of self that he offered the critic Harriette Underhill in a 1917 interview:

> So this form can do other things besides dance in the sunlight. He is learning of the material things which he declares is all that the Western world knows. The Eastern world knows only of the spiritual. "So!" he said, as he placed one little brown fist in the palm of the other hand. "You see this fist, and you would say: what is this fist made of? We would see only this Shadow and we would say: what does this Shadow mean? In my dancing it is my desire to bring together the East and the West. My dancing is not Japanese. It is not anything—only myself."[27]

The feature overflows with condescending orientalism and frank racism. But within Underhill's treatment—and, indeed, in response to it—Ito makes some interesting moves. Invoking the East/West binary, he first characterizes himself as part of the "we" of the East, only to reject this association with a claim of utter individuality. Scholars have taken this quote to mean that Ito wanted to escape this binary and the collapsing of his identity with a Japanese stereotype. Surely, he did. But I think this passage is far more complicated, in part because Ito is the one who introduces the East-West dichotomy, through the trope of a spiritual East and material West. Originating with Sakuma Shōzan's modernizing directive *"tōyō dōtoku, seiyō gakugei"* (Eastern ethics, Western technology), the idea of an East abundant with spiritual riches and a West excelling in material technology had become a commonplace in Japan, but also elsewhere in Asia, showing up in Qing discourse and Indian nationalist writings. With his use of "we," Ito indexes himself as inheriting this tradition of Eastern spiritual wealth. But, he demonstrates this spiritual capacity through what might be understood as a material technology—that of gesticulation—thereby asserting his mastery over the tools of the West as well. Ito deploys this performance to proclaim his individuality. And in the process, he shows himself to be an adept puppeteer, one who can produce visions of both "East" and "West" in accordance with his spectators' desires. Ito's insistence that he is only himself, then, is not, in fact, a refusal of these terms, but an astute performance of his ability to draw from the putative essences of both civilizations, in the creation of a superior artistic capacity. As we will see, this rhetoric drew on the well-developed notion of Japan as a uniquely assimilative nation that could, so the argument went, stand as a mediator between East and West.

"Oriental" Intimacies

For Ito, "the Orient" was a fantasy inseparable from theater. From the splendid stage settings of the 1912 *Shakka* production at Tokyo's Imperial Theatre to Lady Ottoline Morrell's closet of sumptuous garments in London, for Ito, the Orient was a sensuous experience of costume and theatricality. The intoxicating thrill of being in the theater and on the stage, subject to one's own embodied fantasies and aware of being the object of others' gaze, is the foundation of this sense of theatricality and allure. The Orient, for Ito, is a theatrical fantasy of embodiment, in which the dazzling feeling of being on stage affords the perceptual, corporeal opportunity to substitute one body for another. But the Orient, for Ito, was also a theatrical site where his status as an objectified, orientalized performer intersected with his status as a subject of imperial Japan. On both sides of this equation there was slippage between "Japanese" and "Oriental." In this section, I reconsider the early modern dance genre of "oriental dance" and Ito's participation in it, by drawing attention to Japan's own orientalist paradigm *"tōyō."* I argue that in his "oriental dances," Ito was positioned both as a collectible, "oriental" object, but also as an embodied representative of Japan's growing imperial presence in Asia.

Japoniste Collections

As scholars such as Yutian Wong and Priya Srinivasan have demonstrated, "oriental dance" was a genre fundamentally constructed out of whiteness, wherein predominantly white, female practitioners exerted artistic and social agency through their embodiment of the freedoms associated with an "oriental" corporeality.[28] But the genre also involved performers like Ito, who were themselves Asian or from Asia, and whose involvement complicates the genre's racialized representational schema. When Ito became one of the original principal dancers in Adolf Bolm's Ballet Intime in 1917, he joined in a performance of the Orient that fulfilled his own theatrical yearning and participated in an organizing orientalist logic.

The Ballet Intime was founded in July of 1917 by Bolm, a former Ballets Russes principle who had remained in the US after the end of their 1916–17 tour. Though the Ballet Intime's first season took place during the summer theatrical off-season, the company's reception was enthusiastic, and critics celebrated the opportunity to see such different artists assembled together. As *Vogue* described, "For his *Ballet Intime*, Mr. Bolm assembled a number of great artists from that dreamful and meditative world that lies east of the present battle-line in Russia."[29] In addition to Ito, the principals were Roshanara and Ratan Devi, both Englishwomen who, through a mix of personal exposure to India and the effects of performance itself, essentially lived and worked under "Oriental" personas.[30] In the company of these three, Bolm himself also read as "Oriental"—Russia being popularly imagined as somewhere in between Europe and Asia proper. Supporting these principals were the British Mary Eaton and the Danish Tulle Lindahl.

The structure of the company, with representatives "from" different Asian traditions, cohered with the paradigm of the Orient-as-collection, as can be seen in an illustrated feature on the different members of Ballet Intime. This was a practice of ordering the exotic as a comprehensible and categorizable display, seen everywhere from the ethnographic exhibitions at World's Fairs to the arrangement of curio cabinets in bourgeois domestic interiors.[31] In "oriental dance," this collection was staged either across a group of dancers who each specialized in a particular tradition (as in Ballet Intime) or by a single dancer who would take on diverse "oriental" representations in a single program (as in the model of Ruth St. Denis). In both cases, "oriental" dancers insisted on the authenticity of their practice, rooted in personal experience or dedicated research. The genre offered audiences both an aesthetic and an ethnographic experience, in which supposedly authentic glimpses of "oriental" traditions could render the exotic familiar. The Orient-as-collection also offered an epistemology of the Orient: by encountering different specimens

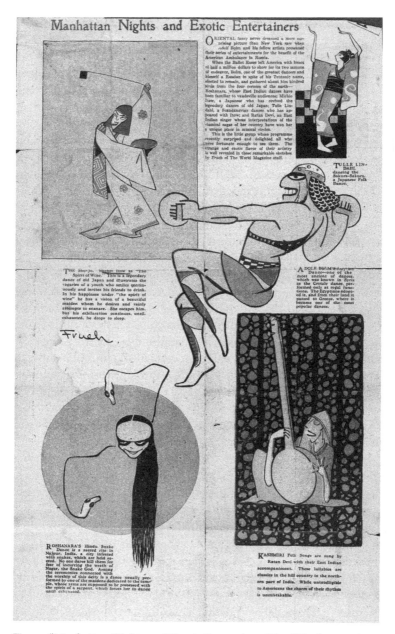

Fig. 11. "Manhattan Nights and Exotic Entertainers," by Alfred J. Frueh, source unknown, 1917. Jerome Robbins Dance Division, New York Public Library for the Performing Arts.

Japoniste Collections

on a single program, spectators could come to know the Orient as a whole through its diverse, assembled parts.

Notably, "oriental dance" offered this epistemology through movement, as embodied knowledge. It was, then, a corporeal corollary to what Thomas Richards has argued was the archival obsession in the ordering of the British Empire—"a fantasy of knowledge collected and united in the service of state and Empire."[32] But collecting knowledge through bodies is not simple. Because "oriental dance" was a genre predominantly made up of white performers, bodily identity was not required as a guarantee of authenticity. Rather, a performance's convincingness was attributed by predominantly white critics to either the dancer's biography and exposure to a given "oriental" culture, or to dedicated research they had carried out in the traditions they represented. This background information (always highly publicized) was then confirmed in the performance itself—the recognizably exotic costumes and gestures served to corroborate and materialize the dancer's claim to expertise. And so, when each dancer performed, their representation, carried out through the body itself, appeared truthful, an authenticity seemingly guaranteed by the body, even as it was actually produced by the genre's constitutive theatricality.

In Ito's case, because he was already "Oriental," the significations of "oriental" representation were laminated onto his body, settling on him as hyper-significations, layers of "real" upon bodily "real." And this was a "real" that not just his spectators, but Ito himself embraced, and understood as a meaningful characterization of his identity. This is what Michelle Carriger teaches us to expect of theatricality: "Theatricality (representation untethered to truth value) precedes truth, thereby structuring which knowledges will be accepted as knowledge."[33] That is, it is the seeming artificiality and excessiveness of theatricality that are the source of its transformational and meaning-making power. Moreover, the collusion between theatricality and embodiment helps explain Ito's own identification as an "Oriental." Between the allure of theatrical spectacle and the fantasies it allowed Ito to step into, and the embodiment which appeared to authenticate and naturalize his claims of intimate understanding of "the Orient," Ito began to understand himself as an exemplary representative of not only the fantasy world of "the Orient," but of its "real" corollary—Asia.

Here the importance of Ito's experience in "oriental dance" for his later allegiance to imperial Japan's New Order in Asia becomes evident, as the dance genre's representational logic cohered with the particular ideology of orientalism in Japan. As Stefan Tanaka has shown in his foundational study, beginning in early Meiji, Japanese intellectuals recognized the need to challenge Euro-American notions of a civilized, modern West (and a decayed, preindustrial East) by developing a countervailing paradigm of a regional Eastern culture—*tōyō*.[34] In penning a history to support this construct, these scholars accepted both the framework of Western thought that asserted a narrative of civilizational development, and the notion of "the Orient" as a place of exotic alterity and an idealized but outmoded past. *Tōyō* offered Asian nations their own civilizational path and narrative of progress, and in this narrative, Japan could emerge as both preeminently modern *and* paradigmatic of this civilization. Japan thus belonged to *tōyō*, but also developmentally stood apart from it. For Ito, the paradigm of *tōyō* allowed him to position himself as included in the Orient, a native informant, and to be outside of it, as a mediating curator.

Ito's positioning—of, and outside of *tōyō*—materializes across the wide range of his "oriental dance" activities in New York. When Ito performed as part of the Ballet Intime, he stood as the representative of Japan, alongside Roshanara and Ratan Devi's representations of India, Bolm's representation of Russia, and featured guest artists. In this case, he fulfilled the principle that Japan was part of *tōyō*, a close member of the geographic, cultural, and historical fantasy known as the Orient. But Ito also carried out projects in which he (and Japan) stood apart from "the rest" of Asia, or served as its paradigmatic, and therefore exceptional, leader. In February 1922, Ito organized a series of "Oriental Evenings" at Central High School in Washington, DC, which featured educational lectures in addition to a program of dances, each evening representing a different nation—Japan, India, and China. In June of the prior year, Ito gave a dance recital at New York's Princess Theatre that featured a typical program of embodied representations of Japan, Siam, Mexico, "the Gypsy," and China. In both of these programs, only some pieces explicitly engaged with Japan. Instead, pieces that seemed to reference a broad geography suggested that all these representations might be subsumed under the aegis of "Japanese." In his role as curator, Ito thus positioned Japan as the exemplar that stands apart; having inherited *tōyō*'s essence, Japan is framed as administrator and mediator between Asia and the West.

Ito developed a robust repertoire of "oriental" dances in the 1920s. But, notably, an even greater number of his "oriental" pieces were choreographed for dance partners such as Tulle Lindahl and Angna Enters. For his first New York recital, in December 1916, Ito choreographed "Sakura Sakura" to the *Nutcracker's Chinese Dance* for Lindahl. From one perspective, this piece is

Japoniste Collections

one more instance of the geographic and stylistic mélange that is orientalism's calling card. From another, we see the logic of *tōyō* at work: the "Chinese" music is subsumed as Japanese under the dance's title "Sakura Sakura" (Sakura, or cherry blossoms, being emblematic of Japan, both domestically and internationally). Here, Japan has not simply absorbed China, but also takes over the West's "oriental" epistemology of China, a wresting of control signified in both the use of music from the *Nutcracker*, and in the setting of the choreography on the Danish Lindahl. Meanwhile, some of Ito's other partners, such as Kohana and the Russian Sonia Serova, presented their own choreographies within his programs, a structure resembling the "Oriental Evenings," in which Ito represented the curatorial, administrative role for other "oriental" presentations. Through his partners' bodies, the imperial imperative took shape as a choreographic imperative. Moreover, as Kushida Kiyomi has shown, Japan soon had its own robust genre of "oriental dance," which may have been precipitated by the work of Teiko Ito (Yuji's wife), who visited in 1934. By the outbreak of the Second Sino-Japanese War in 1937, "oriental dance" had become a mainstay of the major revue theaters.[35] Through these and many other dancers, the paradigm of *tōyō* became an embodied epistemology that—even as it may have looked exactly like Western orientalism—contained Japan's counterargument and its own claims of supremacy.

The genre of "oriental dance" thus structures a particularly embodied form of imperial access that takes on complex meaning when carried out by a Japanese dancer such as Ito. Nayoung Aimee Kwon and Janet Poole, both theorists of Korean literature, have argued for a reconsideration of *ch'inil*, an idiom describing Korean acts of collaboration with colonial Japan, to take seriously the tense implications of the term's literal meaning: "intimacy."[36] Kwon redefines intimacy "as an unstable play of affects informed by desire, longing, and affection—all of which coexisted with the better-known violence and coercion undergirding empire."[37] The intimacies of empire that Kwon traces—in Korean writers' ease in writing in Japanese rather than Korean, in their wish to be recognized by Japanese literary societies, and in their conflicted strategies of self-representation— speak of personal desires for success, for acceptance, for self-recognition, funneled through the structures of Japan's imperial violence. Though *ch'inil* describes the position of colonized, abjected Korea, this is necessarily an intimacy felt by the colonizer as well, though on very different terms.

To understand "oriental dance" as a kind of colonial intimacy is to envision the absent bodies whose clothing is then filled by the imperial dancer.

It is to attend to the kinds of presumed closeness and the sense of access that allows for this substitution. For the majority of "oriental" dancers, their lauded authenticity was predicated on relationships—with teachers, domestic workers, husbands—which comprise forms of intimacy in which one body teaches another the physical positions and bodily movements that make up a dance, while also inhabiting different positions of power. Thus, Roshanara learned her first dances from the family nursemaid,[38] and Ruth St. Denis arranged for private lessons on each stop of her and Ted Shawn's 1925–26 tour of Asia.[39] These are intimacies in the sense that Kwon and Poole have delineated (though from the other side of the equation), and they are forms of proximity and access facilitated by class, race, and indeed, as Laura Ann Stoler has established, empire.[40] But unlike many of his peers, Ito's representations of other "oriental" traditions cannot be traced to any particular relational moment. Instead, Ito's intimacy asserts itself as inherent in his position as Japanese, positing not only that he has a right of entry to other "oriental" cultures, other "oriental" bodies, but also that, as a Japanese subject, he *already knows* the rest of the Orient. It is with this understanding of intimacy that we might recognize the significance of *tōyō* as an *embodied* practice. In Ito's "oriental" dances, where he could position himself as both of and beyond the Orient, the theatricality of these danced fantasies induced a kind of corporeal knowledge and sense of self. In these performances, it was the fantasy of intimacy itself—the idea of a regional interconnectedness as tightly bound as family—that undergirded these acts of bodily substitution and costumed, theatrical possession.

Selling and Sublimating Japonisme: *Pinwheel Revel*

Ito's primary focus, and the sphere in which he continually negotiated the meanings of "Japanese" and "Oriental," was concert dance. But Ito was also active in more commercial outlets, ranging from large Broadway productions to private engagements in the drawing rooms of society women or as entertainment on New York's elite charity circuit.[41] Ito's Broadway activities, for which he usually provided original choreography and dance training, included productions such as *Eyes of Buddha* (1921), *Ching-a-ling* (1927), and the seemingly obligatory *Mikado* (1927) and *Madame Butterfly* (1928). Ito was not unusual, among early modern dancers, in working in the commercial theater; what is obvious, however, is that in Ito's assignments he was also

Japoniste Collections

implicitly being asked to provide "oriental" authentication via his own Japaneseness. And Ito evidently enjoyed these projects; their scale—in budget, spectacle, and audience—appealed to his long-standing enjoyment of theatrical grandeur, as well as to his belief that artistic dance belonged everywhere.

Ito's commercial activities have frequently been treated as excusable, but unimportant, deviations from his artistic work—a distinction he sometimes embraced, in line with elite modernism's general differentiation between high and popular culture, and in line with many early modern dancers' efforts to establish their work as art, rather than as mere (sexual) entertainment. Likewise, part of the appeal of Japanese aesthetics to Western consumers was the fantasy that Japanese art-making took place outside of industrialized, alienated modern production, allowing, as Christopher Bush has shown, for the Japanese-produced thing to be imagined as the "exemplary anticommodity."[42] Ito understood how this fantasy attribution could translate to live performance: Japaneseness, staged as an ineffable aestheticism, could be used to legitimize as "artistic" otherwise roundly commercial forms of entertainment. This power, he recognized, was key to the valuation of "Japaneseness" as its own kind of commercial product. Ito's canny use of sublimated, but always signaling, Japaneseness is most evident in his own large-scale production, the 1922 Broadway-style revue, *Pinwheel Revel* (also called *Pinwheel Review*).

The concept for *Pinwheel* was to bring Greenwich Village uptown, for curious audiences more accustomed to Broadway fare. Starting around the 1890s the Village had become a locus for the New York avant-garde, the New Woman, and a gay refuge.[43] These cultural dissidents rubbed shoulders with recent (primarily European) immigrants, leading to the neighborhood's reputation as a cosmopolitan melting pot, where languages, customs, and mores were all undecided. The confirmed appeal of Greenwich Village's counterculture artistry soon led, particularly in the theater, to an exportation to Broadway of Greenwich Village productions/companies that could capitalize on the neighborhood's reputation. This included the *Greenwich Village Follies*, the Washington Square Players, and the Provincetown Players. Indeed, the Provincetown Players' move uptown was occasioned by the 1920 runaway success of Eugene O'Neill's *Emperor Jones*, for which Ito originated the role of the Congo Witch Doctor in a prime instance of racial fungibility in theatrical casting.[44]

Pinwheel was envisioned as part of this uptown export. To carry out the business side of this endeavor, Ito partnered with the prolific Broadway producer Richard Herndon. Worried, however, that "solemn dances, in large numbers"[45] would not sell tickets, Herndon and then Ito importuned producer and comedian Raymond Hitchcock to underwrite the show and appear as its comic host. What finally opened was a nearly four-hour program of concert dances interspersed with sideline commentary and comedic sketches by Hitchcock and comedian Frank Fay. The *New York Tribune* described the show: "The program indicates an Indian-Spanish-Yiddish Bat Theater. It includes character and classical dances, pantomimes, voice, novelties and folk-songs."[46] Ratan Devi (under the name Ragina Devi) performed items from the "oriental dance" repertoire; Ito's brother Yuji sang; Yasashi Wuriu performed a traditional Japanese dance. The program also contained music visualizations, rhythmic settings, animated tableaux, and interpretive dance numbers, including the premiere of *Ecclesiastique*, which would become an important piece in Ito's concert dance repertoire. Although the production was quickly trimmed to a more manageable length, it closed after a month.[47] The *Tribune* called it "a sober and erudite dancing festival,"[48] and Gordon Whyte, writing for *Billboard*, commented, "It is novel and very, very artistic with a big capital A. If that's your idea of a good time, you will have it at the 'Pin Wheel.' Otherwise you had better keep away."[49]

The production's artsyness was thus loudly proclaimed—both the basis of its allure, and its potential for producing boredom. Its artistry was also code for the elements of Village culture that caused midtown audiences anxiety (and interest)—most obviously, its reputation for queer sexual freedom.[50] This concern was apparent in Hitchcock's nightly framing of the show with the story of its origination: it was, we are told, Ito's tearful pleading that convinced Hitchcock to join the show: "Ever susceptible to the plaintive sobs of the Japanese, he was unable to withstand the importunities of Mr. Itow."[51] Or, as *Variety* put it, "Hitchy just can't stand tears."[52] Here, Hitchcock's tender responsiveness to Ito is immediately disavowed through his very acquiescence: the circulation of affect that is suggested as homoerotic through the effeminizing presence of tears works; that is, it achieves its intended effect of moving Hitchcock. But in yielding, Hitchcock steps back into a more stably hetero-masculine role, as the sideline commentator who lampoons and burlesques, and who, from this position, insists that he is outside of the corporeal, emotional artistry taking place center stage. Similarly, Fay's job was primarily to act as an audience plant, a role that by its beleaguered, indignant nature is "straight." Indeed, all of the descriptions of Hitchcock and Fay's antics suggests that their presence served as a comedic masculine straightening device wrought upon the queer sincerity of the dance program.

Japoniste Collections	113

This framework was reiterated in one of the show's most popular numbers. As *Variety* described:

> The following number was one of the best bits of the evening. It was called "Languor, Ecstasy and Languor." Really an idea-art among tramps. Actually a vein of burlesque, for the tramps could only be nances. The morning music of the birds awakens six hoboes, all in white, but in rags. They come from behind the hedge, one by one and dance in pairs or ensemble to classical music. There was no doubt about the way this number got across, the house giggling all the way. For the close, each "bo" returned to his natural state and lay down to rest.[53]

The male tramps, seemingly the opposite of the city's burgeoning numbers of female modern dancers, perform their own dance to birdsong and classical music. The lampoon of the production's own serious dance numbers is carried out through a burlesque of gender and sexuality. Not only are these tramps "nances" (a contemporary term for effeminate men), they are engaged in homosexual intimacy, as suggested by their dancing in pairs. That the audience "got it" and giggled in response suggests the touristic pleasure—both titillation and unease—that spectators found in *Pinwheel*'s staging of the Village bohemia. Such moments were, however, neutralized through the production's general reliance on scantily clad female dancers, whose presence was intended to satisfy a putatively male heterosexual gaze. The *New York Clipper*, for instance, described a dance performed by Margaret Pettit, "who did a breath-holding bacchante garbed in a few leaves which looked every minute as though they were about to drop to the floor."[54] And as *Variety* commented of the production's costumes, "Enough of the bare leg and bare feet to meet the appetite of Broadway is a fact. Costumes of the drapery kind, and not much of them, never fail to have slits, that the freedom and view of the entire leg may be had."[55] The production's primary dramaturgy and published critical opinions all privileged the spectator as male, heterosexual, and anxious about queer intimacy. But we are free to imagine various queer spectatorial positions present in the audience, for whom stagings of male-male intimacy or female skin might have offered other pleasures, even from the conservatism of a midtown Broadway house.

Among these representations of sexual taste and titillation, the signification of Ito's Japaneseness to the production's reception is overdetermined. In the show's origination story, Ito's Japaneseness is linked to the act of importuning and to the eliciting of effeminate tears, as well as to a sense of irresistibility, given Hitchcock's acquiescence. Meanwhile, in reviews of the show, "Japaneseness" as either an identity or an aesthetic marker can only be recognized in critics resorting to descriptions commonly used in discussions of Japanese aesthetics. For instance, *Life Magazine* singled out the "reproduction of Degas color tones" in the costuming and setting for one dance number, and observed of the production as a whole, "It is made up almost entirely of extremely modern dance numbers, some of which are reduced to terms of such simplicity and economy of effort as to be rather dull, and others of which are unusually fine."[56] Ito's skills of pictorial arrangement, his attentiveness to color, and the descriptors "simplicity" and "economy of effort" (though not entirely positive here) might all be taken as signs of the discourse of Japanese artistry. But they also mark the production's general artsy impenetrability, in which Ito's Japaneseness was absorbed into the broader characterization of Village bohemia as tantalizingly, confusingly foreign.

While *Pinwheel* was a commercial failure, this made it appealing for dance critics—a just-emerging professional category. The *Times* wrote, "But Michio Itow, who is responsible for most of the dance numbers, has provided a number of extremely lovely moments as well as not a few that seemed rather footless. So much of it all is good, however, that it seems rather a shame that it isn't better."[57] The general consensus was that Herndon had been mistaken about the necessity of the comedic bits; the dance was, in fact, the best part of the show. And so, after splitting with Herndon, Ito reopened it at the Little Theatre (now the Helen Hayes), in August of 1922. *Life Magazine* observed, "In its new form, it is frankly without comedy . . . and is much more as it should be. . . . [With] unusual dances [such] as the Faun and Nymph, [. . .] the extraordinary dancing of Josephine Head and Phyllis Jackson, and the work of Michio Itow himself."[58]

It was, in the end, *Pinwheel*'s financial failure and its original generic ambiguity that led critics to esteem it as a win for "Art." As the dance critic John Martin was to write eight years later, in a discussion of Ito's wideranging activities, "Sometimes Ito is engrossed in turning out a beautiful and artistic failure in the way of a musical revue, such as the 'Pinwheel' of cherished memory."[59] The contradictions found in the production were, I think, characteristic of Ito. Always called to give his audiences what they wanted and expected of him, Ito gave them *everything* they wanted, all at once— scantily clad girls and nods to same-sex attraction, modernist choreography and revue kicklines, solemnity and silliness, "Broadway" entertainment and

Japoniste Collections   115

"Japanese" aestheticism. This was, then, another form of the collection, and of Ito's attentiveness to the desires that collections hold. What often seemed the disorganized and overly ambitious result of his enthusiasm for large-scale theatrical productions might also be understood not merely as a refusal to be pigeonholed, but as a capacity to provoke multiple, and often contradictory desires—and to be remembered, in the aftermath, as somehow satisfying them all.

Fetish Subjects

Ito made his modern dance reputation through his solo and group choreography. But some of the most striking archival traces of Ito are photographic and written remains that are not documentations of his dance practice at all, but rather are records of his performance of self, as a nexus of desire. I close this chapter by lingering on two of these—a photograph from Nickolas Muray's studio series on Ito, and Ito's memoir recollection of his episodic relationship to the famous ballet dancer, Vaslav Nijinsky. Both of these help us think about how Ito navigated being a racialized, male dancer in the US. At times he acceded to being perceived as, and indeed constructed himself as, a kind of fetish object; the persistence of this emphasis on his own enduring materiality might, in the end, have been a practice of survival.

That Ito was constructed by the US press as a sort of Japanese art object is unavoidable. Among many examples is this from the *Baltimore Sun*: "He is a slender Japanese boy, as clean cut as an ivory netsuke."[60] The *netsuke*, that sought-after Japanese collectible, is a miniature sculpture, small enough to fit in your pocket. Its weight reassuringly bumps against you as you walk; its cool, hard contours offer an inviting surface to rub your fingers against, privately, within the draped folds of your trousers or jacket. The *netsuke*, then, is the paradigmatic Japanese fetish object for the Japanophile. The *Baltimore Sun* critic's characterization of Ito as a *netsuke* evokes the rigid representational paradigm of the effeminized, infantilized Asian male in white supremacist discourse, a discourse that Ito was subject to in the United States.[61] For example, in 1917, a reviewer for *Vogue* magazine wrote:

> The Japanese are a tiny race; and, in consequence, their art is tiny. . . . But the Japanese, though physically small, are astonishingly alert. . . . We should, therefore, expect to find in the folk-dances of the Japanese these two har-

monic notes of imaginative diminution and astonishing activity; and this expectation was satisfied by the performance of Michio Itow. The dances that he showed were all imagined on a little scale and executed with superlative alertness.[62]

The review's lexicon—"diminutive," "agile," "alert," "swift"—rolls through the standard stereotyping phrases by which East Asian subjects were pinned down, a vocabulary that, though frequently marked by romantic racialism, could quickly shift into a negative register, signifying childishness, untrustworthiness, and effeminacy. These dominant images were part of the legal, economic, and social structures in the nineteenth- and twentieth-century US that, as David Eng has influentially shown, formulated Asian American masculinity as both racial and sexual difference.[63] In Ito's case, his work as a dancer made these tropes seem even more overdetermined. As Yutian Wong writes, "Ito was viewed as an acceptable 'Oriental' as long as he inhabited an attenuated masculinity. Doubly effeminized as a male Asian dancer, Ito was further asexualized through descriptions of his dancing."[64]

And yet, the characterization of Ito as a *netsuke* is anything but asexualized. Indeed, it seems likely that some of Ito's allure lay in the tense relation between a dominant discourse of asexualized Japanese masculinity and his evident appeal to people of both sexes. Such an apparent contradiction helps contextualize, for instance, *Vogue*'s recommendation of Ito as a dance artist who would be suitable for the "discreet hostess" to summon to her parties as "home entertainment."[65] Like a *netsuke*, which offers private aesthetic and tactile thrills, *Vogue*'s framing of Ito might also be understood as the presentation of a fetish object, a figure who could be imagined to supplement the various lacks and anxieties held by his patrons.

The fetish, as a concept, emerges through formulations of religious primitivism, then economic commodity worship, and then psychoanalytic sexual perversion. As Anne McClintock has traced, the fetish took on particular explanatory power in the emergence of European mercantile culture in the seventeenth and eighteenth centuries, as European traders sought to establish systems of valuation that simultaneously enabled trade with Africans while affirming European superiority. McClintock highlights the formative role of imperialism in securing the fetish "as the embodiment of an impossible irresolution."[66] As she and others have delineated, this repetitive scene of imperial encounter produced racial fetishism, the ambiguous desires that make up what Leslie Bow calls "racist love." But, as Bow goes on to delin-

Japoniste Collections 117

eate, the fetish in Asian American racialization is not only an expression of objectification, symbolic castration, and fantasies of racial/sexual dominance. It is also an ambiguous and ambivalent site of pleasure and self-making for the Asian American subject. Bow points to a fraught continuum of Asian American engagement with the fetish, from Anne Cheng's reading of Nancy Kwan's performance as Linda Low in *Flower Drum Song* as a form of self-fetishization to various examples of "Asian Americans as the *makers* of fetish objects,"[67] who, in their "seeming self-objectification, [. . .] offer a twist on racial-sexual voyeurism."[68] To recognize Ito as just such a maker of the fetish is to understand him as not merely a collectible object, one among many dancers whose putative exoticism drew white spectators, but rather, as a collectible object who collected desires in turn. The fantasies by which racial fetishization forms its attachments thus run alongside those self-making fantasies, held, and projected, by objectified subjects themselves.

The contours of these fantasies take shape in a series of photographs of Ito taken by the portraitist Nickolas Muray. These images manifest Ito's own ability to attract, and to hold, the desires of those around him. Muray was a Hungarian-born photographer and Olympic saber fencer, whose Greenwich Village studio was a key site in the neighborhood's legendary atmosphere of bohemia, sexual permissiveness, and funneling of popular culture into modern art.[69] His own long affair and friendship with Frida Kahlo resulted in a series of stunning photographs that represent an extraordinary project of self-fashioning and collaboration. Muray was also passionate about modern dance; he frequently attended dance concerts in New York, and wrote reviews for *Dance Magazine*. This interest is also apparent in the numerous photographs of dancers within his oeuvre—both well-known performers and anonymous subjects—whose frequently nude, sculpted bodies offered specimens of human physicality. Among such subjects were Ted Shawn, Ruth St. Denis, Martha Graham, Mikail Mordkin, and Doris Humphrey. Ito's inclusion in this oeuvre marks both his success as a dancer in the New York scene, and his involvement in the Greenwich Village art world, in which erotics and aesthetics each sublimated the other.

The series taken of Ito uses two gold-foiled, chest-high flats, suggestive of short columns, as background, and in about half of the photographs, he is nude. In one of the photographs, Ito stands facing sideways, but with his torso turned out to the viewer and his downstage arm drawn back, almost as if he were pulling the string of a bow. His fingers instead graze his own chest, delicately resting there and casting a shadow on his skin. His upstage arm is

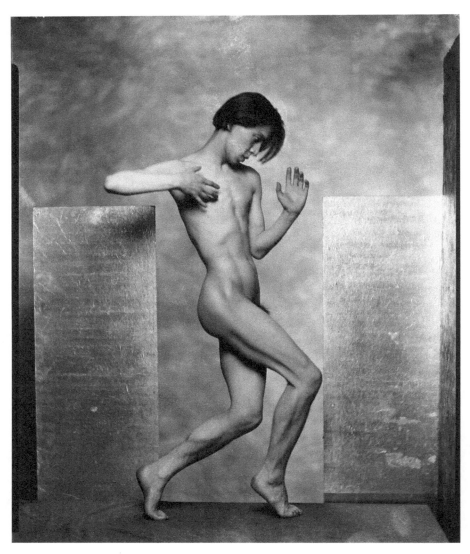

Fig. 12. "Michio Ito," photograph by Nickolas Muray, ca. 1922–1930, courtesy of the George Eastman Museum, © Nickolas Muray Photo Archives.

Japoniste Collections

bent up with palm out and open, and his head bends gently down, so that his eyes seem to look not so much at his hand, but through it. His legs are bent, both heels raised, as if in a stylized runner's position. Not only does the pose suggest extraordinary balance, but it shows off every single line of muscle and tendon, his front hamstring looking less like flesh than carved stone, and his calves rippling with sinew. The chiseled line of his downstage thigh also serves to mostly obscure his crotch; only a whisper of pubic hair is visible, blending into the shadow cast by the twist of his torso.

In this photograph, Ito might seem almost more sculpture than human. With the light gleaming off of his taut skin and every line of musculature perfectly rendered, the gold-foil columns that frame his body evoke folding screens and thus read as signifiers of Japaneseness here. Muray's depiction of Ito, a gleaming, tense statue, can be read as just such a Japanese fetish, an adoring objectification through aestheticization. And yet, this photograph is not as narrowly orientalist as it might first appear. The gold columns were Muray's standard studio prop; they appear in many other portrait series, and both Ito's nudity and sculptural pose are characteristic for Muray's oeuvre, in which dancer-as-statuary was a common theme. Moreover, Ito is assuredly in control of his posing; across the series, bodily positions appear that are reminiscent of his dancing and choreographic method. Ito then is a co-creator in this image—not just the photograph itself, but the effects of desire and representation brought forth by it, pointedly through a dance lexicon.

The photograph, in this case, might be a lot like Linda Low's mirror and Cheng's reading of Kwan's performance in it—a reflection, incontrovertibly bound up in gender and racial norms, that nevertheless provides a site of image- and self-making. That is, Muray's photographs of Ito might involve the kind of mirrorlike awareness that Kwan/Low uses in her performance of feminine self-sufficiency and pleasure. As Cheng writes, "Pleasure is to be found in the very specularization of the self. The three-way mirror acts as a literalization of what is going on specularly in that scene: not just *how I see myself* or *how others see me* but *how I see others seeing me*."[70] In contrast to Kwan/Low, Ito never looks at the camera in this series. Nevertheless, he is minutely aware of the camera; his sense of its gaze is a deep part of the suspenseful, expectant aspect of these photographs. Instead of looking at us with his eyes, seeing us see him, it is as if he looks back with his entire corporeality and its expansive, kinesthetic awareness.

The strange power of the fetish is to hold us. And Ito does hold us, in his charismatic, tense magnetism. As Rey Chow has suggested, collections are attachments; they are objects that produce an emotional bond often seen as obsessive, fetishistic, and excessive.[71] This is a story usually told with a focus on the collector, acquirer, or admirer of the object—but what of the "object" itself? If we think of Ito as a man positioned as a collectible object within a white-supremacist cultural logic of imperial-racial possession, then he is also one who reveals this logic by collecting desire in turn. Thus it is possible to imagine how Ito captured attachments, drawing desirous looks to himself, accumulating the sheen of being in demand. This was, of course, a precarious valuation, contingent on the associated estimations of his cosmopolitanism, the Japanese reputation for aesthetic expression, and his performance of a domesticated exoticism. But this tense, taut photograph discloses his ability to modulate these projections into a position from which he could take possession—if not of himself, then of the desires of those around him.

• • •

If Ito performed himself into a resonant fetish subject, then he did so with an awareness of another dancer who was similarly positioned—the Ballets Russes star Vaslav Nijinsky. Across Ito's postwar memoirs and magazine articles, he penned a series of accounts detailing his relationship with Nijinksy.[72] As discussed in chapter 1, many of these stories may be fabrications, but that is not to say that I consider them to be untrue. Rather, as fantasies, they reveal intimate truths about Ito's own desires. They are discursive performances that reveal the ongoing performance of self that sustained Ito across the exclusions (both literal and figurative, political and artistic) of his career. Moreover, the memoir itself is a form of collection, by which the collector defines themself in the present, through the past. Across the many stories, projections of self, that I have found in compiling my own collection of Ito materials, it is this one that evocatively refracts the many desires that constituted Ito's performance of self—both his own, and those of the many spectators, patrons, artists, and even scholars, who encounter him.

In his narrative, Ito hears the news of Nijinsky's death while riding an elevator in postwar Tokyo with some of his amateur dance students. Stunned, he stands there for a few minutes, until finally, desolated, he walks out into the night, and into a rush of memory and fantasy about the famous dancer. It begins in Paris. Intoxicated by the dancer's performances in *L'après-midi* and *Pétrouchka*, Ito describes his response: "I had reached a peak. I was heated throughout my body, experiencing such thrills for the first time. I left the theater together with the crowd. Outside, a light rain fell. Turning my flushed

Japoniste Collections

face to the rain felt good. The hollow face of the killed Russian doll Petrushka was burned into my memory."[73] Until dawn, Ito walks through the streets crying, his legs aching, his head throbbing. In its language and dramatic rhythm, the episode casts Ito's encounter with the Art of the Dance, and with Nijinsky, as a sexual encounter—which, like the Faun's, is ultimately a scene of auto-erotic solitude.

Vaslav Nijinsky offers an intriguing counterpoint to Ito, and not simply because of Ito's apparent obsession with him. Nijinsky came to define the figure of the male dancer in prewar concert dance. With his striking, almost uncanny corporeality and his Slavic ethnicity, he also became a figuration of "Oriental" embodiment. Indeed, Nijinsky was occasionally called, because of a supposed slant to his eyes, the "Little Jap," a name by which racialization served to manifest the dancer's denigrated class and sexual identities, which were harder to visually identify. Descriptions of Nijinsky slip between the sexual and the racial, trying to pin his extraordinary difference down to some identifiable alterity. As the critic, publisher, and ballet aficionado Cyril Beaumont wrote, "As a dancer [Nijinsky's] work was not of the robust, manly type. Yet neither was it altogether effeminate. Always he appeared to be of a race apart, or another essence than ourselves, an impression heightened by his partiality for unusual *roles*, which were either animal-like, mythological, or unreal."[74] It is hard not to hear in this characterization echoes of Justice John Marshall Harlan's famous categorization of the Chinese as "a race so different."[75] But what is crucial about Nijinsky is how the language of racial exclusion is not only linked to sexuality and gender (a common braiding), but to the language of allure and of artistic iconoclasm. It was these intertwined qualities that Ito had thrust upon him by spectators conditioned by general orientalism and by the very example of Nijinsky, and that Ito also desired and pursued.

As Ito narrates, following his initial experience of Nijinsky's dancing in Paris, his relationship with Nijinsky materializes in two key incidents. The first is a sort of ghostly competition with each other's traces in a reception-hall-turned-rehearsal-studio in Munich. Needing a place to rehearse, he arranged with his hotel's proprietors to use the empty reception hall as a dance studio. He is told he can only come in the afternoons, because "another dancer" has already made a similar arrangement for the morning. The dancer, he discovers, is Nijinsky. Ito arrives one day to see shoe prints high up the wall, traces of the ballet dancer's famously gravity-defying leaps. Taking this as a challenge, Ito goes to the other corner of the room, and with a running head start, flings himself upon the wall, managing to plant one foot higher than Nijinsky's.

> "There, I did it!" I thought, but when I went to look the next day, there, another footprint had landed above it. I became aggravated. I was far from being able to cross that mark, but somehow or other I would have to soar and surpass it. I tried to leap as high, but flipped over and hit my head. So I called for a waiter, saying I wanted him to bring me a ladder, and taking off my shoes, I climbed the ladder, and with a "unh" I laughingly pressed my shoe print onto the ceiling. The following day, I went to see what Nijinsky had done, and in the spot of my shoe print, in German was written, "Idiot."[76]

The two dancers engage in a bodily competition with the traces of each other's presence. Following each other's arc across the room and into the air, heaving themselves into flight, one after the other, they push through space that is thick with the presence of the other body. A choreography of bodily exertion and mischievous cleverness, it is a duet, and a courtship.

The dancers finally meet in New York, a scene that promises consummation, but instead, offers only disappointment and deterioration. Nijinsky, rescued from his house arrest in Russia during World War I and finally permitted to travel, was scheduled to appear at the Metropolitan Opera House. He performs the *Spectre de la Rose*, and with his thrilling leap, captivates Ito. After the performance, Ito rushes backstage and knocks at the door of the idol.

> There was no response. I thought that he wasn't in the room but knocked again. Then in a small voice in Russian, "what is it" "who is it." "It's Ito," I responded, and there was no response. He looked out through the key hole then made a noise and opened the door. When he opened the door a crack he saw me. Seeing me he instantly opened and grabbing my hand pulled me into the room and then quickly closed the door and again locked it. I was so surprised I forgot to even give a greeting. I asked what was wrong and in a small voice he said, "Somebody in my troupe is trying to kill me, he is trying to take my position" and "why did they bring me to America" "Americans are all Bolsheviks." He continued saying nonsensical things, and I didn't know what to say.[77]

Japoniste Collections   123

Finally, Madame Nijinsky and Diaghilev come, banging on the door until they are let in. They are surprised to see Ito, who soon after, "with an ominous feeling," slides out of the room, never to see Nijinsky again.

Ito arrived in New York in mid-August of 1916; Nijinsky's Metropolitan Opera performances took place in the fall of 1916. It is entirely possible that Ito attended Nijinsky's performance, and even that the entire interaction transpired as described. What matters more than its accuracy, however, is the desire encoded in this story, and the way in which Ito stitches himself into a sense of meaningful co-presence with Nijinsky, even as their encounters are fleeting. In this final segment, Ito is a confidante, a fellow dancer whom Nijinsky trusts before others. Pulled into the private-public (and always potentially erotic) space of Nijinsky's dressing room, Ito describes a moment of desperate friendship and charged intimacy in the sweaty period after the dancer's performance and before his full descent into madness. But Ito cannot help this friend, this love, whom he never encounters again.

Critics and aficionados alike read Nijinsky's death-defying (and death-driving) leaps as queer.[78] They register as such within Ito's narratives as well—narratives that place this homoerotic desire in the past, as Ito recalls (and imagines) incidents from his youth, writing from the ravages of his own late middle age and war-torn Tokyo.[79] In this recollection, in New York, the Japanese Ito is the one who can connect with Nijinsky, the overeroticized, overadulated, orientalized dancer. The intimacy coursing between the two is an intimacy of the queered and racialized outsider, whose body, in its performative significations, becomes the vessel for everyone else's desires. But of course, this relationship, this narrative, is a fantasy Ito himself has penned, an expression of his own desires—to leap into modernist genius and historical centrality. But that's the thing. Ito does not leap—not in the narrative, or in fact in his choreography more generally. Ito's gesture is not the gravity-escaping leap; it is something more self-contained, and more grounded. Writing from the post-war period, having *survived*, Ito's dogged self-mythologizing is, in the end, the mark of having made it through. His insistence on individuality, for his students and for himself, through the performance of type, is a doctrine not of modernist genius, but of attentive and attuned performances of self, molded to the contours of collective fantasies—of orientalism, of Japanese artistry, and of the erotics of an art object contained within itself.

CHAPTER FOUR

Japanese America and Fantasies of Integration

California, 1929–1941

> Hundreds of Japanese people are expected to witness the Hollywood Bowl program on Friday evening, August 15th, when Michio Ito, internationally known terpsichorean artist, will present "Prince Igor" with 125 dancers taking part. It will mark the first time this production has been presented, especially Michio Ito's conception of the dance.[1]

In 1930, the *Rafu Shimpo*, a Los Angeles–based Japanese newspaper, announced Ito's newest production at the famous Hollywood Bowl. Proclaiming the artistic significance of this event, it also hailed the "hundreds of Japanese people" that the paper anticipated would attend. The presence of these spectators at the Bowl, and Ito's presence in the pages of the *Rafu Shimpo*, mark a thus-far overlooked aspect of Ito's career: his ties with the Japanese American community in Southern California. Ito's career in Southern California during the 1930s has been predominantly understood through his engagement with the developing modern dance scene in California, and his minor film appearances, most notably by Naima Prevots and Mary-Jean Cowell.[2] But these activities took place alongside Ito's increasing engagement with local Japanese residents and his endeavors to integrate them into the cultural sphere of white arts organizations. This chapter takes up this story.

To date, scholars have not thought of Ito as part of the Japanese American community in California. However, the evidence in Japanese-language newspapers points to a substantial, and complicated, relationship. The attention to Ito found in these pages is notable: in his first six months in California, the *Rafu Shimpo* alone ran forty-six pieces on him, in a mixture of Japanese and English. Other papers, such as the *Shin Sekai*, *Nichbei Shinbun*, *Nippu Jiji*, and even the *Hawaii Hōchi*, also featured Ito. Although coverage slowed

124

Japanese America and Fantasies of Integration

down after this initial period, Ito remained a frequent subject of interest throughout the 1930s. In the *Rafu Shimpo*, coverage of Ito was far greater in the English-language section than in the Japanese-language section, at a ratio of about 13:1. The paper's publishers saw Ito as particularly relevant to the Nisei, at whom the English-language section was aimed.

The Nisei were the second generation; they held American citizenship and thus the promise of futurity for the community at large. Their rootedness in the US was a site of both hope and anxiety for their elders, the Issei, who wanted the Nisei to integrate, but simultaneously to remain "Japanese." The stakes of this balancing act were high: since 1924, all legal immigration from Asia to the US had been closed; in California over the 1920s and '30s, Japanese faced increasing prohibitions on property ownership and leasing, stricter segregation, and a continual narrowing of opportunities to build a successful and secure life in the US. The Nisei, who in theory were rights-bearing citizens, stood as the community's best chance to claim a lasting place in the US. And for the Issei elite in Los Angeles, who dedicated themselves to this effort, Ito seemed like an ideal model to offer the Nisei; he had apparently integrated into white society not in spite of being Japanese, but rather by using his background as the point of entry. Perhaps he could teach Nisei to do the same.

Ito's relationship with the Japanese community developed over his time in Los Angeles; its presence, however, seems not to have been a substantial motivation for his 1929 move to California. Mary-Jean Cowell suggests that Ito had postponed the move from New York, despite being involved with the Hollywood film industry since 1921, because of pervasive anti-Japanese sentiment and the film industry's racist casting and narrative practices.[3] But, she suggests, by 1929 the financial opportunity was too appealing; Ito had been offered employment on the film *No, No, Nanette*, and the onset of the Great Depression had constricted dance patronage in New York. Newspaper notices also reveal that some of Ito's early patrons, such as Mrs. Frank A. Vanderlip, were now in California and eager to support him there.[4] Pauline Koner, who was in Ito's company at the time, recalls that the troupe carried out a cross-country tour in 1929, but having run out of money in San Francisco, the Itos decided to remain in California.[5] It is also likely that Ito went in search of new audiences; reviews from his final years in New York suggest that critics had grown weary of his dance programs.[6] Some mix of financial and artistic opportunity, then, motivated the relocation—his only move since his initial departure from Japan that was not precipitated by war.

In Southern California, Ito became an advocate for the development of modern dance across the region. While the form already had some important champions and institutions in the area (most notably, the Denishawn School, founded in Los Angeles in 1915 by Ruth St. Denis and Ted Shawn), Ito's work to institutionalize modern dance offers a glimpse not only of how the genre took root in California, but just as important, of how dedicated dance criticism emerged there—a phenomenon that has received relatively little attention compared to its parallel in New York.[7] Dance criticism had a role to play in the regional boosterism that Mike Davis and others have highlighted as one of Southern California's major industries.[8] For dance critics, like many other cultural writers in the area, the question of what counted as good artistic dance was also a question of how Los Angeles and the surrounding areas measured up as an alternative cultural center to New York and other major cities. Newspapers' coverage of Ito, then, reveals aspects of both his reception during the period, and the ways Ito stood as a figure for broader fantasies of regional identity held by many of the city's boosters.

The fantasy of integration was central among these. This is a fantasy that can be traced across the pages of both English-language newspapers aimed at a mainstream (white) readership and publications aimed at the Japanese immigrant community. In this chapter, through the dance criticism published in local newspapers and select photographs, I explore the fantasy of national integration, and some of the specific permutations of this fantasy that Ito pursued, or was seen to represent. As Eiichiro Azuma has detailed, integration was a goal that both white progressives and the Issei elite separately strove to realize.[9] For the former group, integration of immigrants into Californian society fulfilled the fantasy of the US as a "melting pot"; for the latter, integration offered a path toward safety and success for Japanese in the US. These two goals intertwined, for Ito, in the community arts movement, which sought to use art as a vehicle for social integration while also establishing Los Angeles as a serious art center. Ito championed his own version of this movement, the community dance movement, as a way to establish dance's centrality to this broader effort.

Part of what made Ito such a compelling advocate for these integrationist efforts was the fact that his body was repeatedly read as a corporeal instantiation of the idea of national integration. I consider how this figuration worked via the Japanese paradigm of *kokutai*, or the national body. The notion of a national body—as an abstract concept, but also as something physically manifested through dance—offers a way of thinking about Ito's ability to

Japanese America and Fantasies of Integration 127

assimilate dance styles and cultural traditions from many different places into his own body. This assimilative capacity had varying meanings for his spectators, especially in light of his own highly publicized marriage to and then divorce from the white American Hazel Wright. The ongoing enmeshment of professional activity with attributed bodily significations was, perhaps, best emblematized by his 1937 Hollywood Bowl production, at which several of his Nisei dancers performed. Reviewers repeatedly read onto these Nisei a slippage between racial and national signification—a slippage that, in hindsight, foreshadows the slippage between Japanese and Japanese American that resulted in the incarceration of most of Ito's students, and his own internment, only a few years later.

The fantasies of integration that the various communities in Los Angeles held about Ito were, in the end, closely aligned with his own sustaining performances of self as a cultural mediator and community-instantiating artist. The importance of these fantasies in the decade prior to the US imprisonment of Japanese on the West Coast cannot be dismissed simply because they were idealistic and/or self-serving. Rather, to recognize them as fantasies is to highlight that precisely as Japan spread its imperial agenda, precisely as the Second Sino-Japanese War began, precisely as laws against Japanese in the US became ever more restrictive, such visions of himself as a historically significant figure were not, as I write in this book's introduction, escapism, but a mode of imagination that tied Ito even more tightly to the sociopolitical order, and to the community formations in which he found himself.

Little Tokyo and a Paradigm for Japanese American Success

In 1935, Ito drew up a proposal for the revitalization of Los Angeles's Little Tokyo district. The *Los Angeles Times* described the effort with typical orientalist condescension, but also interest. Japanese papers were interested not only in Ito's plans, but also in mainstream papers' reactions to this effort. When the *Nichibei Shinbun* covered the proposal, it reprinted the *Times's* entire column:

> Imagine Aladdin and his wonderful lamp arriving in Los Angeles and getting busy.
>
> Imagine him transforming, with magic celerity and keen appreciation of a great opportunity, a sizable part of the city south of the City Hall into a

beautiful little Japanese city—a place of Nipponese architectural charm, with beautiful Japanese gardens, quaint tea houses, a typical drum bridge, colorful lanterns, delightful cherry trees interspersed with weeping willows bordering the streets—a gem of a Japanese city within a great western metropolis and just the locale for appropriately picturesque attire.[10]

Urban revitalization might seem far from modern concert dance. The project begins to make more sense, however, when we recall that Hellerau itself was constructed because of a belief in the three-way correspondence between healthy built environments, healthy bodies, and a healthy nation. It also helps to remember Ito's consistent penchant for wildly ambitious, large-scale projects. Strikingly, Ito attempted, through this plan, to offer the familiar fantasy of Japanese aestheticism not only as a commercial good for the city's benefit, but as something that could concretely improve the lives of local Japanese. In this section, I give context for Ito's engagement with the Japanese immigrant community. His example enriches our understanding of first-generation experiences in California, and of the relations between the Issei and Nisei. Ito's efforts also foreground how much the concept of "integration" and the arts, as a cultural sphere, shaped the discursive efforts of Issei elite to establish a foundation for their community.

Ito's plan is one of touristic fantasy. With its "quaint tea houses, a typical drum bridge, colorful lanterns, delightful cherry trees interspersed with weeping willows bordering the streets," Ito's vision matches the models of "Japanese Villages" in world expositions in both Europe and the US. And, with the construction of the new Union Station by the Southern Pacific Railway Company, Ito's plan noted that all tourists coming to Los Angeles would pass through Little Tokyo, and thus should be induced to spend time there.[11]

Ito's vision of a picturesque village, however, was not merely about constructing "Japanese" facades, like those found on nearby Hollywood backlots. Rather, Ito insisted that this construction was necessary to modernize and improve the living conditions in the district. The Little Tokyo district was one of the primary areas in which Japanese were permitted to live, along with other groups restricted by racial housing covenants.[12] Ito noted that Little Tokyo's buildings did not meet Los Angeles's construction codes, which had been updated after an earthquake in 1933, and that, within a few years, this would probably serve as a pretext to force the Japanese out of their neighborhood unless the buildings were improved.[13]

Ito's argument was not rhetorical invention: the district's housing stock was substandard and overcrowded, and there was little hope of alleviation: Japanese Americans (and other Asians) were prohibited from applying to Los Angeles public housing.[14] Ito called for all of the area's old buildings to be razed and replaced with "new buildings with the most modern facilities to meet our modern needs and beautify them with the most elaborate and unique Japanese architectures."[15] The emphasis on modern facilities was not, in fact, in contradiction with the plan for the buildings' facades to be in a traditional Japanese style. As he observed—I imagine a bit wryly—"The modern architecture of America and Europe, is greatly influenced by the Japanese architecture, therefore, Japanese buildings in this district will not be out of character, they will harmonize with the new buildings planned for the Civic Center."[16] Ito knew well that European and American modern art, architecture, and consumer products had all borrowed liberally from Japanese models in their pursuit of "new" forms. He suggested then that the vernacular of the planned Civic Center was already the vernacular of his vision for Little Tokyo.

To finance this plan, Ito proposed the organization of a new import-export company, the Pan Pacific Financing Co. Ito asserted that "the capital of this Company should be sought among Americans, for this undertaking should be not only for the benefit of the Japanese alone, but for profit should be shared with Americans."[17] We see here Ito's awareness of the balancing act required of Japanese in America, and the necessity of gaining "American," that is, white, support for projects that would support the Japanese community. Ito also takes the role of cultural mediator, and thus asserts that the third aim of the Little Tokyo revitalization project is "To promote good will between Americans and Japanese."[18] We will encounter this sentiment again, in Ito's self-defense during his internment trial, as he sought to explain his activities in Los Angeles and Japan. It was, perhaps, a straightforward articulation of Ito's ambition and sense of himself as a cosmopolitan artist. But it was also a statement of his mode of engagement with the Nisei, and with the Japanese immigrant community at large; artistic expression could be a practice of community definition that produced value for the US, and thus—so the hope went—might be enough to overturn the ever-growing anti-Japanese sentiment.

Ito's Little Tokyo revitalization plan is characteristic of his activities in Southern California in the 1930s. His involvement with the local Japanese immigrant community is a complicated mix of what I take to be Ito's sincere attachment to the community, along with an opportunism that recognized that the presence of this community allowed him to act as a mediator in a

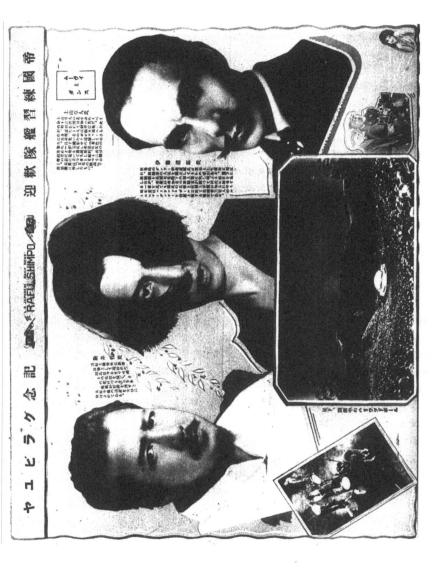

Fig. 13. "Welcoming the Imperial Naval Exercises" ["Kangei teikoku renshū kantai"]. *Rafu Shimpo*, August 23, 1929.

Japanese America and Fantasies of Integration

way that fit with the desires of regional elites to create an "integrated" Los Angeles. Likewise, Ito's early success with predominantly white Los Angeles arts patrons (covered in the next section) helped secure his place within— and his acknowledged usefulness to—the Japanese immigrant community. In August 1929, only a few months after his arrival in Los Angeles, the *Rafu Shimpo* published a special gravure section to highlight the achievements and activities carried out by Japanese immigrants, on the occasion of the Japanese imperial armada exercises. The special section contained pages devoted to local merchants, farming practices, leading businessmen, and so on. One page highlighted prominent Japanese in entertainment, and featured as the exemplars Ito and the film actors Komai Tetsu and Kamiyama Sōjin.[19]

The prominence of these three performers in a special section dedicated to celebrating the achievements of the Japanese immigrant community helps revise common paradigms about the contours of the early Japanese American community—and the ways in which, while Ito's story was certainly unusual, it was not entirely exceptional. Especially on the West Coast, the Japanese immigrant community, and "the Issei" as a figure, has been primarily characterized as made up of laborers, who arrived directly from Japan, worked as farmers, gardeners, domestics, and grocers, and lived in segregated neighborhoods with mounting restrictions placed on their possible livelihoods.[20] Partly for this reason, Asian American dance studies scholar Yutian Wong suggests that Ito was not part of the Japanese immigrant community in Los Angeles, even as she makes a historiographic argument for recognizing him as a figurehead for Asian American dance history. Citing an interview with Amy Iwanabe, a Nisei woman who had wanted to take lessons at Ito's studio, Wong notes that Japanese mothers considered Ito "morally suspicious"[21] and observes that, with his white wife and his ability to access rarefied spaces of white patronage, Ito occupied a very different position than many of his compatriots.

But taking Ito, Komai, and Kamiyama as a trio paints a fuller historical picture of the possibilities for Japanese immigrant life prior to the Asia-Pacific War. Komai was born in Kumamoto, Japan, emigrated to the US in 1907, and remained there for the rest of his life; like many Issei, he was incarcerated at the Gila River War Relocation Center. Kamiyama, meanwhile, was born in Sendai, and traveled to the US in 1919, originally working as a singer and newspaper editor. He acted in a substantial number of Hollywood films during the silent film era, but when the technology shifted to talkies, he returned to Japan at the start of the 1930s and continued his career there. Neither Komai, Kamiyama, nor Ito, either by profession or migratory itinerary, are what is usually meant by Issei, and yet their examples, gathered together in the *Rafu Shimpo*'s special section, evoke the many different patterns of mobility that were, in fact, central to the Issei experience. As Eiichiro Azuma has charted, such mobility was not restricted to artists and the professional class, but was also common to many agriculturalist and mechanical laborers who crossed the Pacific (and sometimes the Atlantic as well) multiple times.[22] This special section also suggests the affective connection that Japanese in America may have felt across class lines—or, at least, that the editors of the *Rafu Shimpo* hoped to foster, in order to create a greater sense of diasporic affiliation.

This broader sense of Ito's relationship to the Japanese immigrant community allows us to understand how community leaders might have regarded him, and have seen Ito's story as relevant to their own. Editors at the *Rafu Shimpo* and other community leaders seem to have embraced Ito because he represented a successful performance of integration, *as a performance of Japaneseness*. This was a strategy that elite Issei were championing more broadly as integral to their community's survival in the US. As Azuma has demonstrated, Issei of the period negotiated the challenge of being citizen-subjects of one nation (Japan) and residents of another (the US) by practicing a "politics of dualism."[23] According to this pragmatic strategy advocated by the community's elites, the most effective way to be Japanese was to carry out successful acts of assimilation. The ability to integrate could thus be claimed as a particularly Japanese characteristic, an assertion that was here used to further immigrants' own agendas, but that, Azuma highlights, we can also recognize as working in parallel with Japan's own ideology of absorptive imperialism, as discussed in chapter 2 and further explored later in this chapter.

This integrative performance of Japaneseness was, in the end, aimed at the Nisei. While the tensions between the two generations, and Issei anxiety over the Nisei, are now a mainstay of Japanese American history, Andrew Leong reminds us that these generational identities were, in fact, emergent at this very moment.[24] (A term such as *Nikkei*, meanwhile, emerged after the war.[25]) Indeed, as Leong has traced, the term "Nisei" (as opposed to *Amerika umare* ["American born"]) was only really picked up in newspapers' Japanese-language sections in the late 1920s. In English-language sections, "Nisei" is quite rare until the early 1930s, when it appears around the planning for the first "Nisei Week" of 1934. Nisei Week, a festival that continues today, was run by the Japanese American Citizens League (JACL) and was created by

Japanese America and Fantasies of Integration

Issei merchants who wanted to draw the second generation to their businesses. The festival intentionally combined distinctive Japanese traditions (kimono, serving tea) with dominant cultural events, such as beauty pageants and fashion shows.[26] Nisei Week, therefore, not only sought to appeal to the second generation, it offered a vision of cultural amalgamation for the Nisei—especially the young women, who played crucial roles in the festival as performers, cultural representatives, and contestants for the title of Nisei Week Queen.[27]

Constructing the Nisei as a cohesive generational identity was a critical project. Increasingly restrictive immigration and land-use laws eroded the possibilities for economic security available to Issei. Their children, however, born in the US, and thus US citizens, held the promise of being rights-bearing subjects, entitled under US law (in theory) to the protections—and opportunities—of citizenship. As Azuma observes, "Issei envisaged a better future not during their own lifetimes but during their children's."[28] Nisei young women, in particular, stood as the overdetermined sign of this futurity, imagined to possess the potential to become ideal citizen-subjects, and to bear future Japanese American citizens. So, while the JACL and other elite Issei used many different strategies as they attempted to shape Nisei into subjects approved by the state, young women's practices of cultural expression were a particular site of this molding. Given these endeavors' fluidity, Ito's dancing served as one vehicle for this evolving project of Japanese integration—an approach that in its obvious emphasis on the body, offered a particularly literal strategy for the shaping of both the ideal Japanese American citizen-subject, and the Japanese community at large.

The Nisei who were drawn into Ito's orbit, taking dance lessons at one of his studios, performing in his large-scale dance symphonies, or working with him on smaller concerts created especially for the Little Tokyo community, might have had a range of previous dance experiences, as Valerie Matsumoto has traced.[29] Many of Ito's students had probably taken lessons in *nihon buyō*, traditional Japanese dance. Perhaps they took lessons at school, or in the youth clubs that were a mainstay of Southern California Japanese youth. Perhaps they ordered lessons on social dance (Western couple's dancing) through the mail, quickly sorting through the household's delivery to snatch away the next installment and study it in private, away from parents' eyes. A few students might have studied some ballet or tap. And perhaps some had no dance experience at all. Ito's dancing, in its musical choices and physical repertoire, was quite different from what most of his Nisei students had been exposed to. Its publicness—not only onstage, but outside of Little Tokyo's enclosed world—concerned some.[30] And yet, it was also more abstract, in movement and musical accompaniment, than most social dance. His dancing had a certain undefinability, which, much as it may have worried some, also helped communicate the sense of Ito as an artistic innovator, and as someone able to perform his way into the white cultural world.

Painterly Dances

From his first arrival in Los Angeles, much of the region's elite embraced Ito precisely for his ability to offer his japoniste modern dance aesthetic as a performance exemplary of the region's own cultural aims. His early dance concerts spoke to audiences more familiar with visual art paradigms and those of Hollywood films. For these viewers, Ito's compositional skill—his use of color, of spatial staging, and of choreographic duration as a way of shaping a sense of the space around the dancers—all helped to confirm his status as a bona fide artist. And, as in New York, these artistic skills were read as characteristic of, and even indicative of, his being Japanese.

Ito's presentations during the spring of 1929 helped to establish his name in the artistic community, and, just as importantly, allowed him to develop relationships with local patrons. The first of these concerts, held at the Figueroa Playhouse in April, was supported by Mrs. Frank A. Vanderlip (his old patroness from New York), the dancer Ruth St. Denis, the actor John Barrymore, and the conductor Leopold Stokowski. The second recital, part of a "May Blossom Festival," took place at the Lake Norconian Club in May, a recently opened resort between Los Angeles and Riverside that drew numerous film and sports stars. The third recital, at the Patio Theatre in Barnsdall Park in June, was hosted by the California Art Club, a large, elite, and traditionalist organization dedicated to promoting landscape and representational painting.

At this last-mentioned concert, a review noted that an astonished painter in the audience exclaimed: "'That guy's an artist!'" The review continued, "This was not a cold bit of judgment but an exclamation drawn from the painter, prefaced by a 'gosh' that was half a 'whew'; and it was about as intelligent a critical remark as could be extracted from any member of that recent Saturday night's fascinated audience, for these quiet people were seeing musical movement of the kind that only appears once in a decade."[31] The reviewer explained that spectators were accustomed to ballet, which stressed the "emotional possibilities of movement." By contrast, Ito demonstrated the significance of the body itself in movement. In quoting a visual art painter's astonishment, this review also indicates that Ito's dancing seemed so effective because of its pictorial composition and painterly use of colors. Other artists, the review suggests, were able to appreciate Ito's work because they recognized in his choreography the tenets of their own media, and were able to see Ito's dancing as pursuing the same artistic aims as their own work.

Alongside this painter's appreciation of Ito's painterly-like dances lay the constant presence of another visual medium that defined how audiences received his work: film. The *Los Angeles Times* review continued,

> In effect these dances are moving pictures. The dancers moved from one complete gesture to another. The passage was beautiful, but it was the arrival at the gesture itself that brought little murmurs of admiration and astonishment from the audience. These gestures were never bizarre or designed to startle, but gave aesthetic satisfaction because they fulfilled one's desire for complete movement, for art that could go logically and inevitably to its extremes without overstepping the possibility of being brought into the controlling design.[32]

The pictorial nature of Ito's choreography inspired the critic to characterize the dances as "moving pictures." The critic's praise of the "controlling design" accordingly imagines Ito's choreographic vision as analogous to the camera's supervisory eye.

Indeed, film was an ongoing background presence for all of Ito's work in Southern California. The string of dance studios that he was able to operate, while indicating his popularity as a teacher, was also the result of a large population of young, would-be stars, who came to Los Angeles hoping to be cast in films and who needed to learn to dance—or at least, carry themselves with grace and control.[33] The film industry was also more directly involved with Ito's Los Angeles career: after appearing in 1921's *Dawn of the East* while based in New York, Ito played roles in *Booloo* (1938) and *Spawn of the North* (1938) and worked as a consultant or choreographer on *No, No, Nanette* (1930), *Madame Butterfly* (1932), and *The Sunset Murder Case* (1941).[34]

In the summer of 1929, Ito presented a series of five evening performances at the Argus Bowl in Eagle Rock, a 500-person amphitheater where performances were always free—as mandated by its founder and patroness, Mrs. J. E. Argus. On the various evenings' programs were two *kyōgen—Somebody-*

Nothing and *The Fox's Grave*—that Ito had translated in 1923 in New York with Louis V. Ledoux, which alternated with restagings of *At the Hawk's Well*. The *kyōgen* featured Lester Horton, Ralph Matson, Thomas de Graffenried, and Komai Tetsu, "a prominent figure in Noh dramas." In *At the Hawk's Well*, Lester Horton performed the role of the Hawk, Charlton A. Powers the Old Man, and Dewitt Bodeen the Young Man. These plays were paired with a substantial program of pieces from Ito's interpretive and "oriental" concert dance repertoire. As always, Ito made sure to publicize the event in Little Tokyo, and the *Rafu Shimpo* observed that "a large number of Japanese were scattered throughout the bowl."[35]

Though these events were smaller in scale than the community dance events Ito would come to focus on, he used them to establish himself as a promoter and organizer of dance in the region. Each concert showcased his own choreography, alongside that of other local choreographers and dancers, some of whom later became principal members of his dance troupe. As one critic noted, "A number of very lovely things were to be seen, and to Ito's credit it must be said that they represented not only his own distinctly stylistic work, but the interpretive efforts of other representative moderns of Los Angeles."[36] Notable figures in his company included Dorothy Wagner, who remained one of Ito's featured dancers throughout the 1930s, and taught at his studio; Georgia Graham (Martha's sister); Estelle Reed, who had studied in Germany with Mary Wigman; the Russian-born Mexican Xenia Zarina, who specialized in "oriental dance"; and Waldeen Falkenstein, who became an important figure in Mexico's modern dance movement.[37] Ito's concerts also featured Hazel Wright (Ito's wife), Beatrix Baird, Dolores Lopez, Edith Jane (whose studio served as an early base for Ito's classes and ticket sales), Arnold Tamon, Anne Douglas, Lillian Powell, Cecelia Mae Fischer, Rosemary Bedford, and Lester Horton (who became a major figure in US modern dance). Ito thus gained a reputation as a cultivator of the Los Angeles dance scene at large, in a reciprocal advocacy that further cemented his own position in the region.

Communities Dancing

An article in the *Los Angeles Times*, covering Ito's arrival in Southern California and the opening of his studio, declared, "He scorns making art incomprehensible, remote, a secret thing for the few, and he accuses those who would,

Japanese America and Fantasies of Integration 137

of hiding ignorance behind subterfuge. Ito is a 'communitarian.' He wants to make this a community of dancers. . . . The main business of Ito's life today is developing this wholly modern idea of communities dancing and the leaders in community life in Southern California are helping him."[38] When the *Los Angeles Times* asserted that Ito rejected "remote" and "secret" art-making, the paper marked a distinct shift in Ito's creative work—in proclaimed tenets, if not in actual practice. No longer was he linked to the esoteric, drawing-room modernism of Yeats and Pound, or to New York's experimental Little Theatre community. Instead, as a "communitarian" Ito would make a name for himself choreographing large-scale "dance symphonies," in which dancers from across the broader Los Angeles region would participate, embodying a vision of community integration and artistic progressivism.

The shift in Ito's choreographic projects, from the small-scale and overtly "modernist" to the large-scale and explicitly community-based, reflects a larger trend in the Los Angeles arts world: the rise of the community arts movement—and Ito's responsiveness to that trend. With roots in the Progressive Era, community arts were upheld by wealthy white patrons who advocated art as a way to integrate immigrants, as an antidote to Hollywood commercialism, and as key to the development of a regional high culture. The Hollywood Bowl, an iconic amphitheater nestled in the Hollywood Hills and founded in 1922, stood as the movement's primary institution.[39] As cultural histories of Los Angeles have emphasized, the community arts movement (sometimes also called the civic arts movement) had its strongest manifestations in music, grounded in the immense success of the World War I–era "community sings." But it also had deep roots in theatrical pageants and artistic dancing as championed by the Theatre Arts Alliance (founded in 1919), which received funding from philanthropist Christine Wetherill Stevenson and the Krotona Theosophical Society for the original purchase of land on which the Hollywood Bowl was built.

The community arts movement offered Ito the opportunity to expand his choreographic practice, in both its material possibilities and its symbolic significations. The large outdoor arenas where the movement's events were staged, with their capacity for hundreds of performers and thousands of spectators, vivified the notion of performance as not simply representing community, but inducing it. In these spaces, Ito expanded his choreographic scale in a way that matched his ambitions and beliefs about dance's world-making capacity. And in the movement's emphasis on the production of a Southern Californian, and even national, community through art-making, Ito found the chance to include members of the Japanese immigrant community in the predominantly white world of Los Angeles arts patronage. In doing so, Ito seemed to materialize, through the very bodies of his Nisei dancers, the promise of political integration.

By the time Ito arrived in Los Angeles, the community arts movement had become a fully established phenomenon, with a seasonal rhythm anchored by the Hollywood Bowl's popular summertime series, "Symphonies Under the Stars," and other venues staging complementary evenings of theater, music, pageantry, dance, and so on. Ito recognized his opening, and set about advocating for dance to be recognized as a crucial thread of the movement. The magazine the *American Dancer*, founded in June 1927 in Los Angeles by artistic dancing advocate Ruth Eleanor Howard, served as a ready partner for Ito's efforts, and dedicated several columns to his endeavor to create a "community dance movement." As an editorial proclaimed, "With the marvelous Community Spirit which is characteristic of California, this state should be the first to pioneer in a Community Dance movement."[40] Ito's approach to creating a citywide movement was modular: he formed small, neighborhood-defined groups of dancers, who could learn and perform together as a stand-alone unit, and then in combination with other groups from across the city. He first formed a group in Hollywood, with sponsorship from musician and activist Artie Mason Carter and Florence Behm (Mrs. Leiland Atherton Irish), who was a principal backer of the Los Angeles Philharmonic and executive director of the Hollywood Bowl. Soon groups in Pasadena and Long Beach coalesced, and then other neighborhoods in Los Angeles started groups as well.

As in the broader community arts movement, Ito fashioned the dance movement around the amateur dancer, who could be readily imagined as a figure of the community at large. And, as the *American Dancer* articles on Ito's efforts suggest, he taught them a version of eurythmics: "Community dancing uses the dancers as instruments of expression. The dancers use a technique which enables them to study and interpret music as melody and rhythm and to give this interpretation a quality or color which is as characteristic as are the various musical instruments."[41] Under Ito's direction, the ideas he absorbed at Hellerau were central to the community dance ethic: "A child, woman or man should go out from the discipline of community dancing and exhibit all the qualities of real education, a strong, healthy perceptive and conceptive power, a power capable of application to all life, equal to the emergencies of any power or thought, and purified by the highest spiritual

Japanese America and Fantasies of Integration   139

ideas."[42] Community dancing, then, was a straightforward appeal to put dancing at the center of civic life, as a force not only of *expression* but of education
and of reshaping the individual's body for the purpose of creating stronger
(physically and spiritually) local and indeed national subjects.

On receiving a commission to choreograph a Pageant of Lights at the
Pasadena Rose Bowl in September 1929, Ito explicitly sought to carry out
the ideal of community integration by including dancers from the Japanese
community. Using the Edith Jane Studio in Hollywood and offering a twice-
a-week ten-lesson course, Ito, through the *Rafu Shimpo*, urged young Nisei
to join. As one notice explained,

> The noted Japanese dancer will personally direct the class. He is very anxious
> to have as many young people as possible in this class. No previous experi-
> ence is needed in order to enroll in this class.[. . .]
>
> A special price is being charged of the Japanese students. . . . Those who
> are skeptical about entering this beginner's dance class are invited to visit the
> first class on Wednesday, July 31st, and then sign up for the next class.[43]

The *Rafu Shimpo* continued to report on the class's progress throughout the
summer, noting that Ito and Dorothy Wagner, who assisted in teaching, were
impressed with the students' "ability and rapid cooperation of their body
and mind."[44] Ito instructed the students in the series of ten movements that
made up the basis of his technique, and at each session also taught a complete
dance. Ito also used the classes as an opportunity to introduce the students
to Los Angeles cultural events outside of the Japanese community. As the
Rafu Shimpo reported, "Instead of holding their regular dancing lessons, the
Japanese pupils of Michio Ito were taken to the Hollywood Bowl on Friday
evening, August 16th, where they saw the entire program for the evening.
Special reserved seats were obtained by the dance artist for these young people."[45] For some students, this was perhaps a first trip to the Hollywood Bowl;
participating in Ito's dance lessons also offered opportunities for movement
across the city.

In taking part in the Pasadena Pageant of Lights, Ito's students joined in
a massive expression of community art. The pageant boasted 150 dancers,
a chorus of 250 singers, and accompaniment by the Los Angeles Philharmonic Orchestra, directed by Modet Altschuler. The program indicates that
Ito divided the program among the different dance groups he led across the
region. *Andante Cantabile* (Tchaikovsky) was performed by the "Los Angeles

Dancers and Orchestra"; Chopin's *Waltz in E Flat Major* was undertaken by the "Pasadena Dancers and Orchestra"; and Chopin's *Waltz in C Sharp Major* by the "Hollywood Dancers and Orchestra." Three movements from Grieg's *Peer Gynt Suite* were carried out by still other groups—"Morning" by "Japanese Dancers," "Anitra's Hall" by the "Hollywood Dancers," and "In the Hall of the Mountain King" by "Ito Male Dancers." After Ito's always-anticipated stage appearance in *Pizzicati*, the program closed with Dvořák's *New World Symphony*, danced by "Hollywood and Ito Male Dancers." This division of the cast into smaller "companies" surely made for more manageable rehearsals and logistics, and also reiterated the pageant's intended purpose of bringing different groups from across the city together in celebration of the Bowl's new lighting system—and of the city at large.

Ito incorporated his Japanese students—eleven of whom ultimately participated—into the pageant in two ways. As the program indicates, the female students performed "Morning," which the *Rafu Shimpo* described as "a Japanese dance." The paper reported that they also joined other "American dancers" from the Los Angeles group, including Dorothy Wagner, Beatrix Baird, and Dolores Lopez, for the performance of *Andante Cantabile*.[46] The male students appeared among the Ito Male Dancers, performing "In the Hall of the Mountain King." The program thus alternated between highlighting the Japanese dancers as a distinct local group—further marked by their contribution being a "Japanese" dance—and incorporating them into other locally defined communities.

Ito's Japanese students vivified the community dance ethos of inclusion most obviously in that their very participation seems only to have been noticed (or explicitly named) by the *Rafu Shimpo*. When racial differentiation receded in the unity of mass movement, "Japaneseness" was instead represented through the dances' subject matter and the production's general artistry. In contrast to actual Japanese bodies, these were indexical signs of Japan that could be inhabited by any dancer, a free-floating representational capacity that served the broader goals of community dance.

Ito's next large-scale production took place the following summer at the Hollywood Bowl. In a performance of Borodin's *Prince Igor*, to be conducted by the famous Bernardino Molinari, Ito again saw an opportunity to involve the Japanese community in the community arts movement. This was another huge undertaking, with 125 dancers performing to a 100-person orchestra, along with singing by the 200-person Mormon Chorus. Ito drew dancers from across the city, enlisting top students from his own schools as well as

Japanese America and Fantasies of Integration 141

those of Arnold Tamon, Lillian Powell, and Edith Jane. Groups from the University of Southern California, and one put together by the Los Angeles Playground Department, were also included. At least five dancers from the Japanese community were enlisted, although ultimately it seems that only one man, Tetsuo Shinohara, performed. Backstage, however, large numbers of Japanese supported the endeavor. Ito's younger brother, the stage designer, Kisaku, came from Tokyo to help with the production's costumes, and several members of the community joined this effort. The Japanese-American Women's Association decorated the venue. With so much involvement of the Japanese community, the *Rafu Shimpo* articulated the sense of importance assigned the production, declaring, "Much of the artistic reputation of the Japanese people depends upon the success of Michio Ito's mammoth production of 'Prince Igor' at the Hollywood Bowl."[47] With so many groups from across the city involved in the production, it was felt that the success of Ito's endeavor would reflect on Japanese immigrants more broadly.

Ito's choreography for *Prince Igor* aimed to satisfy the aspirations of community arts and the expectations of modern dance. Ito divided his dancers into groups of twenty-four. The groups on stage together each performed different movements. Ito was thus able to avoid the static monumentality that would have resulted from a totally uniform choreography at this scale, while still communicating a sense of rhythmic community. However, the *Los Angeles Times* noted that with such range in skill among the 125 dancers, there was an unevenness to the performance: "Only a few of the dancers were sufficiently trained to appear in the much too revealing lighting which was used. Probably the 125 dancers who composed this 'Prince Igor' ballet were inspired by a spirit of community expression but this type of ballet has been done too often by the great European dancers to have the efforts of comparative amateurs appreciated in the same roles."[48] As before, critics turned to the painterly quality of Ito's staging to look past perceived deficiencies, observing that Ito was "more successful in the picturesque effect he achieved with a veiled stage softening the effect of the black-coated orchestra and the color of his dancers' Oriental-Russian costumes than he was with his dance pageantry. With the Japanese skill in simple and suggestive staging, he used chiffon crepe decorated with delicate tracery behind which the music floated with a kind of ethereal beauty."[49] The strength of Ito's pictorial ability shifted the focus from the dancers, and the dancing itself, to the lasting impressions wrought by his stage pictures—received as characteristically "Japanese."

By contrast, and ready to support one of their own, the *Rafu Shimpo's* review was enthusiastic:

> In color and in movement, the dance in its total effect was so captivating that it was some time before the audience returned to their sense of reality as the ballet came to its close. Although the more critical spectators voiced their disapproval on a few minor imperfections, the production on the whole was a great triumph.
>
> In the swift and precise movements, though often uneven individually, the dancers seemed inspired both by the aesthetic impulse of the celebrated director and by the thrilling melody flowing out of the concealed orchestra ably conducted by the noted master Molinari.[50]

The *Rafu Shimpo* thus stood by the premise of dance as community art; what was important was not an individual dancer's perfect execution of the choreography, but rather that music, choreography, and performance had come together in a triumphant whole, signifying Japanese belonging.

Ito's investment in creating a community dance movement provided his Nisei students with opportunities to physically manifest their belonging in the city, and the Japanese community at large understood the potential value of these performances on such terms. Likewise, the large scale of these productions demonstrated to the city and its cultural patrons that dance, like music and visual art, could be a medium on which Los Angeles could build its reputation *and* performatively induce a sense of shared community identity. Though the particular form of the large-scale dance-symphony appears unique to his Los Angeles period, the fantasies that underpinned it—of dance as a mechanism of social formation—connect these efforts both to his earlier education at the Jaques-Dalcroze Institute at Hellerau and to his later proposal for a mass pageant in the Philippines during the Asia-Pacific War, which will be discussed in chapter 6.

Embodying Fantasy

Ito's large-scale dance projects were opportunities for him to involve the Japanese community in the broader Los Angeles cultural landscape. In this recruitment, and particularly in the inclusion of Nisei dancers in his choreographies, he staged a fantasy of integration. While some spectators, such as

Japanese America and Fantasies of Integration

writers at the *Rafu Shimpo*, recognized this, and many others probably did not, the inclusion of young Japanese Americans in these companies did political work. Whether in a segregated group, but framed as part of the whole (just as US Army officials would engineer the service of Japanese Americans thirteen years later with the celebrated—and segregated—100th Infantry Battalion and the 442nd Regimental Combat Team),[51] or mixed into and standing among a generally white corps of dancers, their appearances on stage fulfilled a vision of integration advocated by both white progressives and some Issei elite. Moreover, precisely because of the powers of performativity attributed to theatrical performance, one could read these integrated concerts as heralding a more hopeful political future.

But the stage is not only a site of political reimagining; it is also a site of political remove. At a time when the Nisei were restricted in what restaurants they could patronize, where they could sit in theaters, and which parks, beaches, and playgrounds they could enter, Ito's staging of Nisei integration is a straightforward example of Arabella Stanger's contention that Euro-American theater dance produces "sociopolitical ideals . . . that themselves depend on and conceal material histories of racial violence."[52] Likewise, as Yutian Wong has established, the utopia imagined in Ito's choreographies (as well as his public persona) was not only the ideal of integration, but also the fantasy of artistic cosmopolitanism, the notion that art might enable certain individuals to smoothly cross borders, and to be celebrated for that border-crossing.[53] Ito's choreographic integration, and the visions of inter–Los Angeles harmony that it was taken to embody, thus could be said to paper over the realities of increasingly dehumanizing racialization and to provide aestheticized representations of the US's own national fantasy of itself as exceptional in its ability to integrate "outsiders" into the body politic. As Juliana Chang has highlighted, this is a fantasy particularly underpinned by the narrative of "ethnic succession"—the children, like the Nisei, for whom the promises of belonging in the US might be realized.[54]

Asian American studies has offered both detailed historical analyses of particular moments when the US betrayed its ideals, and trenchant critiques of the very premise of liberal subjecthood on which such promises are founded. Kandice Chuh, for example, has shown that to be recognized as a subject, and thus to seemingly have access to the liberties granted by the state, is only possible by the individual "conforming to certain regulatory matrices."[55] By performing Ito's modern dance in the public sphere of the Hollywood Bowl, the Nisei rehearsed becoming ideal citizen-subjects, in fulfillment of precisely the models held up by both white progressives and Issei elite such as the JACL. They thus entered into the liberal schema of abstract citizenship imagined by the state, and in doing so, were, as Lisa Lowe describes, "'split off' from the unrepresentable histories of situated embodiment that contradict the abstract form of citizenship."[56] Dancing formulated the Nisei as citizens, even as it could not, in fact, meaningfully secure the assurances of liberal subjecthood that modern dance (and the state) seemed to promise.[57]

I want to acknowledge the particular hollowness of performances of integration on the eve of Japanese American incarceration, and to highlight, as the cited scholars and others have done, the ways in which the particular betrayal of Executive Order 9066 was, in fact, the outcome of a racial exclusionism that is inextricable from the history of American democratic liberal subjecthood.[58] But I also want to hold other meanings open, by turning to a photograph taken by the Issei photographer Toyo Miyatake.

The photograph is of a group of young Nisei, dancing under Ito's instruction. They are arranged in a circle at varying heights to form a medallion. Each girl mirrors her partner across the circle, except for the dancer at the top, who stands with arms stretched overhead. In its symmetry and motionless posing, the image suggests a choreography of unobjectionable, pretty poses and group formations. What is striking about the photograph is not its recording of Ito's choreography, but rather, its capture of these girls' faces. Their expressions seem to show a mixture of serious concentration, minor boredom, and amused enjoyment. Only the girl at the top of the circle returns our gaze, but the visibility of nearly all their faces gives the impression that a viewer might be able to imagine their thoughts and feelings, that it might be possible to ascertain their own sense of themselves, at a moment in time that is now overwritten by history. At the same time, for all that the camera seems to capture here, the viewer obtains very little; the girls' faces resist determined interpretation.

I am left wondering: What did it mean for each of these girls to dance in Ito's studio, and to learn some of his dances? What longings are hinted at in these students' poses? Perhaps, as the girl at the top of the circle stares at the camera, she is staring far beyond it, imagining a different life for herself—in Wyoming, or Maine, or New York, as a poet, a teacher, a rancher, a journalist, a cosmetologist, a doctor. Perhaps the girl wearing the pearl necklace dreamed of becoming a Hollywood star; knowing of the actresses who often passed through Ito's studio, perhaps she hoped these dance lessons would be

Japanese America and Fantasies of Integration

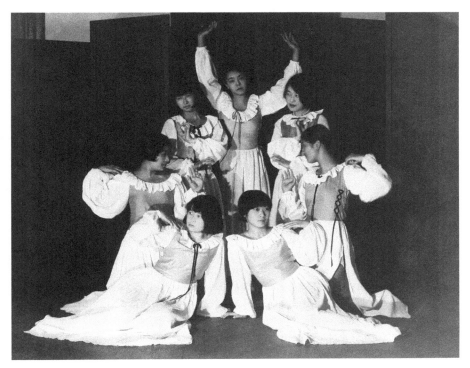

Fig. 14. Nisei girls dancing. Photo by Toyo Miyatake, Toyo Miyatake Dance Collection, courtesy of Alan Miyatake.

a first step toward her own success. Perhaps the one in the bottom right came because she was signed up by her mother, or because a friend was already going. Perhaps the one at the top right, who most clearly has the traces of a smile, found the whole thing a little silly—the solemnity of the accord between movement and music, and her teacher's exhortations to express herself through these dictated choreographies. Perhaps Ito's lessons in modern dance really did feel like a set of corporeal possibilities through which these girls could imagine themselves otherwise. And perhaps not.

These girls might have felt any of these things, and many more. Most important, each of them might have felt more than one desire, in succession or all at once. The point I want to make is: to believe in the promises that America makes to its inhabitants doesn't mean one can't also recognize their partiality, or their particular hollowness for people who are marked, in one way or another, as less-than-fully citizens. That is, to name the exclusionary and violent contradictions that lie at the heart of American sociopolitical ideals doesn't mean we must dismiss them, and the hold they might have had on Ito's Nisei dancers. And while such attachments are certainly a version of Lauren Berlant's cruel optimism, it might be something else as well, something that I am trying to name as particular to fantasy.[59]

If, as is often implied in the term's usage, fantasy is the scene of an impossible desire, it is also, as I suggested in this book's introduction, what binds us to our world, the "real" one, in which we live. It is not just escapism, not just faithless promises and illusory attachments, or merely false consciousness. It is "how we build our claim to solidity in the world,"[60] through our construction of the self within, and as a part of, the social collective. And for my purposes, it is a bodily act; grounded in that which the body knows, and refuses to forget. To characterize Ito's Nisei students as engaged in fantasy, then, means that the material conditions of their sociopolitical positions are part of that fantasy, and indeed, constitute it. In this reading, the Nisei dancing on stage at the Hollywood Bowl carry out a performance not of integration, but of its desire, and the painful, hopeful awareness of integration's unreliability. In this reading, the young Nisei girl in Miyatake's photograph whose hand hovers in front of her chest dreams of how dance might allow her to escape the circumscribed world of Little Tokyo, even as she knows that this is just a dream, and takes pleasure in it as a dream. It is not, then, her secret unconscious that fantasizes, but rather, her arms held taut, and her neck poised at an angle. In this reading, she fantasizes through her body, and takes pleasure in the act of fantasizing, here, among her Nisei peers, in a photography studio in Little Tokyo, a few years before incarceration.

Kokutai: The Integrative National Body

In 1933, Isabel Morse Jones, the music and dance critic for the *Los Angeles Times*, gushed:

> All that nonsense about "East is East and West is West and never the twain shall meet," with due respect to Kipling, is disproven in one artist who lives now in Hollywood. Michio Ito is a Japanese with a European-American educational experience and his art and personal expression are as perfect an emulsion as any chemist could wish for. He was an oriental the first eighteen

Japanese America and Fantasies of Integration 147

years of his life. Then he became successively German, French, British and American as he traveled on his westward way. Today he is a true Californian; enthusiastic, optimistic, dreaming dreams of its future as the center of art and culture.[61]

Making reference to Kipling's worn formula, Jones sees Ito as a materialization of the impossible encounter between East and West, and she stages it not as a meeting between cultural practices, or even two people, but rather as occurring within Ito's performing body. In her eyes, the twain do not so much meet as become absorbed in each other, the parts no longer distinct from the whole. Moreover, Ito becomes "successively German, French, British and American," as if he moves not only through his world itinerary, but through the ethnic and national identities of each place. Jones portrays this as an additive process, a collecting of locally marked "experience" and "expression," such that Ito stands as a perfect cultural "emulsion." Yet she also suggests that in each place, he becomes the quintessential representative of that culture; thus, he is now a "true Californian."

Jones's effusive characterization matches the integrationist significance read onto Ito by white supporters of the community arts movement, as discussed previously. That said, the description of Ito as a sort of international emulsion is striking, and in fact, uncannily matches contemporary Japanese rhetoric about Japan as a "syncretic" nation, in what was known as the "mixed-nation theory." From the 1880s through the 1930s, two theories of the origin of the Japanese people competed to be taken as the *kokutai-ron*, or theory of the national polity. While one of these—the homogenous-nation theory—seems commonplace now, it was the mixed-nation theory, which envisioned Japan as uniquely assimilative, that was especially useful to the imperial government as it sought to naturalize the presence of Japan's new colonies, Taiwan and Korea, within its national imaginary.[62]

Kokutai, a term that could mean "national polity," "national sovereignty," "national essence," or "body politic," might also be taken more literally as "national body," because it is made up of the kanji for "nation" and "body." While the term itself was in use in premodern Japan, its modern formulations drew from European models of theorizing the state, particularly J. C. Bluntschli's *Allgemeines Staatsrecht*. In this German-derived model, the "body" was meant metaphorically as a description of relational organs, where the emperor represents the nation's head and the various governmental departments are understood as its limbs. An alternative formulation asserted that the nation is a natural body, in which the emperor and his subjects are united as parts in a whole. The family as a unit was taken as this argument's building block; just as the family was a unit within which an essential Japanese spirit and paternalistic relations of devotion served as the binding glue, so were these obligations expected to replicate across the scale of family, nation, and ultimately, incorporated empire. In the previous section, I considered what meanings and attachments Nisei might have held in studying dance with Ito, even as they experienced the effects of the US's logic of racial exception. If assimilation was a complicated promise for these young dancers, another model of integration—*kokutai*—suggests how Ito's choreography intertwined both national and imperial visions of bodily absorption.

Kokutai—in all its variations—relies on an implicit image of a body, and it is here that I think Ito's work *as a moving body* is especially important. *Kokutai* is an abstract idea, and in Japanese historiography, it has formed the prefatory dyad to the postwar period's *zeitgeist* of *nikutai*—the fleshly, physically needy and desirous individual body.[63] But despite *kokutai*'s use as a metaphorical abstraction of the ideal relation between a nation and its subjects, it was also always being literalized in representations of the physical body. As Bert Winther-Tamaki, writing on the genre of Yōga, asserts, "the Yōga painter was one who sought to master imported techniques of wresting palpable images of human bodies from the material of oil paint and deployed these body images to serve the sociopolitical ends of visualizing and concretizing notions of the body politic that were more or less supportive of ideological goals associated with the state."[64] If painted depictions of soldiers served to materialize the ideology of the national body, then dance puts acute pressure on the meanings generated by the term *kokutai*, simultaneously so literal and metaphorical. For the medium of dance, temporal and transient—and unlike music, resistant to notation—is often seen as an immaterial art form. But the seeming immateriality of dance is precisely that which makes it seem to adhere so fully to the bodies executing it. Dance thus offers a potent site for the working out of what—or who—can be incorporated into a national body, and Ito served as an exemplary vision of *kokutai*—for both his Japanese American spectators and his white American audiences.

It is instructive to consider here one of his pieces, *Ecclesiastique*, originally choreographed in New York in 1922 to Tchaikovsky's "Andante Cantabile" for the *Pinwheel Revel*, and rechoreographed in California in 1928, when it was set to music by Robert Schumann. In this piece, Ito's Dalcroze-based technique is on full display; imagined as the vivification of a stained-glass figure, the dance moves through several of his foundational poses. In its sense of drama and evocation, Ito rendered the potentially formulaic nature of his position-based technique into a fluid and affective piece. This popular piece had served in New York to cement Ito's reputation as an "interpretive dancer"—that is, not only a choreographer of "oriental dance," but an artist working in the genre that would soon be recognized as "modern dance."

In California, *Ecclesiastique* was performed by Dorothy Wagner. Wagner, a statuesque blond, danced with striking presence, a quality noted repeatedly in reviews (the *Rafu Shimpo* declared that she danced the piece "with the figure of an angel").[65] Carol Sorgenfrei has read Wagner's presence on Ito's stage as a sign of the unassimilability of white dancers into his choreography, which she argues indicated Ito's growing belief in the ascendant imperial ideology of Japanese superiority.[66] But Ito's setting of his choreography on the body of a (hypervisibly) white woman might alternatively suggest the very potency of his ability to master a choreographic, cultural, and indeed national repertoire. Following the insinuations of the mixed-nation theory, Ito's dancing and choreography thus figured an easily integrative national body, one in which the movements attributed to other nations (Germany and the US) could become naturalized within his body—and even set on others'.

In the choreographic success of a piece such as *Ecclesiastique*, I think we see the potency of dance as a figuration of *kokutai*. Ito's success performing his version of Euro-American modern concert dance, reinforced by his ability to set his choreography on white dancers, vivified the possibilities of a body absorbing movement styles that seemed to not match its purported national identity. Indeed, dance itself, when performed as effortless, seamless, and unified, asserts a sense of naturalness that seems to ask, "how could the body move otherwise?" This naturalness is the fantasy of *kokutai*—that the national body, having absorbed alien others, will move with ease, vigor even, to perform as a unified, integrated whole. Moreover, the fantasy of *kokutai* is that subjects devote themselves to the nation freely, without coercion; when they die "for" the nation, they do so of their own free will. Thus, as Takashi Fujitani has shown, the US military's recruitment of incarcerated Nisei was carried out under terms that sought their voluntary, indeed eager, participation. Likewise, the Japanese colonial regime's campaign to recruit Korean soldiers involved a rigorous screening process that not only limited candidates to willing volunteers, but refused those who were economically disadvantaged, to ensure that their enlisting was not driven by economic desperation.[67] While dance certainly can depict constraint and coercion, its fantasy, especially in modern dance, is of free movement. That is, the fantasy of modern dance is that we are simply seeing a body moving freely, propelled by its own internal impetus and volition. Dance's embodiment of *kokutai*, then, instantiates this vision of an uncoerced, "natural" expression of national embodiment through an individual's sincerely moving body.

Ito's ambiguously signifying body, his choreographic absorption of different dance practices, and his success in using a range of young women in his dances all suggested how he could stand as a figuration of *kokutai*, which, as I have shown, was both a national and an imperial concern. But the ease with which Ito seemed to embody this vision of corporeal integration was also—precisely because of its national and imperial implications—a source of anxiety, especially with respect to his marriage to Hazel Wright. Indeed, the question of *kokutai*—of who belongs within a nation's (racially defined) borders—is frequently one that comes down to marriage, as discourses of miscegenation and intermarriage, in both Japan and the US, have shown. So it was that the limits of Ito's assimilative potential seemed to be revealed by the 1936 divorce from his wife, Hazel Wright. Newspapers across the US salaciously reported details of the divorce, playing upon the same Rudyard Kipling formulation that had earlier been used in praise, with headlines such as, "'East is East,' American Divorcee Now Agrees. Japanese Husband Reassumed Oriental Ways, She Says":

> Blue-eyed Hazel Wright, American by birth and, until yesterday, Japanese by marriage, had her own explanation for what Kipling meant by "never the twain shall meet."
>
> Yesterday she obtained a divorce from Michio Ito, internationally known Japanese dancer. Today she told of the slowly developed rift that eventually shattered their marriage. He became Oriental, she more Occidental.
>
> "When I married him thirteen years ago he was absolutely Western in his ways," she said. "Now, as he grows older, he becomes more and more Oriental." The tendency, she explained, "appeared in his clothes, mannerisms, the food he wanted and the companionship he sought."
>
> "Nothing could have been more American than our early life," said Miss Wright. "We were married at the City Hall in New York in 1923, lived in hotels, observed all the conventions of marriage as white races know them. Gradually, he changed."
>
> They have two sons, twelve and eight years old. One, the mother said, was calm, philosophical, intensely proud of his Japanese blood. The younger had the opposite attitude.[68]

Japanese America and Fantasies of Integration 151

There are no accounts offering Ito's version of events; by this time, it seems, he was living with a Japanese woman, Ozawa Tsuyako, who was to become his second wife. The gossipy report nevertheless evokes an image of Ito's life in which his cosmopolitanism, a celebrated emulsion of East and West, slowly dissolved, as if separating back out the constituent elements. The news item makes passing reference to the exclusion laws that had governed the couple's married life: beginning in 1907, US women who married foreigners lost their citizenship; the Cable Act of 1922 rescinded this law, except in cases where a woman married an alien ineligible for naturalization, that is, an Asian man.[69] Wed in 1923 in New York, where there were no antimiscegenation laws, their marriage, although legal, meant the expulsion of Wright from her nation of birth. In 1931, however, the law was amended to allow US women to retain their citizenship even if married to an Asian man; in 1934, the Equal Nationality Act gave to US-born women the ability to provide the possibility of naturalization to their foreign-born husbands (unless they were "aliens ineligible for citizenship"), and to pass on US citizenship to their children if born overseas; this act, however, still aimed in various ways to especially restrict Asian people from settling in the US.[70] Over the thirteen years of their marriage, then, Wright's national status fluctuated as a function of her sex; with nationality constituted as a masculine property, the limits of national borders were drawn across her body. By contrast, for Ito, there was never any chance of American naturalization. Indeed, throughout the report, it is suggested that there is something inexorable about being "Oriental"; although in his youth Ito had performed his way into an American—white—life, according to Wright, as he aged, his Japaneseness could no longer be stifled. In Ito's supposed reversion to his racial essence, the couple's two sons are similarly marked. In Wright's account, one, taking after his father, is characterized as Japanese, while the other is "the opposite." The metaphor of emulsion introduced in the early review by Isabel Morse Jones finds its conclusion, then, in the outcome of his procreation. An emulsion, after all, is not a total dissolution of two liquids into each other; it is, rather, a mixture in which one liquid is present as microscopic droplets, distributed throughout the other. Despite Ito's seeming ability to integrate multiple national cultures within his body, here, with his divorce and the rising forces of anti-Japanese racialization, Ito's cosmopolitan emulsiveness seemed to break, and the constituent elements separated back out, in the bodies of his two sons.

Costume Fantasies

Over the course of his time in Los Angeles, Ito established his reputation as a modern dance choreographer and arts advocate, not only alongside his engagement with the Japanese immigrant community, but in certain respects, through his efforts to integrate the Nisei into the region's white cultural sphere. Even as his divorce unfolded and anti-Japanese sentiment rose, Ito continued staging large productions and leading his schools. In June of 1936 he choreographed a production of Gluck's *Orpheus* at the Redlands Bowl, clearly echoing his early student days at the Dalcroze Institute, where the opera had been famously staged a month before he enrolled in the summer of 1913. In November 1936, Ito staged a ballet for the Los Angeles Federal Music Project's production of *La Traviata*, and in December he presented some of his dances for a children's benefit at the Hollywood High School. In August 1937, Ito staged the most celebrated of his California works: two large-scale ballets for the Hollywood Bowl season, *Etenraku* and *Blue Danube*. These pieces represented a culmination of his efforts in the 1930s to commit himself to the ideal of community dance and its promises of integration. Set against Japan's invasion of China that summer, the production also represented Ito's dogged attempt to maintain his position as cosmopolitan artist. Indeed, these ballets revealed that the fantasies of integration that Ito staged with his dancers were one version of the more fundamental fantasy on which Ito constructed his sense of self: the idea that art-making could produce the conditions and relations for peace, and that he had a role to play in this political brokering.

In the two ballets, Ito set his choreography to classical music—the Japanese *Etenraku*, which newspapers glossed as "Music Coming through Heaven," and Johann Strauss's *Blue Danube*. *Etenraku* was a modern musical arrangement by the conductor Viscount Konoe Hidemaro, of an eighth-century *gagaku*, music traditionally performed with dance in the ancient Kyoto imperial court. The stage was decorated with an enormous gold folding screen, 150 feet long and 14 feet high, that caught and reflected the gleam of the stage lights so that the downstage folds appeared as a series of gold columns running across the stage. The costumes loosely evoked ancient Japanese regalia; kimono-like robes in heavy silks and rich brocade were set off by elaborate headdresses. For *Blue Danube*, Ito designed costumes "in an empire style" in shades of blue silk; the stage lighting used similar washes of blue light to complement the dancers. The pieces featured both Japanese and white dancers. These included Shineo Ono, a dancer from Japan who had arrived

Japanese America and Fantasies of Integration   153

in California the previous year, as well as several of Ito's Nisei students, such as Kazuo Sumida, Lily Arikawa, Cecelia Nakamura, Yoshiko Sato, and Fumi Tanaka, who all appeared in *Etenraku*. From broader Los Angeles, dancers such as Flower Hujer, Ivan Kashkevich, Miriam Dawn, Byron Pointdexter, Barbara Perry, and Paul Foltz were listed as central in the ballets.[71] The *Los Angeles Times* called *Etenraku* "mysterious and exquisite," while *Blue Danube* was considered such a hit that it was reprised on September 24, with conducting by Adolf Tandler, along with two Mozart minuettos, in celebration of the opening of a new pedestrian passageway to the Bowl.

The critical praise and reprise performances at a major civic celebration suggest that the Los Angeles public still appreciated Ito's stagings—japoniste and "European"—and felt that they heightened the city's artistic reputation. On the surface, these ballets appeared to stage—more successfully than ever—the vision of integration that Ito had committed to over the 1930s. But precisely in the ballets' use of mirrored historical referents, and in the use of Nisei dancers to represent Japanese characters, the 1937 production suggested how much the fantasy of integration relied on elisions between race and nation, and aestheticizations of national histories.

Both pieces staged history fantasies, and both suggested that history could provide an access point for the work of embodied integration. Like so many of Ito's earlier pieces, *Etenraku* is another version of the "oriental" fantasy. The choreography effectively orientalizes Ito's own movement vocabulary, along the lines of the gestural repertoire developed by practitioners of "oriental" dance discussed in chapter 3. For example, photographs show the hovering raised knees with flexed feet and torqued torsos, the sharp juxtaposition of head and torso, and the flipped-up hand, which suggest a stylization evocative of notions of an "oriental," and particularly Japanese physicality. The casting, too, with white performers integrated into the group, carries out the expectation that white (especially female) bodies could effectively access the repertoire of this embodied fantasy.[72] As in many instances of "oriental dance," the point of departure for this piece was a historical referent—eighth-century Japan—that provided a "real" foundation for this theatrical scene. But the effect of orientalism, here as elsewhere, is to subject the past to the mechanisms of enchantment and make-believe. From the dancers' costumes to the music, *Etenraku* invoked Japanese history to provide a setting for embodied fantasy.

Seemingly worlds away, *Blue Danube* offered a similar vision. Ito staged a dance of courtship: at the piece's beginning, male and female dancers are

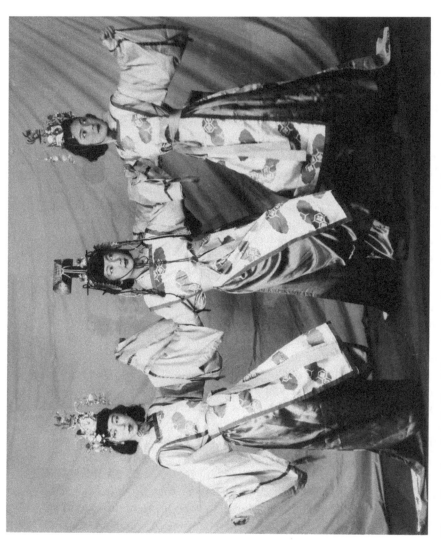

Fig. 15. *Etenraku*, photo by Toyo Miyatake, 1937. Toyo Miyatake Dance Collection, courtesy of Alan Miyatake. Department of Special Research Collections, University of California–Santa Barbara Library.

Japanese America and Fantasies of Integration

separated on opposite sides of the stage, beaming with amorous anticipation. They come together, smoothly sorted into heterosexual couples, and fulfill the promise of romantic love through the repertoire of courtly ballroom dance. The choreography mines both the waltz, and ballet's mining of the waltz. In costumes no less uncomfortable in the August sun than those of *Etenraku*, and with dance steps that had to be learned just as studiously as those of *Etenraku*, *Blue Danube* invokes a "history" that is as much a site of imaginative play as its Japanese counterpart in the program. Paired, these ballets carry out a complicated ideological leveling. For though *Blue Danube* would have seemed "familiar" to many in the audience, and *Etenraku* "exotic," Ito choreographed both as courtly costume dramas, rendering each piece's indexed "past" as a site of historical fantasy and imaginative pleasure.

Ito clearly conceived of the ballets as jointly weaving together the Los Angeles Japanese and white arts communities. A publicity collage made by the Hollywood Bowl emphasized that the evening represented an entwining of two traditions, and two communities.[73] With small central circles for the faces of Konoe and Ito, the rest of the poster features eight photographs, four from each dance. Each photograph zooms in on a small grouping of dancers presented mostly as couples or triplets. While the two ballets at first seem contrasted, the photos in fact contain multiple echoes, revealing similar choreography and atmosphere. The top right photo from *Etenraku*, for instance, in which the dancers point one foot in *tendu* and raise one arm overhead, is echoed in the *Blue Danube* photo on the bottom left, in which the dancers hold a similar pose. Above them, in the middle left, three white women from *Blue Danube* tilt their heads to the right, with arms stretched out low beneath them, and eyes cast to the right corner. A nearly mirror image occupies the photograph diagonally above this one, with three women in *Etenraku*; this time their heads are tilted stage left and the eyes follow suit. The other four photos all present dancers linked together either by their hands or with arms around each other's waist, with one foot raised in a low *attitude*. This movement, a basic ballet position, is shown to be similarly fundamental to forms of Japanese dance, where it is done with a flexed foot. The collage, rather than presenting a mélange of two vastly different dance traditions, suggests a similarity of movement vocabulary, and the ease with which different bodies can take up these positions.

The collage's juxtaposing of the two ballets represented a complicated intertwining of the traditions, nations, and communities. The musical selections represented two "classical" traditions—that of medieval Japan, and that

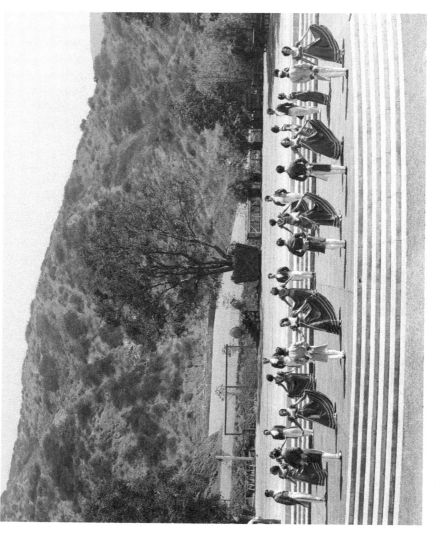

Fig. 16. *Blue Danube*, photograph by Toyo Miyatake, 1937. Toyo Miyatake Dance Collection, courtesy of Alan Miyatake.

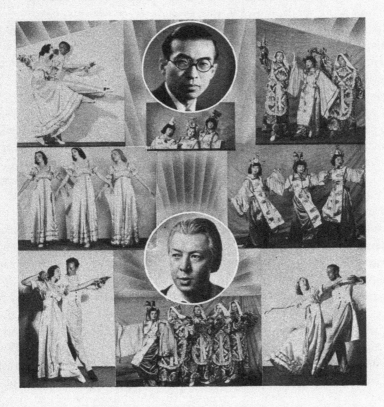

Fig. 17. Hollywood Bowl Publicity Collage, August 17, 19, 20, 1937. Los Angeles Philharmonic Archives.

of Vienna in imperial Austro-Hungary—and with these historical references, emblematized two ethno-racial communities. Thus the bodies of the dancers could be taken as corporeal instantiations of those traditions, even as white dancers performed in *Etenraku* and Japanese dancers performed in *Blue Danube*. More subtle, however, was the tension between the Nisei dancers, many of whom had never before encountered *gagaku*, and the image of traditional Japan they were assumed not simply to represent, but intrinsically to embody. This indexical slippage, of taking the Nisei as figures for Japan, foreshadows the same slippage of race and nation invoked to justify their incarceration four and a half years later.

What the collage sought to communicate via juxtaposed photographs, the paired dance symphonies represented in the bodies of the performers, asserting that dance was a means of community formation—where that community might be local, national, and even international (or imperial). The accessibility of the choreography and the interchangeability of the dancers promoted art as a form of equal access to cultural forms, national histories, and a sense of belonging. The ambiguity of the Nisei's signification, meanwhile, in which they could be taken as both Japanese American, and as Japanese, allowed one to imagine that their participation materialized not simply integration of the Japanese American community with the white, but of Japan and America.

The fantasies staged by *Etenraku* and *Blue Danube* were necessary precisely because of the political background against which Ito presented them. In early July of that summer, the buildup of hostilities between China and the multiplying Japanese forces stationed there erupted in the Marco Polo Bridge Incident, which marks the beginning of the Asia-Pacific War. For the rest of the summer, Japanese forces pressed on in an invasion of China, and newspapers detailed the mounting Japanese brutality in front-page headlines. On July 31, the *Hollywood Citizen News* announced "Helpless Chinese Slaughtered in New Assault on Tientsin. Joyful Invaders Hail Slaughter of Foes." On August 16, two days before the Hollywood Bowl performance, the front-page headline read, "Thousands Killed in Gory Battle for Shanghai. Americans Flee Holocaust."

Ito's Hollywood Bowl presentation emphatically tried to wrench spectators' attention away from these events, insisting that art could be a removed, unifying endeavor. This was particularly explicit in the publicity surrounding the famed conductor Konoe Hidemaro, who in addition to leading the Tokyo Philharmonic, came from an elite political family and was by birth

Japanese America and Fantasies of Integration

a member of the peerage. His brother, Konoe Fumimaro, had just become prime minister in June, a post he would occupy until January 1939. The conductor's presence in California thus could have met with disapprobation. However, promoting art over politics, the *Los Angeles Times* announced in July: "Wise Nipponese: Viscount Hidemaro Konoye of Japan, who comes to this season's Bowl to conduct the Michio Ito Ballet, believes that when music interferes with politics you should give up politics. Before sailing for America he resigned his post in the House of Peers, explaining that his musical duties made membership impracticable."[74] Konoe's renunciation of politics in favor of his music was a gesture that grounded the event's primary claim: that art could supersede war. This was, without a doubt, an intentional strategy on the part of the Japanese government. Indeed, by 1937 Japan had cultivated its reputation as a land of artistry and devotion to craft aesthetics to distract from its growing military capabilities and acts of imperial aggression.

The choice of *Blue Danube* too carried overt political signification amid disavowal of any political meaning. Following the dissolution of the Austro-Hungarian empire at the end of World War I, the *Blue Danube* waltz was embraced as music that was quintessentially Viennese, and therefore Austrian. It thus served the retrenchment into nationalism that so frequently follows the loss of imperial holdings, whereby a newly constructed cultural identity helps naturalize redrawn national borders. Through the 1920s and 30s it served as an increasingly resonant soundscape for the idea of national unity, and after Germany began its attempts at annexation in 1934, as the musical theme of national independence. By 1937, the *Blue Danube* was being put to multiple political purposes at once: still resonant as a celebration of Austria's (withering) independence, it had also become the signature tune of the Fatherland Front, Austria's own fascist party.[75] The *Blue Danube* is famous, however, because it is so catchy; it is beloved as "light music,"— orchestral entertainment perfect for dancing, rather than "serious" art. The *Blue Danube* waltz, then, is a piece of music that encodes political significance, while assuring the listener, with every cello tremor and swelling horn, that this is simply music to joyfully sweep you off your feet.

Etenraku and *Blue Danube* offered to both dancers and spectators the pleasure of choreographic escapism. This escapism worked through the very specificity of historical referent, where places that were currently sites of political anxiety could be recast as locales of stunning mystique and joyful coupling. This effect was compounded, rather than undermined, by the Hollywood Bowl's outdoor setting, with all its local specificity. The open amphitheater, where stage lights met the Southern California summer night sky, suggested not just the venue, but Los Angeles itself as a stage set for these fantasies, and indeed any others. As Mitchell Greenberg, following Jean Laplanche and Jean-Bertrand Pontalis, has observed, "fantasy is not the object of desire, but a scene, a stage setting for the elaboration of desire."[76] *Etenraku* and *Blue Danube* staged both the fantasy of history as escapist retreat, *and* the fantasy of history as a venue for integration. These were settings, then, for the playing out of the many desires held by Nisei, by Issei elites and their white progressive counterparts, and by Ito himself, to claim ownership of these appealing histories and reimagine them as the basis for an idealized future. For Ito especially, the successful work of staging these two fantastical ballets seemed to affirm that *he*, in particular, could present art, and the embodied work of dance, as a strategy of friendship, of shared (movement) vocabularies, shared histories, and shared theatrical enjoyment. For those evenings in August, it might have seemed momentarily, tantalizingly possible for art-making to eternally suspend the oncoming descent into war.

The tensions and political realities that the 1937 Hollywood Bowl concerts tried to choreograph away suggested the ways in which Ito's status as a cosmopolitan artist was beginning to lose its force. A similar shift is visible in the four trips abroad he took during the 1930s, which are treated in the next chapter. While his tours to Japan in 1931 and to Mexico in 1934 were met with enthusiasm for the international, integrationist possibilities his dancing seemed to suggest, subsequent trips to Japan in 1939 and 1940 met with changed spectatorship, as critics began to reject his "foreign" approach. So too did Ito's desire to mediate between Japan and the US become an increasing liability each time he returned home: the FBI began tracking his activities, his trips to Japan suggested he might be a spy, and his efforts to promote integration through Japanese culture appeared as forms of imperial propaganda. The incarceration of Ito and his Nisei dancers only a few years after the Hollywood Bowl event seems to render their desires "mere" fantasies, self-deceiving attachments to naïve political hopes. But if such fantasies were an escape, or a refuge, then they might also be a kind of self-preserving impulse, of a kind we will also see in Ito's wartime notebooks in chapter 6. A complicated mix of inner and outer life, fantasy might have offered Ito and his students a way of continuing to be themselves, as the world around them became unrecognizable.

CHAPTER FIVE

Cosmopolitanism, Masculinity, and National Embodiment in the Borderless Empire

Japan, 1931; Mexico, 1934; Japan, 1939–1940; Japan, 1940–1941

Ito's twelve years in California were punctuated by trips abroad—to Japan in the spring of 1931, to Mexico in the summer of 1934, again to Japan from the end of 1939 to the summer of 1940, and once more to Japan over the winter of 1940–1941. These trips brought him in front of audiences who had their own investments in what Ito's dancing signified. And these audiences, with the exception of the Mexican cultural elite, were predominantly Japanese. Yet, there was notable variety in this reception, as spectators, critics, and at one point, even the Tokyo Metropolitan Police, saw in Ito's dancing body an instantiation of the various affiliations that they held for themselves—or held in suspicion. Across this varied reception, Ito vivified a pressing question: how does a body carry (or seem to carry) race, nation, and culture within it? As this chapter will explore, in his various international trips during the 1930s, Ito became a particularly resonant—and vexing—figure for the mixedness of empire, and the concerns that arose when this mixedness was located within an individual's body.

Ito carried these significations in multiple, contradictory ways: one was his body, which was read as racially/ethnically Japanese—although in Mexico some critics found this to be ambiguous; another was his choreography, which in both its interpretive and "oriental" genres represented several different cultures; a third path of signification was his biography—where Ito was born (Japan), where he was educated (Germany and England), and where he lived (the US) could all be taken as national identifications that he carried with him.

Central to the ambiguities attached to Ito's body were the peculiar circumstances of what Eiichiro Azuma characterizes as Japan's "borderless empire." As Azuma explains, Japan's practice of borderless settler colonialism "lumped together Japanese-governed territories and foreign lands as the undifferentiated object of expansionist fantasies and practices under the all-encompassing language of overseas development."[1] Japan's relatively late start in colonial conquest meant that many territories (such as the US, and then Hawaii) were not only closed to the establishment of formal Japanese sovereignty, but also asserted exclusionary politics propelled by white settler colonialism/racism. Japan's expansion proceeded via private endeavors of settler colonialism, which created a patchwork, "borderless empire" of Japanese subjects, "bound by racial ties and national consciousness,"[2] who were imagined—and imagined themselves—as laying the groundwork for an interconnected, future New Japan.

Azuma's masterful study focuses on the Japanese farmers and agriculturalists who crisscrossed the Pacific, serving as the agents of this borderless empire. These agrarian migrants were the predominant and explicit foot soldiers of this extramilitary colonial project. But in this chapter, I suggest that for many Japanese commentators, both in Japan and abroad, Ito was understood within a similar paradigm, and that Ito's status as a dancer (that is, an artist whose art is *embodied*) elucidates different aspects of this imperial fantasy. What Ito's example suggested was that the borderless empire was not something only to be carried out *through* the migrating bodies of Japanese subjects, but was also something that could be corporealized, *within* individual bodies, as a repertoire of embodied expansionism. That is, the production of a sense of borderless presence could be achieved within the body itself.

The idea of a body carrying within itself some kind of imperial expansionism contains echoes of the concept of "extraterritoriality," a form of "legal imperialism," whereby rather than being subject to the laws of the place in which a person is, that person carries the laws of their own country with them; in these cases, imperial sovereign jurisdiction effectively attaches to a person, beyond the geographic bounds of territorial possession.[3] Extraterritoriality was a principle with which Japan was painfully familiar. It was a key feature of the "unequal treaties" that the US forced on Japan in the 1850s, and eliminating this provision was one of the major motivations behind Japan's effort to have the treaties renegotiated, a process that went on through the 1890s. By contrast, the agents of Japan's borderless empire did not carry extraterritoriality, or any kind of protected sovereignty, within their bodies— thus the precarity of their position. They did, nevertheless, carry something

Cosmopolitanism, Masculinity, and National Embodiment   163

of their nation with them—a sense of attachment, certainly, but also of agential purpose.

In this chapter, I trace the shifting requirements of national embodiment as revealed by the interpretations that his spectators assigned to Ito. In Japan in 1931, Ito was seen as a potent figure of Japanese imperial cosmopolitanism—for many, as a sign of the nation's assimilative capacity, but for some, a disturbing reminder of other nations' incursions into Japan's sovereignty. In Mexico in 1934, two distinct reception formations—Japanese immigrants in Mexico, and Mexican cultural critics—both read Ito according to their own fantasies of what a (masculine) figure of national agency required. For Japanese immigrants, Ito's successes confirmed their own value to the Japanese Empire as subjects living outside of Japan's formal territorial holdings; for Mexican cultural critics, however, Ito seemed to represent a provocative mirror for the national ideology of *mestizaje*, whereby his own corporeal ambiguity and profession as a dancer potentially undermined the masculine power attributed to this ideology. Ito's second trip to Japan, from late 1939 to mid-1940, found a less liberal atmosphere; while critics still welcomed his achievements, his "cosmopolitanism" was now marked as "foreignness," and with this shift, his form of Japanese embodiment was no longer suited to the nation's needs. The chapter closes with a brief consideration of one more trip Ito took to Japan, over the winter of 1940 to 1941, documented via conjectures by the FBI—yet one more fantasy of what Ito's border-crossing body signified.

The period covered in this chapter thus overlaps with that of the previous chapter, which focused on Ito's activities in California in the 1930s. By pulling out his trips outside the US into a separate chapter, I am able to highlight other thematics in his career. Thus, while chapter 4 explored how Ito became a figure for fantasies of integration, here I shift our attention to frameworks of imperialism and masculinity. As will become clear, as in the previous chapter, these are concepts of ideological struggle, which Ito seemed to provoke because his body was so frequently taken as representing some notion of the national body, or *kokutai*. Pulling out these international trips also allows me to take an explicitly reception-focused tack in this chapter. That means that while this chapter gives an account of Ito's activities in each place, I am less interested in Ito's own sense of himself as an artist here, and primarily concerned with other people's fantasies, and how Ito served as an irresistible figure for those fantasies. In this way, this chapter offers a certain rhyme with chapter 3, in which I examined the fantasies of Japan and the Orient, for which Ito became a particularly resonant figure. But whereas the reception evidence in chapter 3 figures Ito within the terms of collection, as a curio or as an individual collector, and thus points to a framing of Asian masculinity as an *object* of (repressed) desire, in this chapter, terms of cosmopolitanism, amalgamation, and foreignness can be understood as working to frame Asian masculinity as a conduit for nation- and empire-making, that is, as a *subject* of world-historical import. Put differently, the fantasies of chapter 3 revolve around the idealization/abjectification of Ito's body as a site of (semi-) private desire; the fantasies here in chapter 5 revolve around the question of how audiences imagined Ito to perform as a masculine subject of history, and indeed, of whether his version of Japanese masculinity was the one needed for this moment in time.

Perhaps precisely because the masculine, as a historical agent, appears as a fraught value in the various receptions examined here, the question of intermarriage also haunts the fantasies swirling around Ito on these trips. Indeed, intermarriage as a sociopolitical issue repeatedly intersects with the interculturalism of his dancing to produce an ambiguity about the exact nature of Ito's national-racial-cultural cosmopolitanism. Notable here is the contrast with the status of intermarriage, or "amalgamation" in the US, where it was a threatening and nearly unspeakable circumstance, and in Mexico, where it was upheld as a foundation for national vigor.[4] In both places, anxiety over patrimony led to elaborately constructed ideologies about the nation's blood essence; in the US, the concept of miscegenation imagined a racial threat to supposed national purity; in Mexico, *mestizaje* articulated a national essence predicated on racial mixing. As we will see, Japan shifted between these two paradigms, as it attempted to elaborate a eugenic paradigm that complemented its own imperial program. As Ito traveled, his own body, his choreography, and his biography seemed to variously signify all of these competing visions for what a cosmopolitan masculinity could mean for the state, as his many spectators projected their own desires and interpretations onto him.

Japan, 1931: Worldly Dancing

Ito arrived in Yokohama on April 10, 1931, five months before the Manchurian Incident and Japan's full-blown invasion and occupation of Manchuria. At the turn of the decade, military and right-wing factions were gaining power, pushing for greater aggression in Asia and a rejection of US diplomatic ties. But many progressives in Japan were still emphatically committed to ideals

Cosmopolitanism, Masculinity, and National Embodiment 165

of international cooperation, and liberal notions of individual and social freedom common during the "Taisho Democracy" (1912–1926) were still part of public daily life. Against this backdrop, Ito's various commentators saw in him a chance to work out what "worldly" meant, as an embodied characteristic, and for Japan. To some critics, worldliness was a form of imperial cosmopolitanism and a sign of Japanese expansion, but to others, such as the Metropolitan Police, it was a sign of the dissolution of Japanese order—and perhaps, even, of Japanese "purity."

Ito's visit was double-billed as a triumphant return for the artist to perform for his own country, as well as a sort of delayed honeymoon. Traveling with Ito was his wife, Hazel Wright, and their two sons, Donald and Gerald. Ito also brought along several dancers, including local Los Angeles dancers Charles Teske and Jerre (née Miles Marshon), about whom little other information exists; Waldeen Falkenstein, who would go on to become a pioneer of modern dance in Mexico; and Teru Izumida, who was one of Ito's Nisei students from the Japanese American community. Over two months, the group presented around five recitals, performing most of the pieces in Ito's repertoire. *Tango* and *Pizzicati*, with which Ito closed every performance, were hailed as masterpieces. Also popular were Hazel Wright's performances of *Habanera* and *Little Shepherdess*, Teske's *Primitive Rhythms*, and Waldeen in *Sonata*. The solo dances were broken up with some of Ito's group pieces—*En Bateau, Ecclesiastique, Etude*, and *Prelude*. Tokyo newspapers noted that Ito's old artist friends—Ishii Baku, Yamado Gorō, and Hanayagi Sumi—all attended performances, as did the Russian ambassador.

The troupe's recitals were evaluated with enthusiastic praise, as well as some jingoism. Touching on the costuming and lighting, and the concept behind each dance, the critic Ushiyama Mitsuru declared, "everything thoroughly surpassed the dance troupes that have visited Japan up until now."[5] Ushiyama had, for example, reviewed performances by La Argentina in 1929 and the Sakaroffs at the beginning of 1931, but he might have also been thinking of the Denishawn troupe, which had visited Japan in 1925 and stopped by again at the end of their tour of Asia in 1926.[6] He continued, "As long as we have Ito Michio, I think we need not feel inferior to any other countries on the world's dance stage."[7] Such a comparison asserted Ushiyama's own informed critical acumen, and placed Tokyo on the map as a frequent site of touring performance. Ito's visit thus allowed critics and the cultural elite to demonstrate their active participation in and affiliation with a global modern culture.

Ito's presence also served as an occasion for an articulation of imperial cosmopolitanism as a valuable performance of Japaneseness. While Ushiyama compared Ito, who had come from abroad, to other foreign dancers, he also included Ito in his rhetorical "we"—the "we" of dance spectators, artists, and promoters of national achievement. Ushiyama's characterization of Ito as performing "worldly dancing" (*sekaiteki buyō*), then, evokes multiple significations. On the one hand, "worldly" carries the valence of "cosmopolitan." In this nuance, "worldly" is a word that reveals an orientation: it expresses an appreciation for other cultural practices, and an affiliation with those who esteem globally circulating artistic products. In this sense, worldly *signifies* almost the opposite of "foreign," in that it signifies a desire to bring distant people, practices, and things close, and to fold them into a fantasy of friendly availability. On the other hand, "worldly" here might also be a literal description of the subjects of Ito's choreography—the "oriental dance" embodiments that made up much of his repertoire. Indeed, Ushiyama goes on to write, "Within his dances there is China, Java, Russia, every country of Western Europe. And of course, his native country Japan proudly offered its spirit to his art via the Noh. Each country's dance essence and dance idiom was skillfully digested, in his creation of a unique dance artistry."[8] This is again the concept of *kokutai* that we saw in chapter 4, an assimilative national body that is not at all metaphorical, but applauded as an effective, performative practice of corporeal-imperial expansion. These two significations of "worldly" are not contradictory; as my discussion of "oriental dance" in chapter 3 showed, the "worldliness" of "oriental dance" embodiments was predicated on an attitudinal "worldliness" of presumed intimacy and access across the globe.

If Ito's worldly dancing offered critics the opportunity to assert a cosmopolitan affiliation, and to see in Ito an embodiment of a particularly cosmopolitan imperialism, questions about the reach of Japan's empire also manifested in more disruptive incidents. On May 5, the troupe performed for a gathering of the International Club at the Tokyo Kaikan. Halfway through, in the middle of one of Hazel Wright's dances, the inspector general and five policemen from the local Marunouchi Station burst in, leaping on stage to arrest Wright and terminate the performance. The Itos were brought to the police station, accompanied by the outraged chairman of the International Club. As newspapers reported the next day, the recital violated a prohibition against "social dancing," since the program contained dances such as *Tango* and *Empire Waltz*.[9] Social dancing—by which was meant, popular forms of Western couples' dance—was seen as a menace to public morality, leading to

Cosmopolitanism, Masculinity, and National Embodiment

frequent raids on dancehalls during the 1920s and '30s. The law cited in Ito's case was the Regulations Concerning the Management of Performance Halls and Performances (*kōgyōjō oyobi kōgyō torishimari kisoku*), which had been in force since 1921, when a series of earlier laws governing theater, entertainment halls, film, and so on, were combined into one. Ito and the chairman argued with the inspector general until 2 a.m., when it was finally determined that the arrest was the result of a series of misunderstandings: prior to the performance, as was required, the chairman of the Tokyo Kaikan had submitted an application for the performance. It was at first refused because the recital included dances such as the foxtrot, tango, waltz, and dances to blues music, which seemed to violate the injunction against social dancing. Four days later, the chairman went to the Public Safety Division and explained that the recital was strictly "stage dancing" in which some dances took social dance as their subject. He thereby secured an oral agreement permitting the recital to occur. Either this information was not passed on or the inspector general later changed his mind about the recital's legality, a "misunderstanding" that resulted in the dramatic raid. Once Ito had worked out the issue and been released, the inspector general and chief of the Public Safety Division announced that new regulations would be drawn up to avoid similar situations in the future. These aimed to simplify the petition process and granted social-dancing exemptions for private banquets and artists performing in their own studios. Citing the uniform regulations of dancehalls, however, they stated that no new halls would be permitted to open.

The incident, though effectively resolved, revealed the tension underlying the presence of Ito's troupe. In a common modernist gesture, Ito's choreography used popular cultural forms—in this case, social dancing—as material for his modern stage dancing. But this distinction was lost on the police, who saw in Ito's recital a threat to public morality. Indeed, though the problem seemed to be the police's lack of sophistication in recognizing different forms of dance, their objection registers the broader threat posed by the dancing body. For while Ito's choreography did not feature men and women pressed up against each other, in the bodily citations of social dancing's postures and choreography, Ito's dancers could be seen to also embody its wantonness, and they did so on a highly visible stage. That the troupe was primarily foreign, and performing foreign forms of dance, was at the root of its apparent threat to public morality. The *Asahi Shimbun* hinted at this when a columnist hypothesized that the troupe might also have violated a rule requiring foreign performers to submit proof of identity. Although a quotation from the chief clerk of entertainment of the Metropolitan Police Department seemed to dismiss this possibility, the hypothesis registered the disruptive nature of Ito's presence.[10] For the troupe, made up of both Japanese and white dancers, performing an array of different national and racial personas in their borrowed dance forms, suggested how national purity or morality could be violated even when one danced alone.

It was, then, perhaps no accident that the police burst in during one of Hazel Wright's numbers. Wright, Ito's white wife and the mother of his two sons, represented a particularly vexed position between two empires. At the point of her marriage to Ito in New York in 1923, Wright became subject to the Cable Act of 1922, which revised the Expatriation Act of 1907 such that US-born women who married foreign nationals could retain their US citizenship, unless their husbands were "aliens ineligible for citizenship"—that is, Asian men. When the couple moved to California in 1929, though their marriage was legal because it had taken place in another state, they surely contended with denouncements of "miscegenation," which in California was illegal. Meanwhile, intermarriage in Japan had been an actively debated issue since the 1880s, a debate that drew on various globally circulating eugenics discourses as well as native theories of Japanese identity. Early on, many intellectuals explicitly encouraged intermarriage with white Europeans and Americans as a strategy of supposed racial improvement;[11] as Japan pursued its assimilation and imperialization (*kōminka*) policies in Taiwan and Korea, intermarriage was also recommended as a way to absorb inhabitants of those countries into Japan;[12] and by the 1920s, for many commentators class was seen as an equal or greater concern in determining "superior" or "inferior" offspring.[13] In 1930, however, the Japan Association of Racial Hygiene was founded, and theories of "racial purity," which had been widely circulating since the 1880s, began to dominate. As Tessa Morris-Suzuki notes, because so many Japanese researchers were educated in Germany, some were receptive to the racial ideas of National Socialism, but because within that paradigm, the Japanese were considered an inferior race, many also rejected that framing.[14] From a legal perspective, Japan's citizenship laws stated that foreign-born women could be absorbed into the polity if their names were entered in the family *koseki*, or registry.

It is impossible to know what position on intermarriage the inspector general of the Metropolitan Police held in 1931. But it seems likely that somewhere between the generic ambiguity of the program's dances and the "racial admixture" represented by Hazel Wright (and the couple's two sons), Ito appeared as a troublesome figure. The relationship between the company's repertoire and the company's personnel, moreover, was not simply one of parallelism; social dance, after all, was such a contentious activity because it seemed not simply to represent, but to actually induce, sexual and reproductive transgression. The police raid, then, sought to halt both the symbolic and performative effects of the company's presence in Japan. Moreover, the raid was an exercise in asserting Japanese sovereignty—over them all, but particularly over Hazel Wright, who legally could not claim the protection of the US government. The shifting grounds on which the police based their raid, then, were perhaps more than a misunderstanding, but spoke to a persistent, but usually thwarted, desire on the part of the Japanese government to make the US attend to it as an equal imperial power.

The contrast between dance critics such as Ushiyama and the Metropolitan Police's reception of Ito suggests competing formulations for Japanese masculinity and its role in maintaining the empire. Ushiyama's comments could be read as envisioning Ito as precisely one of Japan's agents of empire, his bodily capacity for absorbing repertoires standing as a more general capacity of Japanese expansion. It is harder to pin down what the police thought: Ito's marriage to Wright could be a sign of Japanese strength, especially given the gender roles involved; conversely, she could be a sign of Japanese dissolution, exemplified in the couple's choice to present "social dances" on stage. Either way, the strength of their reactions suggest that it mattered that Ito was a Japanese man, whose actions had consequences for Japan's evolving position in the world.

Interestingly, on the return voyage, two other internationally circulating Japanese actors were on board: Sessue Hayakawa and Sano Seki. Fujita Fujio suggests that Ito and Hayakawa already knew each other from meeting in New York;[15] Hayakawa had had immense success as a matinée idol during the silent-film era, playing roles as a sexually alluring villain—roles that propelled him to stardom, but also were seen by Japanese, in both the US and Japan, as contributing to anti-Japanese sentiment. Hayakawa's career paralleled Ito's, not only because of the film star's own transnational circulation, but because, as Daisuke Miyao has shown, his success in the US also hinged on a precarious masculinity, that was successful so long as it was alluring without appearing threatening.[16] Sano Seki, meanwhile, was a major figure in proletarian theater. Like Ito's brother, Senda Koreya, Sano had been moved to political action by the 1923 Kanto earthquake, and the vigilante violence against Koreans in the earthquake's aftermath. In the 1920s, Sano and Senda worked together in proletarian theater; Sano was, in fact, on the ship as a replacement for Senda, as a representative of Japanese proletarian theater organizations at a meeting of the International Workers' Dramatic Union in Moscow.[17] Fujita suggests that on the ship, Sano enthusiastically engaged the company members in conversation, perhaps to distract them from the absence of Waldeen, who while dancing for Ito was also covertly working for the International Association of Theater Workers; she had stayed behind in Japan to contact other proletarian theater workers, and to try to connect with the Japanese Communist Party, through introductions Sano had made for her.[18] The two were to reunite when Sano and Waldeen both returned to Mexico in 1939. The meanings attached to Ito, then, were not unique to him. Ito, Hayakawa, and Sano were all highly visible Japanese artists, whose masculinity, whether for white audiences in the US or Japanese commentators in Japan, implicated varying conceptions of Japan as a nation, and what that meant for its role as a world power.

Mexico, 1934: National Representation, Racial Ambiguity

In June and July of 1934, Ito took a small troupe of dancers on a tour to Mexico, organized by a Mexican entertainment promoter, Jesús Sánchez.[19] The company consisted of Waldeen, who had also participated in the Japan trip, and three other dancers who were active in Ito's Los Angeles studio: Bette Jordan, Jocelyn Burke, and a man who simply went by the name Josef. Hazel Wright accompanied the group but did not perform. The tour was to have significance for Mexico's history of modern dance: it was Waldeen's first visit to Mexico; she found the country so compelling that she remained there for some months, further studying local dances. In 1940 she staged the theatrical dance *La Coronela*, which was recognized as a watershed event that, along with her other pieces, established Waldeen as one of the major cultural figures of the postrevolution period in Mexico.[20]

While in Mexico, Ito's troupe gave around ten performances at the Teatro Hidalgo and the Teatro Arben, with the dancers presenting over twenty pieces in an evening, and adding new material within the program to encourage audiences to return. These works featured Ito's solo and small-group choreography, Mexican-inspired dances by Waldeen, and masked solos by Josef. As had become customary, the final piece on every program was Ito's *Pizzicati*. Ito's reception in Mexico was, in certain ways, of a piece with his 1931 reception in Japan; in both places, he was identified as a potential figure for Japan's imperial expansiveness. But in Mexico, Japanese immigrants saw in Ito an explicit affirmation of the value of overseas Japanese, who, even as they were not part of the formal Japanese Empire, nevertheless had a crucial role to play in representing and establishing Japan abroad. Mexican critics, meanwhile, hailed Ito's cosmopolitanism and appreciated his presence as a sign of Mexico's international importance. But they also heatedly debated what the apparent (racial and gender) ambiguity of Ito's own body signified for his capacity to stand as a national figure.

Mexico had its own burgeoning modern dance scene, a tradition that had begun with Anna Pavlova's 1919 visit. According to dance historian Jose Luis Reynoso, her performances, which had already enchanted audiences in Europe and the United States, allowed Mexico City elites to assert a "homo-topic" cultural affinity with European values, demonstrating their modernity and sophistication.[21] While Pavlova was in Mexico City, however, she also explored the nonelite spaces of the city, venturing into popular performance halls. She incorporated the themes and movements she observed into a new piece, *El Jarabe Tapatío*, which she performed *en pointe*. This piece, which fused modern ballet with native Mexican traditions, served as a foundation for the development of Mexican modern dance, which, Reynoso argues, thereafter developed as a fusion of the universalist ideology of US modern dance with the particularities of Mexican tradition and dance idioms. During the 1920s and '30s, ballet technique remained essential training for modern dancers in Mexico, who following Pavlova's innovation were expected to treat Mexican themes, both on the concert stage and in mass performances.

By the time of Ito's visit, the bloody years of the Mexican Revolution were more than a decade in the past. National identity and its representation, however, remained an active site of contestation. The concept of *mestizaje* (the outcome of colonial racial mixing) was worked out among political leaders and cultural commentators as an articulation of what the nation should valorize postrevolution. For Mexican elites, Ito represented not the possibility of imperial corporeality, as he had for commentators in Tokyo in 1931, but rather one possible vision of national embodiment. Although Mexico was free of active imperial dominion, it was acutely aware of the pressure it faced from US imperial aggression. Indeed, as Jerry García has found, on occasion, Mexico used its positive diplomatic relations with Japan as a way to prick its northern neighbor.[22] Mexico's debate over national identity, then, while seemingly a domestic issue, was in fact shaped by the competing imperialisms surrounding it. Ito's presence put into literal form the idea that national identity is always also a question of international relationality.

If Mexico felt the competing pressures of the two dominant Pacific empires, it also hosted a dispersed array of Japanese migrants within its borders, who were similarly negotiating the question of national identity. But for these migrants, the question was how to position themselves in relation to Japan, when they lived and labored on the other side of the globe, in what was in 1934 a minor outpost of Japan's borderless empire. Mexico had, in fact, been the site of Japan's first Latin American expansion, with the Enomoto colony in 1896. Though it rapidly failed, the effort nevertheless offered Japan several lessons that it quickly applied to subsequent, more successful endeavors in Brazil, Paraguay, and Bolivia.[23] Much of Mexico's appeal, for both the Japanese government and the many migrants who traveled there, was its contiguousness with the US, which offered postexclusion migrants passages to slip into the US, and opportunities for US-based Japanese to operate businesses and own properties from across the border. Indeed, after 1924, when opportunities for both migration and land ownership in the US were closed, Mexico became a particularly resonant setting for fantasies of settlement, ownership, and success. Meanwhile, as Japan grew as a world power, Japanese migrants residing in Mexico City in particular understood themselves as part of a vocal network of overseas partners of the Japanese Empire, who were able to use their business and cultural endeavors to complement the agrarian empire-building that their rural counterparts offered.

For the merchant- and professional-class writers in the *Mehiko Shinpō* who aimed to speak for Japanese in Mexico broadly, Ito's internationalism was valuable, first because his artistic success abroad signified as cultural capital to the Mexican elite. And second, Ito's success, especially in its assimilative dimensions, signified the value to Japan of all its citizens working and living abroad. An early feature on Ito explicitly identified him as cosmopolitan, and recognized the wide appeal of such a figure: "Ito seems a bit old-fashioned at first, but because his refined, gentlemanly style as a cosmopolitan does not have the slightest sense of condescension or pretentiousness, he cannot fail to make a good impression on everyone."[24] This critic's fantasy of cosmopolitanism, which Ito so adeptly embodied, was a fantasy of a kind of ease and affableness; the *kokusai jin* is someone who can fit in anywhere and get along with anyone. But Ito was also deemed cosmopolitan because other "cosmopolitans"—figures from the international community in Mexico—

Cosmopolitanism, Masculinity, and National Embodiment

took an interest in him. Thus he was invited to a ceremony celebrating the founding of the National Bank, at which were present diplomatic ministers representing Britain, France, China, Colombia, Ecuador, Cuba, Poland, Denmark, Honduras, Santo Domingo, Paraguay, Nicaragua, El Salvador, and Uruguay.[25] Alongside these significations, Ito represented a dense node of foreign cultures through his background and training, evoking various associations of Japan, Germany, England, and the US, and he could be felt to transport all those cultures to Mexico, as one artistic agglomeration of international culture. Writers in the *Mehiko Shinpō* thus saw in Ito a solution to their sense of Mexico's peripheral status: "This is a rare opportunity for we who live in Mexico City, which has a slightly neglected view of culture from the world."[26] For these critics, Ito had brought the world with him, carrying this amalgamation within his body, and vivifying the possibility of Japanese success abroad.

As was the case with commentary by Japanese in California, *Mehiko Shinpō* critics were ready with positive evaluations of Ito's artistic accomplishments, but because so much political and cultural weight was assigned to the success of his presence, they also worried a great deal about whether his artistry would be appreciatively received. Several writers grumbled about the raked stage at the Teatro Hidalgo, which created issues with the lighting equipment and thus interfered with the all-important cast shadow in *Pizzicati*.[27] The numerous mentions of this issue reveal an understandable anxiety about Ito's reception, anxiety fueled not only out of national pride, but out of a recognition that spectators had little experience with this kind of art. Indeed, one critic, who admitted that he himself had previously only seen Shochiku-style entertainment and *kabuki*, was nevertheless entranced by Ito's dancing, exclaiming, "It's a poem without sound!"[28] Another fretted that many of their fellow Japanese would not appreciate the significance of Ito's visit, or his art, asking: "For the Japanese people who are only accustomed to popular erotic revues, is it possible for these countrymen to have understanding and interest in the truly artistic dancing of Ito Michio's troupe, and especially the unique charm of his subtle Japanese expressiveness and fine gestures?"[29] This critic's comment makes apparent the class divisions within the Japanese migrant community. As Azuma has shown, professional-class Japanese in the US frequently worried that their working-class counterparts would disrupt the image of a cultured, artistic Japan that was central to their strategy for fighting racism in the Americas.[30] Moreover, in this review, it is implied that if Japanese could not appreciate Ito's dancing, Mexican spectators similarly might not. The resounding call for Japanese in Mexico to support Ito was a matter of national pride, and was a way to assert a specific, trans-Pacific vision of Japanese identity as cultured and internationally engaged.

Ito's visit was thus overwhelmingly understood as an opportunity to unify readers in their identity as Japanese, and to specify what such an identity meant for migrants' relationship to Japan. Ito's utility in this regard was of particular value in disseminating a positive sense of Japaneseness to the second generation, who, it was feared, felt less of a connection to Japan, and in many cases were the products of intermarriage.[31] Thus, almost as soon as he arrived, the newspaper organized an event, especially aimed at the second generation, "An Evening of Conversation with Ito Michio," proclaiming that Ito was a "Japanese in the world" of whom they should be especially proud.[32] The paper declared that because Ito had gained success living "amongst white people," hearing about his experiences was of the utmost importance for developing the awareness of young people living abroad.[33] Journalists covering the event all dwelled on Ito's status as a racial outsider, and they all declared the evening an unmitigated success.

The event's success seems to have been due to Ito's ability to speak inspiringly about Japan itself, and to evoke a sense of pride and achievement in being a Japanese abroad. Several articles noted that Ito spoke of his own trip to Japan three years prior, and found in his anecdotes the proof they needed of an ineluctable national tie: "This veteran, having lived overseas for twenty years, amongst a different race and pioneering a unique artistic territory, got flushed cheeks and his eyes glistened once he started talking about his homeland, Japan. Those who listened to him truly understood how deep was his patriotism for his country."[34] Having left Japan at a young age, Ito suggested that he, like the youth in the audience, had been ignorant of Japan's treasures. But, as his own experience demonstrated, such ignorance and absence from his home country could not interfere with his sense of belonging, and the sense of attraction and comfort he felt there. Ito's message thus implied that to be Japanese was to always be at home in Japan, even when it was not one's home.

Indeed, Ito's value as a role model was his personal understanding of what it meant to be a Japanese abroad. As one journalist wrote,

He preached in tones filled with enthusiasm and sincerity about the great determination of the Japanese and the overseas brethren [*zaigai dōhō*] marching in the vanguard, which made a deep impression on all who were present. That determination was based on their sense of their great responsibility to perfect the individual by balancing the spiritual and material and to construct a new civilization that balances Eastern and Western civilizations. That is to say, he offered encouraging calls, born out of his own belief in his utter devotion to perfecting dance through the harmonization of oriental and western dance.[35]

Clearly, Ito knew his audience. In his talk, as reported by this journalist, Ito drew on the paradigm of Japan's ability to balance the spiritual and material, and thus "Eastern" and "Western" civilizations—a paradigm that he had used to describe himself in an interview with the *New York Tribune* in 1917 (chapter 3). This ideology asserted that Japan was uniquely capable of unifying, or putting into balance, the world's two clashing civilizations, through the creation of a new civilization, made up of people who had balanced these aspects within themselves. Hailing his listeners as "overseas brethren" (*zaigai dōhō*), Ito presented himself as someone who truly recognized the extraordinary responsibility they were carrying out.[36] Indeed, Ito recognizes the civilization-constructing labor of his listeners because he is one of them, carrying out the same work, but through dance. In the journalist's syntax (in the Japanese), the characterization of Ito "perfecting dance through the harmonization of oriental and western dance" parallels the individual who perfects himself through a balance of the spiritual and material. Both Ito and his listeners are in the vanguard—a word that simultaneously registers military and artistic advance.[37] This writer, then, thought of Ito—as a dancer, choreographer, teacher, and cultural figure—as doing the same work as the Japanese settler-colonial farmers whose labor was considered the linchpin of expansion. Especially in the face of US racism and exclusion policies, Ito could serve as a different kind of vanguard, one whose art offered a kind of diplomacy and nonaggressive advertisement in regions anxious about Japanese presence.

• • •

Spanish-language writers for Mexico City newspapers, including *El Mundo, La Prensa, Universal Grafico, El Nacional, El Universal,* and *Excelsior,* also understood Ito's visit as an opportunity to assert national identity. They did so through the same demonstration of cultural acumen as did critics in Japan during Ito's 1931 tour. But, in the aftermath of the Mexican Revolution, Ito's presence also provoked a more tense set of negotiations over the relation of ethnic identity and artistic style, and over constructions of masculinity in the service of national character.

For critics writing in mainstream Mexico City newspapers, eager to demonstrate their cultural cosmopolitanism, the trope of japonisme served as an established and internationally recognized paradigm by which to appreciate Ito's recitals—a version of Reynoso's homotopic cultural affiliation. Thus Ito was enthusiastically greeted as the "Spiritual Ambassador of Japanese Rhythms in the West."[38] Reviews repeatedly commented on the "fineness" of his artistic sensibility, his "oriental" mystique, and the stunning simplicity of his interpretations. One writer noted that Ito's *Spear Dance* seemed "to have been torn from a screen in Japan"[39]—an evocation of artistry through comparison to Japan's graphic arts, which, we might recall, was a mainstay of his reception in New York and California as well. Japonisme, then, was not just a language for interpreting Ito's recitals; it was also a strategy of asserting fluency with international currents of artistic valuation. It was for just such a reason that the papers exhorted Mexicans to attend the performances. Empty seats, they suggested, would not reflect badly on Ito, but rather, on Mexicans who did not know to go see "culture" when it arrived at their door.[40]

While japonisme allowed critics to place Ito within a recognizable discourse, his dancing also seemed to contradict the model for modern dance established since Anna Pavlova's 1919 visit. As one writer observed, noting that the majority of Ito's pieces were accompanied by music composed by Chopin, Debussy, and Brahms, "despite his Asian origins, Ito's predilection is for Western dances."[41] If Pavlova had localized modern dance by setting her choreography to recognizably Mexican musical accompaniment, Ito's preference for classical Western music challenged these expectations. But that is not to say that the critic expected Ito, like Pavlova, to turn to Mexican music to make his dancing particularly appealing to local audiences on tour. Rather, it seems that the critic expected Ito's music to be Japanese, so that the implicit "localizing" of modern dance performed by the sheer presence of Ito's racialized body would be mirrored in a formal choice, such as the musical accompaniment. This, of course, is a version of the binary of ethnic particularity and white universality that, by the 1940s, was to become a common paradigm in dance viewership, not just in the US, but in many places across the globe.[42] But in this particular context, the comment also alerts us to a sense of ambiguity in how to "read" Ito, that was not only about his formal choreographic and musical choices, but, ultimately, a troubling ambiguity of his very body.

The conservative music and literary critic, Carlos Gonzalez Peña, was

Cosmopolitanism, Masculinity, and National Embodiment

the most outspoken about Ito's seeming implacability, and the anxiety this caused: "The name is exotic, Michio Ito. They say it's Japanese. The truth is that, seeing him dance, we are convinced that his eyes aren't oblique enough to guarantee his ancestry. I don't know whether in Japan, this obliqueness is general, or just partial. Either way, isn't he something of a *mestizo* Japanese?"[43] Gonzalez Peña's evaluation of Ito dances across linguistics and physiognomy in an effort to pin down his racial character. Ito's name, which *sounds* exotic, might be Japanese, but Gonzalez Peña holds out the possibility that it could be something else. While he first insists on physical characteristics as a guarantee of racial identity, in the next breath he dismisses the assessments of physiognomy. Both name and eye shape, seemingly markers of ancestry (Ellen Samuel's "fantasies of identification"[44]), are suspect to Gonzalez Peña, who knows too well how such tokens might be misread. And so, he lands on the only explanation for Ito's apparent ambiguity that makes sense to this Mexican critic: Ito must be *mestizo*.

Gonzalez Peña's use of the term *mestizo* entangles Ito in a key contemporary Mexican nationalist discourse. *Mestizaje*, a concept combining biology and culture, was the ideological affirmation of the *mestizo*, or mixed-race product of colonial conquest. Rooted in the conspicuousness of the racialized body, *mestizaje* indicated as well the concomitant blending of indigenous and European culture. During the period of the Mexican Revolution and its aftermath, the term *mestizaje* was embraced as an articulation of a political movement and of a modern racial and national identity. Gonzalez Peña's hailing Ito as *mestizo*, then, created a racially explicit gloss on other characterizations of Ito as cosmopolitan. For in the critic's evaluation, it is not simply the overall diversity of performers in Ito's troupe, his blended dance style, or his international circulation, but rather the ambiguity contained within his very body, that constitutes him as a figure of embodied cosmopolitanism—and therefore, of national potentiality. Cosmopolitanism here is an ambiguity, even illegibility, caused by the historical circumstances of international encounter and collision. For Gonzalez Peña, this ambiguity, as a signal of hybrid vigor, offers the same national political potential as the concept of *mestizaje*.

However, as the review continues, it turns out that Gonzalez Peña cannot hail Ito as a "*mestizo* Japanese," because something is not quite right. The problem is that Ito is not virile enough, a problem that is indistinguishable, it seems, from the fact that he is a dancer. He writes, if the male dancer is to appear naked at all, it should be to show off "his manly torso, sinewy legs, athletic chest, rude gestures. What's more—the beautiful outline of his calves . . .

flexible arms, and eyes and mouth in a smile that says, 'I want to see you here. That's it. Now over there.'"[45] In Gonzalez Peña's fantasy, the powerful naked male dancer overpowers his feminized, if not female, spectator, asserting raw dominance. Male nudity is only acceptable as an expression of power, a power that can then be understood as a reflection of the emergent nation as well. As Robert McKee Irwin has shown, in postrevolutionary Mexico, conceptions of masculinity broadly shifted from that of the upper-class dandy to a more rural, hypermasculinized *machismo*.[46] Critics such as Gonzalez Peña, though of the urban literati class, demonstrated a commitment to the revolutionary spirit through their embrace of the *machismo* ideal. Indeed, Diana Taylor points out that the reclaimed racial and cultural identity of the *mestizaje* ideology was staked out on the denigration of the female—the gendered bodies that had suffered the original acts of colonial sexual violence.[47] While it seems likely that Ito's Japaneseness—even if to Gonzalez Peña this was an ambiguous, *mestizaje* Japaneseness—contributes to the critic's sense that Ito lacked virility, it is Ito's status as a dancer that confirms and makes this explicit. The threat posed by Ito's profession is pointed to a few lines later when Gonzalez Peña similarly dismisses the dancers Nijinsky and Marius Petipa of the Ballets Russes as "alarmingly feminine." Pervasive associations of the Ballets Russes with homosexuality *and* with orientalism made dance an overdetermined site of (racialized, misogynistic) homophobia. Ito's work as a dancer necessarily produces, in Gonzalez Peña's eyes, an effeminized body that, it is suggested, effects a sort of racial degeneracy, rather than the racial ascendancy that the critic desired.

The Mexican press, however, was not monolithic in this interpretation. In fact one critic, writing prior to Gonzalez Peña's feverish review, had quite the opposite view of Ito's dancing: "What are we going to bet that neither our 'ballarinos' nor our 'ballarinas' have gone to admire Michio Ito and his marvelous choreographic 'troupe' at the Hidalgo theater? . . . If they had gone, the national dancers would know that to do Classical Art, it is not necessary to be effeminate metaphorically or materially."[48] At stake here is still the question of national masculinity, and the fear that dancers are particularly threatening to this figuration, but now Ito is upheld as a model of (hyper)masculinity in dance, who can serve as an inspiration for the anxious nation. Following Gonzalez Peña's criticism, this debate heated up, as another journalist explicitly went after the conservative critic's racial logic and homophobia:

> I do not believe that the best way to identify a Japanese, especially when one recognizes our ignorance about his country, is to look precisely at the oblique-

Cosmopolitanism, Masculinity, and National Embodiment 179

ness of his eyes. It would have been more natural to resort to more valuable characteristics, e.g.: the psychology of Mr. Ito. Also, I do not think it is vitally important to know the origin of a prominent artist. And if we are being fair, what is the point of putting issues of sexuality into art and trampling over the artist's intimate person in the process?[49]

Taking a swipe at Gonzalez Peña's hysterical need to know, this critic draws boundaries around what the artist can be taken to represent. He asserts that an artist's sexuality is private, and even that national origin should be disregarded in artistic evaluation. Nevertheless, he adds that nationality might be gleaned, not from phenotype and external appearance, but from psychology and internal essence. This critic, then, is assuredly also invested in the nation-defining principles of *mestizaje*, but seems to recognize that if the foundational fact of *mestizaje* is a sort of racial illegibility, then true *mestizo* embodiment must be a matter of internal essence.

This critic thus sounded a note that echoed aspects of Ito's reception in the *Mehiko Shinpō*. Like the Japanese writers who asserted that migrants' shared experience living in extraterritorial lands formed the basis for a particular kind of Japaneseness, for at least some Mexican writers, national essence could not be a matter of surface legibility. Rather, national identity—and perhaps as important, an individual's perceived value to their nation—was a matter of a certain interiority, something that could be imagined as a shared essence, and something that, though visually unidentifiable, was given apt expression by Ito.

Conspicuously Foreign: Japan, 1939–1940

In September 1939, Ito again went to Japan, this time alone. As the Tokyo press reported, the trip was in honor of his parents' fiftieth wedding anniversary. For the celebration, Ito, his brothers, and his sister-in-law Teiko (a New York Nisei married to Yuji, and herself an accomplished dancer) put on an elaborate recital, which included a performance of *At the Hawk's Well*. The trip also offered an opportunity for Ito to reaffirm his ties with Japan, a commitment he had frequently spoken of during his 1931 visit. As usual, he did so through his creative work, choreographing a production of the ballet *Prince Igor*, and, with his brothers, presenting a massive historical drama, *Daibutsu Kaigen* (The Great Buddha's Awakening). This event, staged as part of a national festival, placed Ito squarely within cultural efforts supporting

Japan's rising nationalism, foreshadowing the artistic-political negotiations that would occupy more and more of his career. In contrast with his earlier trips, on this visit to Japan, while Ito was still appreciated to the extent that his dancing could signify imperial capacity, on the whole he was now deemed too foreign to effectively embody the nation's agenda.

As with his earlier tour of Japan, the press eagerly covered Ito's activities; their greatest praise went to his productions of Western and "Oriental" work. This focus suggests that in Japan, Ito's merit lay in his demonstration of mastery over foreign material—to be taken as a clear sign of the success of a representative of Japan abroad. In early November 1939, he staged at the Nichigeki Theatre a version of the *Prince Igor* ballet he had choreographed for the Hollywood Bowl in 1930. His choreography followed Diaghilev's 1909 innovation by presenting just the "Polovstian Dances" section of the Borodin opera; critics noted, however, that Ito's choreography departed from that of the Ballets Russes. As a reviewer in the *Asahi Shimbun* observed, Ito's choreography was "more or less made up of Americanized novelty; in its treatment of the group dance it shows a wonderful talent, as uninhibitedly oriental rhythms joined together with the chorus, gradually and steadily becoming more frenzied in a climax of a magnificent and large-hearted group dance, whose overwhelming intensity created a terrifically deep impression."[50] The reviewer appreciated both how Ito had put an "American" stamp on the piece, making it fresh again, and how the choreography took advantage of the music's orientalism to produce a stirring climax. Similar themes were stressed in press coverage of the Ito recital organized for their parents' anniversary in December. While a critic recognized many of Ito's solo dance pieces from his concerts eight years earlier, he singled out the "oriental dance" pieces such as *Lotus Land* (danced by Teiko), *Pagoda Queen*, and *Persian Impression* for their "polished technique and grasp of precise rhythms."[51] The Ito siblings' joint effort on *At the Hawk's Well*, translated into Japanese as *Taka no ido*, was applauded. This time, Michio played the Old Man, Senda took the part of the Young Man, and Teiko danced the role of the Hawk. Yūji was in charge of costumes and music, Kisaku oversaw the set and props, and Michio directed. That the famous Yeats had used noh as inspiration for his play was already a point of pride; under Ito's direction, the play "successfully formed a harmonious fusion of poetry, music, drama, and dance, an elegant total work of art."[52] The reviewer's evaluation of the recital suggested that in bringing his successes home for production among family and friends, Ito was able to fully perfect his work, an assertion that the dancer and his dances rightfully belonged in Japan.

Ito envisioned the production of *Daibutsu Kaigen* as a similar demon-

Cosmopolitanism, Masculinity, and National Embodiment

stration of his continuing ties to his homeland. The production was hailed as marking a new phase for *shingeki* (modern Western-style drama in Japan), enabling the genre to move from small "little theaters" to a grand stage and scale. The script, by playwright Nagata Hideo, presented in five acts a massive historical drama narrating the eighth-century construction of the Great Buddha at Nara. With a cast of 250, Ito had delayed his return to America to oversee the production, enlisting, as usual, Kisaku for stage setting, Yūji for music, Teiko for dancing, and Senda to help with directing and to supply actors from his company, the New Tsukiji Theatre. Ito explained in the *Asahi Shimbun* what drew him to the script, and his vision for the production:

> When I read "Daibutsu Kaigen," it made me realize that the state of national unity that enabled the construction of the Great Buddha back then is truly a mirror image of contemporary Japan. Although I intended to return to America once I created a satisfying work in Japan, given this unique opportunity, I'm determined to do everything I can to create a work that lives up to the expectations for such a celebratory project. I intend to use gagaku, to do a new, modern-style choreography, and to organize everything through symphonic rhythms into an effective spectacle, to give the world of shingeki a new phase.[53]

Recognizing that the festival would offer the resources for the type of ambitious spectacle he enjoyed creating, Ito tied his artistic vision to an articulation of national unity, both past and present. Pairing his modern choreography with classical Japanese music, as he had done so frequently in his career, Ito asserted his dancing as a medium of cultural renewal. And through this creative intertwining, Ito also explicitly affirmed his devotion to his homeland, Japan.

Daibutsu Kaigen was presented within an arts festival, part of the year-long celebration of the founding of Japan 2,600 years earlier by the mythic emperor Jimmu. This foundational myth became, in 1940, the basis of a countrywide cultural movement, drawing participants of all ages and classes, with massive governmental support. Asserting 660 BC as the year of Japan's founding allowed the nation to claim an unbroken imperial line that predated both Chinese civilization and the Christian era; this claim became a key part of wartime ideology, as it articulated a history of national continuity, cultural purity, and civilizational priority.[54] *Daibutsu Kaigen*, which dramatized a key moment of Japan's early history, thus seemed an ideal work for this moment of performative national unity.

However, Ito's approach to the staging—a blend of old and new, Western and Japanese, though representative of his own vision of national belonging, was out of step with the prevailing cultural sentiment. While a critic writing for the *Asahi Shimbun* praised the accuracy of the period costumes and Kisaku's grand sets, and was even willing to excuse some historical inaccuracies in the narrative, he complained about the foreignness of Ito's choreography: "Regarding the directing by the dancer Ito Michio, his drama does not have as many dance elements as expected. I found a glimpse of these elements in the casting of the Buddha sequence, and in the memorial service procession, but the presentation was done in a foreign style. But since he has been educated almost entirely as a foreigner, there's no use criticizing this."[55] What Ito had grandly envisioned as an effective spectacle of "symphonic rhythms" instead struck this viewer as conspicuously foreign, and therefore, inappropriate. Ito's plan for "symphonic rhythms" indicates that he was mining his education at the Dalcroze Institute (as well as his California "dance symphonies"). It is likely that, had the reviewer perceived the dancing as recognizably German, he would not have objected so strongly. Instead, "foreign" here, means "American."[56] While Ito's choreographic Americanisms might have been fine for an obviously fantastical and foreign piece such as *Prince Igor*, such nonnative intrusions were unwelcome in a nationally symbolic event. Moreover, in the critic's final dismissal, it is clear that his disapproval is not simply of Ito's choreography, but of Ito's education and his life abroad. In the critic's view, there was no longer a need—or a place—for American cultural practices in Japan; and in dismissing the choreography, he also disavowed Ito's place in his own nation.

Senda Koreya later commented of the production's negative reception, "Indeed, this was probably the majority opinion in that time of rampant intolerant nationalism; for four cosmopolitan brothers . . . in the celebration of the '2600 Years of the Imperial Era,' to be left to their own wills was, in the end, a strange bit of chance."[57] Using katakana (an alphabet primarily used for foreign loan words) for the words "nationalism" and "cosmopolitan," Senda emphasizes semantically and typographically both the affiliation with the foreign that the brothers shared, as well as the way this attitude made them stand out. Only a few months later, in August 1940, Senda was arrested along with thirteen other *shingeki* practitioners for communist sympathies.

Ito, however, continued to espouse principles of international cooperation through cultural exchange. Right before leaving Tokyo, he made plans to open a dance school in Nagoya, with the intention that his students there and at his Hollywood studio would spend part of their time in exchange at

Cosmopolitanism, Masculinity, and National Embodiment   183

the other location.[58] He also continued to style himself as a force for political diplomacy: when he left Japan, he brought with him two white peacocks that he intended to present to Mrs. Roosevelt.[59] (It is not clear whether this was his own initiative or part of a broader diplomatic strategy on Japan's part; one also can't help but wonder whether Ito shared his ship cabin with the birds.) Ito also came back to California with substantial sums of money; neighbors (and the FBI) noticed that Ito went from being an always-in-debt dance teacher to living quite luxuriously, with a flashy car, servants, and new bank accounts. As I will discuss in more detail in the next chapter, it seems apparent that at least some officials in Japan, like many of the critics in this chapter, saw Ito as not only a dancer, but as an individual who carried political possibilities. Not just the significations of his body, but his habit of moving across the globe, and his own eagerness to be at the center of things, made him someone who could act (or could be used?) as an agent of history.

Coda: Japan, 1940–1941

As I have traced in this chapter, in Japan in 1931, in Mexico in 1934, and again in Japan in 1939–40, Ito became a potent figure for other people's fantasies, as spectators, critics, and even his own family members saw in him a personification of their own and others' desires for how a body appears to signify nation and race. As a counterpart to his activities in California, these trips help to round out a sense of how he continued to perform himself as a cultural mediator during the 1930s. What becomes evident across these sites of reception is that Ito's persona as a cosmopolitan Japanese, and his increasing involvement with the Japanese community in California were not just a result of his own engagement with them. Rather, Japanese commentators in Japan, Mexico, and of course California increasingly identified Ito as someone who was not just useful for their local purposes, but as someone who could be made to figure something more ambiguous, and more capacious, about Japan itself, as a nation and as an empire.

It turns out, Ito took one more trip to Japan, from September 1940 to February 1941. But unlike on his previous trips, neither the Japanese nor the American/Japanese American press covered any part of this visit, other than his arrivals in Japan, and then back to the US on his return. This trip is also, disconcertingly, not mentioned in Fujita Fujio's otherwise comprehensive biography. All I have been able to find are the FBI's conjectures about Ito's activities: according to the findings listed in the documentation of Ito's trial before the Enemy Alien Hearing Board, on this trip, Ito brought with him "certain documents which he had received in Washington . . . for the purpose of delivering the same to the Japanese Minister of Economics."[60]

This is another kind of reception and constitutes yet one more fantasy of Ito. As always, "fantasy" here does not indicate the "truth" or "falsity" of this information; rather, it points to the desires that fuel this way of seeing Ito. To the FBI and the Internment hearing board, such pieces of information adhered to an already-rabid desire to imagine Japanese and Japanese Americans as fundamentally untrustworthy to the US, because they could not be other than innately, unmovably loyal to Japan. As in his previous trips, Ito's body and biography become sites for national and racial attachments—both those that the FBI imagined of Ito, as well as, implicitly, these bureaucrats' own visions of what being "American" must look like.

To understand the FBI's report about Ito's trip as fantasy is also to foreground the deeply consequential, material results that fantasies can produce. Far from being disconnected reveries, fantasies such as the FBI's intersected with Ito's own fantasies—of being a cultural mediator, of being at the center of things—and yielded all too real effects. The night following the Japanese bombing of Pearl Harbor, the FBI raided Ito's Los Angeles home and arrested him as an enemy of the state. He spent the next two years in a series of Department of Justice Camps, ripped from his family and the modern dance and Japanese immigrant communities in which he had thrived. But living with other political internees and forming a new sense of community, the turn to Japan that was hinted at during his career in the 1930s became a robust commitment to Asia, as Ito sought to make sense of his internment and ruptured cosmopolitanism.

CHAPTER SIX

Pan-Asianism between Internment and Propaganda

The Asia-Pacific War, 1941–1945

In his 1946 book *America and Japan*, Ito devotes a chapter to his plan for an international cultural institute he called the Theatre of the Sun. The kernel of the idea, he writes, emerged in the summer of 1921 when he participated in an artists' colony held at the estate of the sculptor Gutzon Borglum in Connecticut. With sixteen of his students gathered in residence, everyone did as they pleased, engaging in whatever artistic activities they desired. The one rule of the colony was that they were to avoid contact with the outside world, so that they would be free to pursue their art and enjoy the simplicity of nature. Ito writes:

> However, there was one exception. This was the Japanese man employed as a cook. Every day he had to go to the town to buy groceries. And so he alone had contact with worldly affairs. One day, I had gone into the kitchen, where the cook was reading a newspaper. When I saw this, I could no longer simply pass by, letting him be. As I was so close, the cook, with a hint of surprise, quickly hid the newspaper. "In truth," he began to explain to me, "when I was in town buying meat, someone wrapped it with this newspaper. Certainly I never would have bought it." I smiled and said, "It's fine, I don't care how many newspapers you read. Incidentally, how about letting me read it a bit?"[1]

The newspaper contained news of the naval disarmament conference that President Harding was then in the process of convening, and Ito read the paper with great interest. That evening around a campfire with the other students, Ito revealed his own transgression, and relayed the political news. From then on, the isolation of the colony was shattered; every night they all gathered to debate the possible terms of peace, each in turn eagerly offering plans for how they would enact a meaningful and lasting peace.

From these discussions, Ito hatched his own plan, which he later called "the Theatre of the Sun": the major nations involved in the peace talks would each donate the cost of one battleship, and this fund would support an international dance school that Ito analogized to the Red Cross—able to enter any country, it would bring together youth from across the globe in the harmonious study of dance. This international engagement with art would foster cooperation and understanding, and with the youth of every nation involved, both the impetus and manpower required for war would disappear. Borglum encouraged Ito to go to Washington with his plan, and, according to the narrative, so he did. He met first with the Japanese ambassador, Shidehara Kijūrō, who, explaining that Japan was present at the disarmament conference simply as an observer, asked Ito not to interfere. Undissuaded, Ito then met with Harding himself. Harding, Ito writes, was kind and admired the plan, but characterized it as a plan "for the future," whereas the conference was an effort to deal with the past. With Harding's rejection, Ito decided to change his approach: "After returning from the White House, as I thought about it, and the sort of things I had said, I decided, why not ask a fellow Asian, who might better be able to understand. And so I went to the Ambassador of China."[2] In Ito's account, the Chinese ambassador was indeed supportive, and helped Ito to organize an art exhibition of work by artists from Japan, India, and China, which the ambassadors of China, England, and Spain attended. It was from this experience, Ito writes, that he decided "it would be my life's work to promote peace through the stage."[3]

It is hard to know how much of this story is invented. The art exhibition he references is surely part of the "Oriental Evenings" he organized in Washington, DC, in February 1922. Fujita Fujio suggests that Ito simply sent a letter.[4] The story about his audience with President Harding is referenced in a 1928 *New York Tribune* article[5]—so whatever happened, Ito began to share it quite early. Perhaps, then, this is one of those events that seems impossible but, like so much of Ito's life, really did take place. As with Ito's other fantasies, what is important here is the expansive vision of choreographic cosmopolitanism that he advocates, and his unshakable and sincere belief in dance as a means of changing the world. What we also see in this story, from the encounter with the Japanese cook to the positive reception of his project by the Chinese ambassador, is Ito's turn to Asia, not just as a source of "oriental

Pan-Asianism between Internment and Propaganda   187

dance" material, but as a site of political allegiance. In the version of the story that Ito penned in 1946, he was also asserting that his vision for the Theatre of the Sun, and his belief in a cooperative Asia, long predated the war, and so could be recuperated for the postwar period. But, as we will see, despite its purported aims of world peace, Ito adapted his Theatre of the Sun scheme quite effectively for the war. We can recognize in this versatility the persistent continuities of Ito's adherence to a notion of Japanese cosmopolitanism, even during his experiences of violent rupture and dislocation caused by the war.

In the earliest hours of December 8, 1941, in the aftermath of the bombing of Pearl Harbor, the FBI raided Ito's Los Angeles home and arrested him as an "enemy alien." He spent the next two years in four Department of Justice Camps. Kevin Riordan has offered an evocative reading of Ito's internment "trial," arguing that his profession as a dancer and international artist were read as the ultimate evidence of his untrustworthiness as a dangerous foreigner.[6] Indeed, during his internment trial, Ito's defense of his activities was characteristic: he explained that he was working toward peace among "the world brotherhood of men." The naivete of such a statement makes it easy to dismiss, but I think we should take Ito at his word. The very meetings with Japanese army officials, which would have looked so suspicious to the FBI, are evidence of Ito's total investment in his own fantasy of world peace through art-making—a fantasy that sustained him throughout the war, even as he endured internment, repatriation, and the final years of Japan's total war mobilization.

After Ito repatriated to Japan in 1943, he spent the final eighteen months of the war trying to construct a new life for himself, even as conditions grew increasingly dire. With the help of family connections, Ito founded the Greater East Asia Stage Arts Research Institute, an organization that aimed to produce performances across the "Co-Prosperity Sphere." However, with the exception of one production, none of these plans came to fruition. The Greater East Asia Stage Arts Research Institute is thus a performance endeavor that exists only on paper, in the form of thirteen documents held at Waseda University's Theatre Museum. Similarly, what remains of Ito's experience in US internment camps are two notebooks that he filled during that period, and some letters he sent to his wife, Tsuyako. These archival remains are the parallel traces of the US incarceration of Japanese and Japanese Americans, and of Japan's imperialism in Asia.[7]

The internment notebooks and institute documents seem to clearly belong to two different aspects of the Pacific War, which have been held apart due to the distinct disciplinary formations of Asian American studies and Asian studies. Indeed, this division has shaped some of the most important English-language scholarship on Ito. On the one hand, Yutian Wong, a dance scholar who has been central to establishing the field of Asian American dance studies, has argued that Ito, precisely because of his incarceration, expulsion, and exclusion from the US and from the American modern dance canon, is a necessary starting point for Asian American modern dance history.[8] On the other hand, Carol Sorgenfrei, a scholar of twentieth-century Japanese theater, has argued that in response to the failures of interculturalism, Ito turned toward the growing Japanese fascism, to embrace what she calls "Japancentrism," an ideology that asserts the uniqueness and superiority of Japan, in order to position it as the universal representative for all of Asia.[9] I think both of these essays are fundamentally correct in their treatment of Ito. But, after spending years scrutinizing Ito's notebooks, I don't think we can make so clear a division between Ito's experience of internment and his participation in Japan's imperial project.

The internment notebooks at Waseda University's Theatre Museum have been assigned the catalog numbers J21 and J22, and in the finding aid, they are both tagged as "Camp Livingston"—the third of the camps in which Ito was interned. But the content of these notebooks is not easily categorized: some portion of their pages were almost assuredly written after Ito's repatriation. This mixed-up-ness is more than a vagary of the archive. It means that we cannot separate the two parts of Ito's wartime experience—his incarceration by the US government on account of his race, and his participation in Japan's imperial project of Asian dominion. Ito's wartime experience, then, is where Asian American and Asian studies converge and must intertwine, a meeting that is part of the emergent field of Global Asias. The unknowability of these documents and the provisional status of their contents also produce opportunities: in drawing together usually distinct disciplinary formations, and in reading across these two halves of Japanese experience of the Pacific War, we are able to glimpse aspects of Ito's career that exist only in the realm of fantasy. If throughout this book, I have insisted on taking Ito's fabricated stories seriously, here I will propose that an unrealized festival pageant proposal counts as a crucial part of Ito's career, meriting methodological acts of imaginative reconstruction, to conjure performances that never were.

Internment[10]

In the days immediately following the bombing of Pearl Harbor, more than 7,000 Issei leaders in the Japanese community in California and Hawaii were rounded up by the FBI. The capture of these (primarily male) individuals had been planned as early as 1935 to provide hostages in case of war with Japan, and by spring of 1941 precise lists had been drawn up by the FBI and Department of Justice.[11] Suspected of espionage and accused of being incapable of loyalty to the US due to their race, these Issei were detained without warning, ripped from their families and communities for the duration of the war.[12]

The FBI and US Justice Department had been investigating Ito since at least the spring of 1940. In September 1939, Ito had gone to Japan to celebrate his parents' golden wedding anniversary, and he stayed all through the fall, winter, and spring, returning to the US in June of 1940. Ito left the US again at the end of August 1940—a quick turnaround that certainly might have been explained by his teaching schedule at his Hollywood studio, but that evidently raised the FBI's suspicions. Meanwhile, Hazel Wright was also looking for Ito. As she explained in a letter to the Secretary of Labor, Ito was hundreds of dollars behind in his court-ordered $15 a week child-support payments.[13]

Whether in response to Wright's queries or for some other reason, on September 7, 1940, Lemuel B. Schofield, the special assistant to the attorney general, sent an order to the Los Angeles branch of the Immigration and Naturalization Service (INS) to withhold Ito's reentry permit until contacted by an FBI agent.[14] Nevertheless, when Ito returned from Japan on February 8, 1941, he successfully reentered the US, at which point he was issued an Alien Registration Card, in accordance with the newly passed Alien Registration Act, which required all noncitizens to register and be fingerprinted, and made it a criminal act to contribute to the overthrow of the US government.

The FBI waited, building a file on Ito that would condemn him as "extremely dangerous to the security of the United States."[15] The FBI's case, presented at Ito's internment trial on February 13, 1942, hung upon his apparent activities and associates, all of which, so they argued, pointed to him being an unregistered "foreign agent." He was accused of spreading propaganda, possible espionage, and working on behalf of a foreign government without clearance. On his return from Japan in 1940, the FBI noted that an informant, who had purportedly obtained information from Ito's son Jerry, reported dramatic changes in Ito's financial situation: prior to his 1939–40 trip, he was often in debt, with one frequently overdrawn bank account that never held more than $200. However, after June 1940, he offered $18,000 in cash to purchase the house he had been renting at 7268 Franklin Street; meanwhile he used another property, 1753 Highland Avenue, Hollywood, as his business address; he "entertained lavishly" and employed several servants. The file asserts that on July 22, he had opened a new account at Bank of America with an initial $1,000 deposit, but also had a "large roll of bills with him and . . . these bills were probably placed in Ito's safe deposit box inasmuch as he used only one of the bills to open the account." The report notes that Ito "has displayed considerable wealth since his return, [and] has not engaged in his pretended business of operating a dance studio."

At the center of the case was Ito's role in the organization of the Pan Pacific Trading and Navigation Company—a company founded with the goal of serving as the sole trading partner between Japan and the US for mineral ore and gasoline. Its listed officers were three men named John F. Dolan, Manuel G. Brassell, and Anthony M. Langren, who together capitalized the company in Nevada, in the spring or summer of 1941, for $300,000,000—an extraordinary sum of money. (In today's dollars, it would be around $6.24 billion.) It appears that half of this sum was to come from Japan and the other half from the US, with Harry Chandler, the *Los Angeles Times* publisher and real estate magnate, being a primary investor. Whatever Ito's role in this company was, it appears that he hired a white US citizen to assist in obtaining the company's contracts and governmental clearances, and to more generally promote pro-Japanese sentiment in the US. This man, Frank Y. McLaughlin, had been the head of the California WPA in the 1930s, and it was perhaps through Ito's own involvement in WPA projects that he had first met McLaughlin. Ito reportedly agreed to pay him $5,000 a month. When Ito was arrested, a copy of a set of letters between him and McLaughlin was found, in which McLaughlin offered to "act as an agent of the Japanese Empire." In Ito's response, he asserted that he was not "an agent or representative of the Japanese government" and did not expect McLaughlin to be able to become one "until that government reaches the conclusion based on your efforts, which we both believe will be successful, that you should be so engaged."

At the time of his arrest, the FBI reported that Ito had a list of the names and US addresses of several high-ranking military Japanese, who were perhaps involved in or being solicited for this endeavor: General Isoda, the military attaché of Japan; Colonel Endo, a Japanese army inspector; and Colonel T. Nishi, the Japanese military attaché to Mexico. In his trial, Ito confirmed that he had been given this list while he was in Japan, and had met with at least one of them to try to improve the relationship between Japan and the US. He also had in his possession copies of several telegrams: one sent by Ito in July 1940 to an official at the Nippon Keizai Renmei (the Japan Financial Federation); a set of three telegrams sent by Harry Chandler of the *Los Angeles Times* to various officials and businessmen in Japan; and a copy of a letter from Paul Dietrich, a Bank of America vice president, to E. G. Kojima, care of Chandler, confirming that he had made an introduction for Kojima to J. L. Curtis, of the National City Bank in Tokyo. This paper trail appeared to match a series of calls and visits that the FBI tracked: in August 1940, prior to his departure for Japan, Ito made several calls to E. Gitaro Kojima, who seems to have been working for the Pan Pacific Trading Company initiative, and was in close contact with Harry Chandler; Kojima was already also being investigated by the FBI. After Ito returned to the US, the FBI's informant recorded that Ito made calls in March of 1941. One was to Sakomizu Hisatsune, a leading official in the Japanese Ministry of Finance;[16] another was to Kubo Hisaji, a leader in the Japanese film industry who had apparently already been deported from the US in 1934 for attempting to bribe an immigration inspector, but who was also in 1938 the chief negotiator with Hollywood studios, allowing for limited film imports to Japan after a total ban in 1937.[17] When Ito visited Washington, DC, in May 1941, he placed more calls: to the Japanese Embassy, the military attaché, and to Kojima. The paper trail and call log appeared to correlate to the movement of money. Within Ito's file are several mentions of him transferring money from his Bank of America account to various Japanese individuals who may also have been associated with the Pan Pacific Trading and Navigation Company. While there was obviously a great deal of money involved in this venture, Ito's claim that his involvement was motivated by a desire to "cement friendly relations between this country and Japan" is not unconnected. Some of the principal agents and investors in the company, at least on Japan's side, were enthusiastic about it precisely because they were invested in maintaining US neutrality vis-à-vis Japan's war with China, and hoped that fostering strong economic ties between Japan and the US would effectively guarantee that the US would mind its own business.[18]

Whatever Ito's ties to this trading company may have been, he appeared to have damning associations with certain Japanese military figures. While the FBI noted that his brother-in-law had been a general in the Japanese army until his death a year earlier, the real concern was Ito's relationship with Tanaka Gunkichi, a major in the imperial army who had been imprisoned for a year in Japan for his role in an attempted coup d'état in February 1936. Tanaka had been identified as a member of the Black Dragon Society, a paramilitary, ultranationalist group that was primarily focused on preventing the expansion of the Russian Empire, but that was active in several countries, including the US, where it promoted Pan-Asianism. In January 1941, Tanaka came to the US, with letters of introduction to major film studios, for the purpose of purchasing 20,000 cameras and projectors for the Japanese government. At this time, Ito was in Japan. But when Tanaka visited, the FBI reported that he stayed at 7268 Franklin Street—Ito's house.

Even as the FBI collected information, the turf war with the INS seems to have continued. On November 18, 1941, Lawrence M. C. Smith, chief of the Justice Department's Special Defense Unit, requested from the INS a copy of Ito's alien registration form and additional information about the terms of his repeated entries to the United States. Smith noted that Ito was behind on his child-support payments, and his request included this note: "We should appreciate it if you would advise us as to any possibilities of deportation or other action under the alien laws, should it seem desirable after a consideration of all aspects of the case."[19] But the INS took their time, and in an internal memorandum, one official confirmed with another that the INS did not share their files with other agencies, and so would not provide the Justice Department with the requested documents.[20] Accordingly, on December 4, the INS sent a return letter stating that they had no extra information to share, but that all of Ito's entries to the US had been lawfully made, under the terms of his original 1916 immigration. They wrote, "This office has no extra copies of the subject's Alien Registration Form. . . . However, if you wish, this office will lend you its copy."[21]

The growing FBI and INS files on Ito secured his detention in the first round of arrests after the bombing of Pearl Harbor. He was taken from his Hollywood home to a local Hollywood prison, and the next day moved to the Federal Correctional Institution on Terminal Island, in the waters south of Los Angeles. On December 19, he was moved to Fort Missoula, Montana. There he, like the other Issei men in this group, was tried before an "Enemy Alien Hearing Board," and on February 26, 1942, he was ordered interned. After four months, Ito was moved to Fort Sill, Oklahoma, and then in the fall of 1942, he was moved to Camp Livingston, Louisiana. Finally, after being granted repatriation, Ito was transferred to the Santa Fe, New Mexico, facility on June 7, 1943, where he was reunited with his wife, Tsuyako, who had been incarcerated at the Heart Mountain Relocation Center in Wyoming.

On September 2, 1943, they boarded the M.S. *Gripsholm* in New York, and then on October 19, transferred to the *Teia Maru* in Goa as part of a prisoner exchange. Finally, on November 14, 1943, they landed at Yokohama.

As I elaborate below, Ito's wartime notebooks contain only a few, brief references to his experience in the camps. We must rely on recollections provided by others who were interned to piece together a sense of what the experience might have been like. For instance, we might look to the interviews conducted by Paul J. Clark, especially one with the Reverend Seytsu Takahashi, whose own path through the internment camps closely matched Ito's.[22] Takahashi's account reveals the sheer terror and grim resignation felt by the Issei. At several moments, especially moving from one camp to another, they were convinced that they were all going to be killed, and indeed, had to watch as on a few occasions their compatriots were either shot or committed suicide. Similarly, Carol Bulger Van Valkenburg has documented the serious physical and verbal abuse internees experienced at Fort Missoula, especially during the loyalty hearings.[23] This pervasive terror was accompanied by the inescapable boredom of prison life. Between these emotional states, the men organized themselves into self-governed units and developed friendships that sustained them during what many feared might be permanent imprisonment.

Ito's notebooks from his period of internment contain a wide-ranging, almost motley assortment of reflections, transcribed passages from other texts, and philosophical compositions. There is page after page of notes on the human anatomical system, passages on human anthropology, and transcribed theories on the development of man and human civilization. There is a long section wherein Ito imagines his own birth and his coming into consciousness, and then he recounts memories from his childhood in Tokyo. Ito writes long compositions on the origins of dance; he writes of Dalcroze and rhythm, and of dance across cultures. At a few points in the J21 notebook, he goes back through his previous notes and rewrites them all, editing the language and making a clean copy.

The notebooks contain few concrete references to the camps. This silence is itself reflective of Ito's experience, and the state of suspended, anxious terror under which internees spent the war. For while the internment camps were, technically, prisoner of war camps, and therefore subject to the terms of the Geneva Convention, the threat that prison guards might confiscate an internee's possessions and read anything he had written was all too real. Unlike most of Ito's writings, which were explicitly written for an immediate readership, in the internment notebooks Ito writes under the threat of an unintended audience, with potentially deadly repercussions.[24] These notebooks thus offer a performance of self-censorship—a precise modulation that is all the more interesting given the ways that the political situation does appear in these documents.

Within the notebooks, there are three scattered references to life in the camps. On one page, Ito references telling a story to the other men in the barracks that made everyone laugh.[25] Another set of pages records haiku written by his fellow internees. On another page, Ito jotted down the words to a song the men had composed, in the form of a *yosahoi bushi*, a parodic counting song that uses alliterative wordplay to make jokes, usually about sex[26]:

一ツ出タワイナヨサホイノホイ

One out *yosahoi no hoi*

人里離れたミゾラにて　ホイ　男ばかりの侘住い　ホイホイ

In middle-of-nowhere Missoula *hoi* nothing but men in this wretched place
hoi hoi

二ツ出タワイナヨサホイノホイ

Two out *yosahoi no hoi*

深き御縁に連れられて　ホイ　打しも打されぬ方ばかり　ホイホイ

Taken suddenly away *hoi* surrounded by superb and well-known fellows *hoi
hoi*

三ツ出タワイナ・・・・・

Three out *yosahoi no hoi*

みえやていさいぬきにして　ホイ　男同志の磨き合い　ホイホイ

Dispensing with pretensions and appearances *hoi* just rectification among
men *hoi hoi*

四ツ・・・・・
　世の成り行きをよそにして　ホイ　長期修養面白や　ホイホイ

Indifferent to the course of world events *hoi* interested only in long-term
　self-improvement[27] *hoi hoi*

五ツ・・・・・
　何時も心を朗かに　ホイ　体大事に●致しましょう　ホイホイ

Always keeping our hearts cheerful *hoi* well, let's take care of our bodies *hoi
　hoi*

六ツ・・・・・
　無理を成さるなお年寄　ホイ　芝居の大諸見にやならん　ホイホイ

Older men, don't strain yourselves *hoi* you've got to see the entire play *hoi
　hoi*

七ツ・・・・・
　泣いても笑うても御同様　ホイ　戦すむまで居るやならん　ホイホイ

Whether we cry or whether we laugh, it's all the same *hoi* We've got to stay
　here until the war ends *hoi hoi*

八ツ・・・・・
　やけを起すな若い方　ホイ　今の苦難が身の薬り　ホイホイ

Young men, don't get desperate *hoi* now suffering is our (body's) medicine
　hoi hoi

九ツ・・・・・
　子供女房もまめな様に　ホイ　神や佛に念じましょう　ホイホイ

Like our devoted wife and kids *hoi* well let's pray to god and Buddha *hoi hoi*

十ツト・・・・・
　とうとう許しの出る迄は　ホイ　皆な仲好く暮しましょう。　ホイホイ

> Until finally we are pardoned *hoi* let's all just get along happily together *hoi hoi*

The standard *yosahoi bushi*'s (heterosexual) sexual intimations are parodied here in the relationships formed under the circumstances of this homosocial isolation, where the men can only be rivals for each others' affections. These men are the leaders of the Japanese community (the "superb and well-known fellows"), and so, rather than the expected sexual satisfaction, they provide "self-improvement"—a substitution that surely parodies the notion of American reeducation that the camps espoused, even as it probably describes the various activities with which the men passed their days. If, as other pages in the notebooks suggest, Ito also spent time in the camps thinking about his early education at the Jaques-Dalcroze Institute for Eurythmics, then this song, too, offers a kind of rhythmicization of institutional life. But rather than the carefully attuned and technically precise rhythmic expression of the Eurythmic dancer, here, the song marks the mundane synchronicity of a group waiting together. Against this stultifying waiting, the *hoi hoi* bursts in again and again, requiring the singer to contract his stomach muscles in a pulse of expelled air, a reminder of his fundamental corporeality.[28] The singer offers the perspective of older men (Ito and his peers), who watch the "desperate" younger men but take a more philosophical approach. For them the goal is to survive, to "see the play's many parts," and to find some odd kind of comfort in each other as they await a pardon from capricious fate and the US government.

The notebook offers brief glimpses of Ito's life—the grim humor, resigned camaraderie, and small diversions that punctuated his experience of the camps' isolation and brutal disruption of his previous life. By contrast, far more of the notebooks' pages reference the global situation and Japan's imperial project. Three pages in J21 explain why in 1939 the United States abandoned the Japan-US trade treaty that had been in effect since 1911. Ito first attributes the renunciation to pressure from Great Britain, which was "becoming more and more uneasy about its rights in the Orient."[29] He insists that after the Manchurian Incident, as the "Chinese government raised cries of help to the US," anti-Japanese propaganda finally turned American public opinion, which soon came to "emotionally regard Japan as an aggressor."[30] Ito closes this passage by observing that because of America's interceding in British-Chinese issues, there is now no issue on which America and Japan can find agreement.[31] There are also pages dedicated to a sort of pedagogical

Pan-Asianism between Internment and Propaganda 197

lesson about the origins and purpose of imperial Japan, with subtitles such as "The Creation and Development of the Imperial Bloodline"[32] and "The Ideals of Imperial Japan and World Peace."[33] These lessons unfold in a question-and-answer format—a format Ito frequently used in his postwar books as well, with the questioner characterized as a wholly ignorant but eager-to-learn outsider. There is discussion of Emperor Jimmu, of the founding myth of Japan and its supposed 2,600 years of continuous imperial rule. There is instruction about the meaning of *hakkou ichiu* ("the eight corners of the world unified under one roof") and the *sanshu no jingi* ("Three Sacred Treasures"). The lesson asserts that since its founding, Japan has been a nation committed to peace and justice, and its fundamental mission is to spread peace through the world. These pages are surely part of the story of Ito's turn to Asianism, but it is hard to pin down precisely where he stands in relation to this content. Ito seems to identify with the Questioner role in the dialogue, as if he is working at mastering the catechism of Japanese imperial ideology. But there is no external commentary, no breath of his own reactions to the material.

In these notebooks, then, lie the crux and stumbling block of Ito's position both as someone subjected to the racialized violence of US internment *and* as someone who signed onto Japan's imperial project. The primary issue is: what can we take these notebooks to *mean*? This is where the cataloging of Ito's notebooks begins to matter. It is tempting to place a sort of interpretive dividing line between the notebooks labeled "Camp Livingston" and the documents labeled "Greater East Asia Stage Arts Research Institute." That is, it is tempting to treat Ito's experience of internment separately from his collaboration with Japan's imperial government, a distinction that would then neatly slot each event into its expected disciplinary framework. But the notebooks are not so easily categorized. And the confusion they produce productively entangles the disciplines of Asian American studies and Asian studies, and the histories that seem to distinctively belong to each field.

With some confidence, I think that the first half or two-thirds of J21 are pages Ito wrote while interned. Within these pages are the three concrete references to the camps, as well as the long discussions of imperial ideology and Ito's explanation for US abandonment of the Japan-US trade treaty. With perhaps a bit less certainty, I also think that J22 was probably *not* written in the DOJ camps, but rather, was a notebook Ito filled once he had repatriated to Japan. In part, this conclusion rests on the kind of material transcribed in each notebook. J21 contains many pages on which Ito has laboriously transcribed long sections from the writings of the Japanese New Thought leader,

Masaharu Taniguchi. It seems plausible that someone had brought these materials into the camps. J22, by contrast, begins with two pages of transcription from Taki Ryōichi's 1937 article "On Dance in the Orient" (Tōyō ni okeru būyō ni tsuite).[34] Later, Ito has transcribed a few pages from volume I of a Japanese translation of the Danish actor Karl Mantzius's *History of Theatrical Art*, which was first published in Japan in 1930. There is also a passage, in English, from Edward Gordon Craig's 1908 "The Artists of the Theatre of the Future." While it is always possible that these theatrical texts made their way into the internment camps, they seem more likely to be texts he could only have accessed back in Japan. More directly tying J22 to Ito's being back in Japan is a very early draft of his plans for the Greater East Asia Stage Arts Research Institute, in the form of a list of potential teachers/researchers, a few of whose names ultimately can be found in the planning documents he submitted to the Greater East Asia Ministry. That said, even J21 bears marks of being a notebook Ito used on returning to Japan, and even after the war: it contains a long transcribed article from the *Asahi Shimbun* in August 1953 discussing the hydrogen bomb.

The notebooks' mixed-up-ness might be the result of historical conditions (paper scarcity both in the camps and in wartime and postwar Japan) or personal idiosyncrasy (did Ito turn to an open page at random, and then use the remaining empty pages as he found them?). The result of their indeterminacy is that his internment experience cannot be divided from his collaboration with Japan's imperial project. During the war, the US government insisted that each internee's status be measured by the question of "loyalty"— whether they would fully pledge their allegiance to the US and whether they were willing to renounce any loyalty they might have had to Japan. The question of loyalty is still frequently used as a shorthand to emphasize the innocence of incarcerated Japanese, or conversely, to describe figures such as Ito as those whose "loyalties shifted." But loyalty seems an insufficient concept for understanding the entanglement of texts and ideas found in Ito's notebooks. Rather, the notebooks are a scattered record of ideas with which Ito attempted to make sense of his experience, and to construct an understanding of political events that he could reconcile with his long-standing beliefs in cosmopolitanism, in the notion of universalism, and in the power of art to effect these utopic states.

What emerges in Ito's notebooks is also some part of the process by which he found a way into Japan's imperial project, and elaborated a role for himself within its expansive vision. As we will see, under the call of "peace

Pan-Asianism between Internment and Propaganda   199

and understanding," Ito could join Japan's political program with the sense that it offered the best opportunity for him to continue his danced practice of embodied cosmopolitanism. From within the guarded perimeters of US Department of Justice camps, Japan may well have seemed like the natural successor to the ideals of danced cosmopolitanism that the US had so suddenly and painfully rejected.

Japan in the Final Years of the War

In November 1943, when Ito landed in Yokohama, he returned to a drastically changed country—one operating under a new ideological apparatus, as well as administering a massive geographic expanse. Japan's "New Order in Asia" emerged out of its increasing use of Pan-Asianism as a justifying and mobilizing ideology for its imperialism. Early in the twentieth century, Pan-Asianism had several different strains and various supporters from countries across Asia.[35] There had even been a period when Pan-Asianism truly seemed like a viable movement by which Asian nations could together resist Western hegemony and colonization. For instance, following Japan's 1905 victory against Russia, Jawaharlal Nehru commented, "For little Japan to defeat one of the greatest and most powerful of European Powers surprised most people; in Asia the surprise was a most pleasant one. Japan was looked upon as the representative of Asia battling against western aggression and, for the moment, became very popular all over the East."[36] By the late 1930s, however, the strong currents of an inter-Asian Pan-Asianism had faded, and the 1930s saw the ascent of Japan's use of Pan-Asianism to justify its imperial project. From the 1931 Manchurian Incident and subsequent occupation of Manchuria and foundation of Manchukuo in 1932, to Japan's 1933 withdrawal from the League of Nations, to the Konoe government's 1938 declaration of a "New Order" in East Asia, and the promulgation of the "Greater East Asia Co-Prosperity Sphere" in 1940, Japan adapted Pan-Asianist ideology to proclaim the need for Japanese leadership over the rest of Asia, in the name of inter-Asian community and as a challenge to Euro-American imperialism.[37] Even as Japan carried out its brutal Asian conquest, Pan-Asianism continued to serve as a compelling ideology, recruiting and motivating individuals to offer their talents to the imperial project. Writing of the economic development of Manchukuo, historian Louise Young observes, "Because such imperial projects were multidimensional, the mobilization of support among their divergent interests required an inclusive vision that promised something for everyone."[38] Pan-Asianism was one of several mobilizing visions (or fantasies) that allowed the Japanese to align themselves with the vast project of imperial occupation, administration, and war-making.

This capacious ideological construct was needed to justify imperial Japan's vast territorial expansion. Although Japan's empire-building had been underway with the acquisition of Taiwan, Korea, and Manchuria before Ito first left for Europe in 1912, at the peak of its territorial control in 1942, the Japanese Empire covered much of East and Southeast Asia.[39] The vast territorial expanse of this conquest only begins to hint at the brutality and oppression carried out in the name of "co-prosperity." Such well-known episodes as the 1937 Nanjing Massacre, in which Japanese soldiers raped as many as 80,000 people and killed as many as 300,000 over a period of six weeks; the 1942 Bataan Death March, in which as many as 80,000 Filipino and American prisoners of war were forced to march until they died; the "comfort woman" system of sexual slavery involving an estimated 200,000 girls and women; and the lethal human experimentation carried out by Unit 731 in China throughout the war, are only some of the most spectacular and briefly summarized instances of the Japanese Empire's extraordinary violence. This brutality was carried out alongside ongoing campaigns of cultural erasure and coercion—from the forced assimilation of Koreans that demanded the widespread adoption of the Japanese language, to forced Shinto worship and courses in "moral education" for all schoolchildren in Micronesia.[40]

By the time of Ito's return, the early wave of victories had turned, and Japan was desperately attempting to defend its vast territory and to administer governmental control of these regions—an effort for which it was unprepared. Ito was welcomed back to Japan and given preferential treatment, but his long absence insulated him from the desperate confidence that supported many Japanese in the final years of the war. Ishii Baku recalled that on his return, Ito declared to him that the United States would win the war.[41] Ito wrote as well, in a new notebook, "With their overwhelming material resources, the American and British enemy will either obliterate our empire or demand unconditional surrender."[42]

This third notebook offers us one more view into Ito's experience of the war. It is smaller, a composition-style notebook, cataloged under the call number J30. Its first page is titled "Greater East Asia Stage Arts Research Institute Dance Laboratory." It is dated the first day of Showa 20—January 1, 1945—New Year's Day. The page contains a list of participants, including

Pan-Asianism between Internment and Propaganda

their given and stage names, their birthdays, addresses, and phone numbers, and then, at the bottom, notes for a rehearsal scheduled for January 29. This notebook, then, is clearly from the final year of the war. Whereas the "Camp Livingston" notebooks contain only a few concrete references to Ito's immediate situation, in this notebook, nearly all of its pages contain content that explicitly references not only the war, but Japan's imperial agenda and the role of art in supporting this vision.

In rest of this chapter, I turn to this notebook and the series of planning documents for the Greater East Asia Stage Arts Research Institute to consider how we understand Ito's contribution to imperial Japan's war effort. If Ito's "Camp Livingston" notebooks—whether or not they actually date to his period of internment—have the status of meditative, diary-type writings, the materials considered in this section can be primarily understood as blueprints—planning documents related to theatrical production. But, as I will detail, it is not clear that any of these performances ever occurred, or, in fact, that Ito even truly thought they would. These, then, are performance fantasies, scripted as much toward irreality as toward material realization.

This J30 notebook includes perhaps the most detailed choreographic notation to be found among Ito's papers. The drawings for this unnamed dance call for around twenty dancers, and denote general movement patterns across the stage that would be accompanied by lyrics, which either the dancers or an unidentified chorus would sing. The curtain opens on three steel-factory workers who throughout the piece are each respectively associated with a chant to "polish!" "cut!" "strike!" Their movements corresponding to these calls, related to the production of steel, signify the war effort at large. Enlisting the productive power of "the arms and legs" of the factory laborers, the three dancers are joined by their fellow workers with the repeated affirmations that "we too, we too produce" and "we too, we too fight," the lyrics suggesting movements in unison. "Production" and "assault" are tied together as the lyrics in the first section describing the "hot winds" of the scorching steel factory furnace soon call up the divine winds of the *kamikaze*. Referencing the popular image of "human bullets flying along,"[43] two opposing groups of ten dancers each move toward each other from stage left and right, then all as one group take a step upstage, as the "ten thousand go to the factories for war." The women together take a step upstage as they call out "Certain Death," to which the male dancers, with their own step upstage, respond, "Certain Kill." Then all together the group progresses downstage as they "join the battle in the factory." The dance ends as the lines of dancers, the "human bullets, ramming our bodies," step downstage and then toward the center, chanting "we men too, we women too, we men too, we women too."

As the three workers of the beginning of the dance merge into the anonymous group of workers, Ito's choreography enacts the primary function of war mobilization. Individuality is submerged into the group, as the war effort equalizes even gender—both men and women march into the factory, dedicating their bodies as so many human bullets. Uncomplicated group formations, and movement that is often restricted to single steps across the stage, suggest a choreography that shies away from dancerly virtuosity, instead embracing the regimented approachability of everyday movement. The lyrics of the song, the movements of the dancers, and the music's beats (which Ito has also fully written out in the sketch) are all synchronized—the rhythm of war brings everyone into a unified tempo, measure by measure, beat by beat drawing the group toward battle.

I don't know whether this dance was ever performed. It seems, however, precisely tuned to the range of theatrical production possibilities available to performing artists in the years of total war mobilization. These included a wide range of genres: modern music and dance revues, topical treatments using older forms such as *kabuki* and *rakugo*, *shingeki* dramas, comedy skits, and circus.[44] These performances took place in city centers, but increasingly, via the Mobile Theatre Federation (led by Ito's brother, Kisaku), they were exported across the country and across the empire. Indeed, even in the final years of the war, when the major urban theaters were requisitioned to serve as factories, military headquarters, and so on, mobile theater was still recognized as crucial to disseminating propaganda and fostering patriotic, imperial identification. Moreover, in a self-sustaining cycle, when mobile theater performers returned from abroad, they frequently contributed their ethnographic observations to scripts, choreographies, and musical depictions of Japan's colonized peoples, representations that then circulated across Japan (to inform Japanese about their new, though inferior, "brothers") as well as back out across the empire (to model for local spectators what the ideal colonial subject should be).[45] With substantial sums of money available from the government, and new audiences in the factory, the battlefield, and the colony, performing artists found that the war offered significant opportunities to pursue their creative work, albeit under closely defined parameters, and in the service of Japan's imperial violence.[46]

Within these options for public performance, performing artists in Japan and across the colonies contributed their creative labor and performing bodies to the imperial project throughout the war. For instance, in theater, one of Japan's most prominent dramatists, Kishida Kunio, served as chief of the Division of Culture of the Imperial Rule Assistance Association.[47] And even among proletarian *shingeki* (new, Western-style theater) practitioners, some of whom were imprisoned for communist loyalties, the postwar consensus was that everyone had participated in the war effort in one way or another.[48] Similarly, in the dance world, concerts for the general public had been banned; as Hoshino Yukiyo notes in her study of Korean and Taiwanese dancers who performed in Japanese companies during the war, "the only way to dance was to go to the front lines or to a military factory to entertain soldiers or laborers."[49] Going to work for the war was not simple opportunism; the power of Japan's imperial endeavor was how broadly it appealed to a wide variety of subjects. For example, Choe Seung-hui (known in Japan as Sai Shōki), a renowned Korean dancer trained by Ito's friend Ishii Baku, was like Ito, inspired by the idea of a Pan-Asian aesthetics, so much so that she devised a new modern dance form that she called "Eastern dance."[50]

Across these examples, from the most central Japanese cultural figures to colonized subjects, participation in Japan's imperial project has been predominantly treated—by many of the artists, their postwar colleagues, and by historians—as a matter of volitional war responsibility. But as Nayoung Aimee Kwon discusses, the binary of "collaboration" and "resistance" is a reductive and obscuring framework for understanding the web of colonial interrelations and fraught artistic production that took place during Japan's imperial era.[51] This is true of Ito as well. As discussed in chapter 3, Kwon offers the concept of "intimacy" as a way to fathom the fundamentally intertwined desires and coercions structuring artists' work in this period. Likewise, what we find amid the bureaucratic details of Ito's Greater East Asia Stage Arts Research Institute proposals is that after a nearly thirty-year career in Europe and the US, in which Ito understood himself as cosmopolitan because of both his international itinerary *and* the representational claims of his "oriental dance" choreography, Japan's fantasy of benevolent, multicultural imperialism seemed like the most promising site for continuing to pursue his cosmopolitan ideals. Most particularly, Ito's long engagement with the genre of "oriental dance" as an *embodied* epistemology of the Orient served as the foundation for his embrace of Pan-Asianism as a vision of cosmopolitanism. Likewise, the broader ideology of modern dance, especially as he absorbed it at the Jaques-Dalcroze Institute in Hellerau, asserted the potential of modern dance to not only repair the individual but to renovate society at large. This was an ideology that helped to assert the importance of dance in the construction of Japan's New Order in Asia. Ito's career-long desires and the terms by which he understood himself as an artist thus seemed to find compelling articulation in aspects of Japan's imperial efforts. As with so many others, coercion, opportunity, and desire operated here in intimate proximity.

The Greater East Asia Stage Arts Research Institute

Certain of Japan's defeat, Ito nevertheless flung himself into the war effort. He responded to the calls for total mobilization by drawing up plans for the Greater East Asia Stage Arts Research Institute (*daitoa butai geijutsu kenkyūsho*). With a name that clearly echoed the Greater East Asia Co-Prosperity Sphere, Ito envisioned it as an institution for mobilizing performing artists across the empire, and as a center for Asian youth to come together for training in cultural arts. It was, in many ways, a reinvention of his earlier vision of a Theatre of the Sun, which was itself a re-envisioning of the Dalcroze Institute at Hellerau. However, reflecting his own turn to Pan-Asianism, as well as the demands of wartime mobilization, Ito's Greater East Asia Stage Arts Research Institute recast the internationalism of Hellerau as a Pan-Asian cosmopolitanism, in which his own experience as a worldly modern artist mirrored the position of Japan as a modernized nation and leader of the New Order in Asia.

The institute seems to have been active from the early spring of 1944 through March of 1945. An abandoned beauty parlor owned by a friend from Ito's Los Angeles days served as a rehearsal space, and for his newly established dance studio. Ito's efforts were short-lived; by the spring of 1945, American firebombing had destroyed the office and rehearsal space and Ito fled to the countryside with his family and some students and performers. With only one production actually realized, evidence of the institute exists in the series of plans Ito drew up to outline its purpose and organization. Two of these were submitted to the Greater East Asia Ministry, and have been stamped "Secret." The others remained in his personal papers, circulated, perhaps, among the other involved artists and his brothers.

Ito's endeavor was supported by high-ranking officials in the government and army. This patronage, even at such a late stage of the war, reflected the fact that his proposal drew on and fit with other cultural propaganda activities carried out across Japan's empire. Government officials had attributed

Pan-Asianism between Internment and Propaganda 205

Japan's earlier difficulty in controlling China in part to the fact that little effort had been made to convince the local populace of Japan's liberating cause. Therefore, in 1941, a new policy of cultural propaganda, based on the Nazi *propaganda Korps*, called for battalions of civilian *bunkajin* (men of culture) to be attached to Japan's armies in Southeast Asia. These writers, painters, musicians, filmmakers, and other culture-makers had the responsibility of persuading indigenous populations to willingly join in the creation of a new Asia. Under these auspices, significant funding was devoted to theater and dance that hewed to the required messages of Asian unity and Japanese benevolence.[52] For instance, in Indonesia, the journalist Takeda Rintarō established the Theatre Direction Center (*engeki shidōsho*), which mobilized local dramatists and performers to create new touring productions.[53] And in the Philippines, the writer Kon Hidemi organized a dance revue that culminated in a grand finale in which all the performers waved Japanese flags and sang the *Aikoku Kōshinkyoku*, or Patriotic March, a song used in Japan's occupied regions as a substitute for the local national anthem.[54]

Ito swiftly solicited the involvement of prominent artists for his institute—especially those who were already involved in various government and military cultural initiatives. For instance, both Takeda and Kon had returned to Japan by the end of 1943, and they became involved in the institute's activities. Ito also structured the institute around the concept of mobile theater units, which were central to Japan's cultural strategy, both domestically and abroad.[55] Not coincidentally, one of Ito's younger brothers, Kisaku, was the bureau chief of the Japanese Federation of Mobile Theatres, the main organization overseeing this mobilization. Ito also secured the support of several notable artists and intellectuals, such as his friend the composer Yamada Kōsaku, playwrights Kishida Kunio and Kubota Mantarō, and scholar of Indian literature and Sanskrit Tsuji Naoshirō. Less expected, perhaps, was the involvement of another of Ito's brothers, the *shingeki* director Senda Koreya. Senda had been arrested for communist beliefs in 1940, and released from prison in August 1942 after committing *tenkō*, a public recantation of his communist beliefs.[56] His release stipulated that he refrain from working in the theater or continuing his past activities. And so, he used Ito's institute space at night for secret rehearsals for the newly formed Haiyū-za (Actor's Theatre). Senda also seems to have served as a sort of secretary for his older brother; Fujita Fujio argues that some of the Greater East Asia Stage Arts Research Institute planning documents are clearly written by Senda, under the name Ōmura Kentarō.[57]

Ito's own tendencies, combined with the significant official support he received, help explain the scale of his plans for the institute. While most artists simply lent their talents to propaganda performances and comfort tours (which Ito did as well), in the grandest articulation of his plans, Ito envisioned the Greater East Asia Stage Arts Research Institute as a way of reorganizing society, and Asia. Indeed, the details of Ito's explanation reveal how thoroughly the project was enmeshed with historical and philosophical discourses about Pan-Asianism. For instance, his characterization of the Research and Education Section as creating an "intellectual treasure store" references, in particular, Watsuji Tetsurō's formulation of Nara as the endpoint of the Silk Road, an assertion that made Japan the repository of the intellectual and cultural achievements of the world.[58] The quixotic grandeur of this vision, yet another example of the modernist impulse to remake society as *Gesamtkunstwerk*, suggests how Ito saw, in the war and imperial Japan's geographic expanse, an opportunity to realize his abiding vision of performance as a force of social rehabilitation.

Ito's proposal for a grand festival pageant in the Philippines provides the clearest instance of his efforts to accommodate Japan's imperial project to his fantasy of cosmopolitan, "oriental" ethnographic performance. Ito proposed the pageant as a celebration of the first year of Filipino "independence." Ito's choice of the Philippines as the site of his festival reflected its status as a major site of military and cultural contest during the Pacific War. The Philippines had been a Spanish and then a US colony, until on December 8, 1941, Japan invaded it in a series of battles that lasted through May 1942, occupying the country until the summer of 1945. During this period, the Philippines, like Burma, occupied an ambiguous category in Japan's Co-Prosperity Sphere. To substantiate the claim that Japan's imperialism served a broader, nobler goal of Pan-Asianism, Japan granted the Philippines independence in October 1943. In reality, however, administration and military conditions were under Japanese control, albeit carried out through local officials. This arrangement was meant to exemplify the idea behind Japan's vision for a New Order in Asia, in which Asian nations, free from Western dominion, were united in partnership under Japanese leadership.

The Philippines national pageant exemplifies Ito's ability to marshal resources and cultivate people in positions of power. And it highlights the ways Ito repeatedly tied his choreographic projects to national concerns. The Philippines national pageant, however, did not happen. The only records we have of this project are the documents in Ito's Greater East Asia Stage Arts

Pan-Asianism between Internment and Propaganda

Research Institute plans, two of which are dedicated to the pageant proposal. This unrealized project is another of Ito's fantasies. And it is precisely as fantasy that Ito's Philippines national pageant demonstrates how his belief in the renovating possibilities of modern dance structured his embrace of Japan's imperial ideology and its project of creating a New Order in Asia. I draw on the institute's documents, as well as details from his technique, his dance education, and past experiences, to produce a description of an event that occurred only in Ito's mind. This is what I see:

The festival was supposed to take place in Manila. However, as I imagine it, as with the Geneva pageant and the Dalcroze Institute itself, Ito envisioned a location slightly removed from the city, where nature asserted itself as part of the backdrop—and was thus incorporated as a national property. I picture the ground cleared for a stage with two levels of platforms and sets of ramps and stairs on both sides. The playing space would be both this explicit stage and the cleared area running into the audience, so that spectators would feel the depicted history as their own. Reflecting Adolph Appia's contributions to the Hellerau experiments, when performers massed themselves on this stage, the lines and shadows created by their movement would transform their bodies into an additional source of architecture, molding the empty air into meaningful space.

Ito embraced the pageant genre for its capacity to enact a performative instantiation of national community. This ideological work was woven into Ito's vision for the Philippines pageant's dramaturgy, its participants, and the process of its creation. For instance, the pageant's content consisted of an episodic presentation of the history of the Philippines up to independence:

> ... before the Spaniards came, then the era of Spanish rule, the era of American rule, [and then] under the Great East Asia war, the four stages of the era of the construction of a new Philippines [. . .] the tyrannical rule of Euro-American colonial dominion, the growth of a national (*minzoku*) sentiment among the Filipino people, the history of the hardship of the independence movement, and the awakening of the Greater East Asia Co-Prosperity Sphere through which, with Japanese support, independence was achieved.[59]

The episodic structure, presuming an ignorant spectator, presented history as teleological drama. The pageant's content thus imparted educational significance to an explicitly bookended narrative, whereby the nation's history became familiar and preordained.

I imagine that each stage in this national history would be a scene beginning and ending in a tableau vivant, as in the Geneva pageant. Each scene would include representational pantomime along with more abstract choreography to suggest the emotional import of the action. I imagine that, as in his California dance symphonies, Ito would have broken the hundreds of members of the movement chorus into smaller groups. Each group would perform its own simple, graphic choreography in unison, alternately filling the space with a sense of massed movement and still presence. As in the *Orpheus* at Hellerau, protagonists would emerge out of these groups, with the collectivity reforming behind them. And, true to Ito's Dalcrozian training, there would be close correspondence between the pageant's dramaturgy, the performers' rhythmic movement, and the music, to induce strong emotion in the spectators.

The national pedagogy achieved by the pageant's content was to be complemented by its participants and production process. Ito called for the festival activity to be led and carried out by locals: "Filipino writers, musicians, actors, dancers and so on will be mobilized and trained, from the drawing up of scripts to the entire creative process, so that as much as possible is done by Filipinos themselves. . . . This plan's chief executive should, of course, be Filipino, a local member of the cultural elite [*bunkajin*], who can directly make contact with artists, as it is essential that they make the final decisions."[60] Highlighting the abundant artistic, cultural, and organizational capacity of the local populace, Ito emphasized that community participation was essential to the performative staging of national collectivity. I imagine that, as had been the case in California, Ito particularly saw this as an opportunity to train young local dancers, who could then perform solo interludes within the program, demonstrating in their artistic presence the corporeal potential of Filipino youth.

Just as surely as the proposal envisioned a choreography of Filipino national collectivity, however, it disclosed Ito's position as a subject of imperial Japan. In his dramaturgy, the expression of national allegiance doubled as an expression of colonial allegiance. Thus, Ito writes that the institute would "sponsor the artistry of stage artists from every area of Greater East Asia and, at the same time, encourage awareness of themselves as independent peoples, with their hands raising up the New East Asian Culture, with deep emotion for both the 'sun' and 'Japan.'"[61] In this formulation, local Filipino "awareness of themselves as independent peoples" overlaps with, and even engenders a "deep emotion" for, imperial Japan, the presence of which is doubled in the

Pan-Asianism between Internment and Propaganda

reference to "Japan" and to its national symbol, the "sun." To express this coupling of national and colonial identification, I imagine elements of Ito's own choreographic repertoire and method repurposed for this moment. Perhaps he would have used a straightforward sequence of codified positions from his technique, in which the arms, raised overhead but bent at the elbows, move through a flourish with the hands. Performed with the dancers' faces beatifically lifted upward, the scripted sentiment "with deep emotion for both the 'sun' and 'Japan'" would be corporealized in broadly legible movement, as the abstract positions of the Ito technique became explicitly representational. Ito's plan for the pageant thus choreographed the simultaneous performance of two different collective identities—that of the Philippines as a nation, as well as that of the Pan-Asian spirit unified under the protective sphere of Japan's Greater East Asia.

It is here that we see how Ito's interest in the pageant form combined with his long involvement in the genre of "oriental dance." In calling for local Filipino artists to spearhead the pageant's various creative elements, Ito used "oriental dance's" ethnographic method, which insisted on regional specificity and expertise, to undergird its fantasized representations. In this approach, the best way to celebrate Filipino "independence" would be through the exhibition of Filipino culture, as represented in (and by) dance. But, as I argued in chapter 3, for Ito, "oriental dance" is also always the Orient of *tōyō*, in which Ito's ability to produce this event, to organize its hundreds of artists and contributors—indeed, to be able transform a national history into "art"—is the mark of Japan's supposed superiority and historical responsibility to lead the rest of Asia.[62] And it is here, as a fantasy of performative, embodied imperial community, that we also see how this project seemed to offer Ito a sincere vision of cosmopolitanism, in the hundreds of bodies massed together in representation—and literal instantiation—of a collectivity.

Ito's proposal for the Philippines festival pageant was never carried out. American forces began to retake the territory by mid-1944, and in later documents, Ito suggested that a different festival be planned for Shanghai. From our vantage point, what is perhaps surprising is not that the festival did not take place, but that it received so much support to begin with. As Senda wrote in his autobiography:

> But the army and government people, especially my *senpai*, the former Finance Minister Sakomizu Hisatsune and Minobe Yōji, why did they back up Michio? Was it as a reward for "dodgy dealings" in America? Or did they,

at their wits end, latch onto Michio's dream as a last-ditch effort? Or giving up the war as hopeless, did they think it would help when it came time to make peace with America? Allowing this cosmopolitan to speak his dreams, or awaiting some sort of opportunity, even today we don't know [why they supported him].[63]

Did these officials embrace Ito's plan precisely as a kind of fantasy—a vision of a reality that was no longer to be, and so could only exist as theater?[64] It is easy to dismiss Ito's vision as implausible; the deteriorating conditions of the war made such an expenditure of human and material resources almost unthinkable. And yet, the pageant was also by no means impossible. Ito's prior experiences had consistently demonstrated surprising allocations of funds, time, and people to such grandiose projects. The very origin of his dance education and of his wartime proposal—the pageants and festivals connected to the Dalcroze Institute at Hellerau—were themselves extraordinary instances of the attainability of such visions. Indeed, though it might seem a wasteful absurdity, the needs of wartime empire to justify itself had authorized and seen to fruition many other similar efforts of performance propaganda.

Ito's proposal for the Philippines pageant, then, anticipated the project's failure at the same time that it took seriously the possibility of its enactment—and even more so, took seriously the significance of its ideological promise. For what is striking about Ito's proposal is the way it ties Japan's imperial agenda to his own fervent belief that choreography might remake the world by calling into existence a sense of embodied collectivity. This was a belief that was foundational to the Life Reform Movement enacted at Hellerau and to the origins of early modern dance in both Europe and the US. In the dislocations and reversals in status that marked his experience of the Pacific War, Ito picked up the thread of this belief in the ideology of Pan-Asianism.

Ito's commitment to this belief meant that he was willing to accommodate himself to a variety of political regimes over the course of his career, insisting on the power of art even in the face of extraordinary violence. We saw this in California in 1937, when he triumphantly staged *Etenraku* and *Blue Danube* as celebrations of community, while reports of the Nanjing Massacre ran on the same newspaper pages as reviews of his concerts. And this political agnosticism meant that when Ito returned to Japan, he could pen an invective-filled article in the magazine *Engekikai* describing the barbaric and uncultured essence of American life;[65] he could choreograph an explicitly fascist war dance, even as he predicted Japan's defeat; and he could outline a massive arts institute operating across all of Japan's colonies. In the final years of the war, Ito could understand all of these activities as in service to an ideal of artistic universalism that would outlast and overcome any particular political situation. Thus could Ito work alongside political realities, without seeming to see them. The force of fantasy itself, and the tantalizing possibilities of (hegemonic) world-making that fantasy promises, allowed Ito to persist in a willful, unrelenting utopianism.

We should, then, read Ito's proposal like his other published narratives— that is, as a performance of self. This is especially so because the mass-pageant form is a genre in which self-actualization occurs through self-narration. Moreover, the imagined status of Ito's pageant crystallizes the tantalizing promises that Pan-Asianism seemed to offer Ito and so many other artists during the war. For in this fantasy of a reordered world, an individual's own private dreams could be tied to those of the empire, suddenly articulated as not merely personal, but serving a broader social, regional community. The appeal of this vision was precisely how it transformed individual desires into national-imperial ones.

The Imperial Revue

Although short-lived, the Greater East Asia Stage Arts Research Institute produced one piece, a musical drama with the theme of Greater East Asia. This production was performed for three days in January 1945, at the National New Theatre. Shima Kimiyasu, an old colleague of Senda Koreya's from the proletarian theater group Mezamashitai, contacted the institute on behalf of two dancers, Ootomo Chiharu of Takarazuka and Mitsuhashi Renko of the Nichigeki, who had recently formed a new dance group, New East Asia (shintōa). With Ito as the overall director, together they developed a piece featuring the major territories of the Co-Prosperity Sphere. The production was divided into three parts—one representing Japan, one China, and the third, Southeast Asia. Tying together the sections were dance interludes from Tahiti, Thailand, and India.

With a short rehearsal period and limited resources, the script was cobbled together from preexisting sources, and performers gathered from different troupes. The Japanese part consisted of a verse drama written by Kurihara Kazuto, along with the newly composed noh *Miikusabune*, which the Haiyū-za had performed in August of the previous year as part of a trial performance announcing the opening of the troupe.[66] The Chinese part was a drama written by Shima Kimiyasu, *Kikyō Monogatari* (The Story of the Chinese Bellflower), about the Great Wall of China. Takeda Rintarō, who had been dispatched to the front as a journalist, contributed a musical drama script about Java. Music was composed by Hattori Tadashi and another of Ito's younger brothers, Ousuke. Since the dance group New East Asia was made up of women, male members of the Haiyū-za and the mobile theater troupe Mizuho also participated in the performance, and female dancers from Takarazuka, Shōchiku, and the Nichigeki supplemented the ethnic dance segments. With paper for newsprint nearly nonexistent, none of the newspapers reviewed it. Senda Koreya only briefly evaluated the production, commenting in his autobiography:

> The dances and ballads of India, Thailand, Java, and so on, were from the repertoires of the Takarazuka and Shōchiku's Girls Opera, and well as from the Nichigeki, and so the troupe members of Shintōa considerably mastered the material. However, given the raw material, the scripts, and the preparation time, Michio's dream of surpassing a simple presentation of ethnic dances and songs was impossible to realize. At that time, in January of the year of defeat, it ended as nothing more than an unusually elaborate and theatrical show.[67]

This production suggests a structure similar to the one outlined in Jennifer Robertson's analysis of the Takarazuka Revue's wartime performances. It is, in fact, likely that the production was inspired by Takarazuka's 1943 *Children of East Asia* (Tōa no kodomotachi), which also used a tripartite structure featuring Manchukuo, China, and the Southern Region to celebrate the future of the New Asian Order. As Robertson explains, in *Children of East Asia* and other wartime productions with titles such as *Saipan-Palau: Our South Seas* (1940), *Mongol* (1941), and *Only One Ancestral Land* (1943), Takarazuka's revue form celebrated the different forms of exoticness embodied by each locale. Yet its presentation of these nations as a series of theatrical scenes asserted a flattened similarity of relation—all belonged to the Japanese Empire.[68] Indeed, given that this revue borrowed so many performers from Takarazuka, such similarity is not surprising. But we also see in this production's imperial curation the ethnographic structure of "oriental dance" programs that was so familiar to Ito. The juxtaposed arrangement of this revue was yet another way to represent the overlapping collectivities of nation and empire imagined by Japan's New Order in Asia.

Pan-Asianism between Internment and Propaganda

Though this project was realized, I am nevertheless drawn to what didn't happen. Senda's note of regret pulls our attention to the imagined choreography behind the staged performance. As he writes, it was Michio's dream to "surpass a simple presentation of ethnic songs and dances." From the entries in Ito's notebooks and the planning documents of the Greater East Asia Stage Arts Research Institute, it seems likely that he had hoped to present a form that would truly embody the inclusive internationalism that he attributed to Pan-Asianism. The revue, a form that is inherently fragmented, was perhaps fundamentally inadequate for this vision. It was, however, a genre that would become a mainstay of Ito's work in the postwar period of the Allied Occupation of Japan. As a choreographer, director, and producer at the Ernie Pyle Theatre (the main entertainment venue for Allied personnel in Japan), the capacious nature of the revue again offered Ito a way to cast his modern dance practice as central to the construction of a cosmopolitan society.

CHAPTER SEVEN

Being Watched

Making New Bodies for a New Japan, 1945–1955

On August 15, 1945, Japan surrendered to the Allied Forces, and on September 2, the Allied Occupation of Japan began, led by the United States. Two years later, in July 1947, Ito published a small volume titled *Etiquette* (Echiketto). Like many other publications from the early postwar period, it endeavored to teach its readers new modes of behavior suitable for American-style democracy. Yet unlike most straightforward manuals, Ito enfolded his pedagogy within a narrative about a young aspiring dancer, Makiko. One day, "S—Sensei" (a thinly veiled Ito), hears a knock on his office door. He receives the visitor with a "Come in," and the door cautiously opens to reveal Makiko. Trembling with nervousness, she requests permission to become his dance student and to join his troupe. During the war she had worked in a factory, but passing by his dance studio every day, she was filled with desire to become a dancer, until finally she found the courage to approach him. S—Sensei readily agrees, and then asks:

> "By the way, when you entered the room, do you recall how many times you bowed?"
> "... ..."
> "It's actually not polite to bow so much."
> "Oh! I'm sorry."
> "Hey there, you're bowing again. That makes seven times I think."[1]

Makiko turns red, and S—Sensei, smiling, changes the subject. But when Makiko turns to go, she again bows, another eight times, before finally leaving the room.

The episode epitomizes the problems that Ito's manual aims to address, and the complications that this chapter explores. Makiko's Bourdeusian hab-

Being Watched

itus, shaped by traditional Japanese protocol and further stunted by her time laboring in a war factory, is outmoded and hollow. Her mechanical bowing reveals a body that cannot control itself, and that performs motions empty of meaning. Ito must teach her—and his readers—new corporeal habits that will enable Makiko to move her body freely and with intention, a corporeality that will allow her to engage with the new social expectations of democracy and internationalism.

During the Occupation, Ito positioned himself as an expert who could teach his fellow Japanese, particularly young Japanese women, the bodily comportment and internal attitudes that would enable them to engage the postwar world as cosmopolitans. He did so through three primary venues. At the Ernie Pyle Theatre, the primary entertainment venue for Allied personnel, Ito staged numerous productions through which he offered an appealing vision of a new Japan, and in the process, taught the theater's dancing corps how to inhabit this reimagined nation. He penned articles in women's magazines teaching comportment, with a particular focus on walking. And he coached fashion models in how to pose and present themselves with an abstracted individuality necessary for the work of inspiring postwar consumption. In all of these outlets, Ito used both the practice of modern dance and its ideologies, as inherited from his own training at Hellerau and experiences in the US, as the foundation for corporeal remaking.

Many Japanese felt the need for this remaking. Postwar Tokyo was a devastated landscape: whole neighborhoods and the people within them had been incinerated by the firebombing campaigns; emaciated children, amputee returning soldiers, and desperate women roamed the streets, lining up for food, attempting to purchase goods on the black market, and finding shelter amid the rubble. Across the country, this physical landscape was mirrored by a psychological one: most Japanese had lived their entire lives as participants in Japan's imperial program, which had reached into the private corners of mundane life: children recited imperial prescripts at school in front of a portrait of the emperor; youth groups put together care packages for soldiers at the front and raised money for ambulances; government censorship, the Peace Preservation Law of 1925 (which allowed for widespread arrest), and a jingoistic press produced a public sphere that overwhelmingly celebrated the military's accomplishments and exhorted the public to do the same. And as the war went on, Japanese people, in both urban centers and rural villages, sacrificed material goods and their loved ones to the national cause. For the many Japanese who had been promised that this was a holy war (whether they believed it or not), the sudden defeat produced feelings of disillusionment, betrayal, and hopelessness.

The Occupation, then, was simultaneously a shameful subjugation, but also the possibility for something new. And many Japanese eagerly desired many of the Occupation's early promises—civil liberties, democratic government, consumer freedom, and material abundance. Indeed, in some cases, such as the decision of the Supreme Commander for the Allied Powers (SCAP) to protect the emperor from being accused of war crimes, many Japanese felt that the Occupiers were too hesitant to make the changes that would truly renovate the nation.

In this general atmosphere, women stood as harbingers and ready adopters of the massive political and social changes that accompanied the arrival of the Americans.[2] In far greater numbers than their Taisho-era *moga* (modern girl) predecessors, women embraced the new opportunities and behaviors made possible by the Occupation, as they worked, consumed leisure activities and material goods, and simply occupied public space, sitting, standing, and walking outside. In focusing his attentions on young women, Ito brought his belief that dance was a force for remaking individuals—both corporeally and spiritually—to bear on subjects who were assigned a great deal of symbolic meaning in terms of what the Occupation signified. In tracing their possible responses to this bewildering period, I ask what the Occupation's ideals—of freedom, liberal subjecthood, and cosmopolitan beauty—might have meant for these young Japanese women, under the gendered and racialized structures of the Occupation and the lingering structures of imperial Japan.

In this chapter's attention to the young women Ito trained, there is a parallelism with chapter 4's consideration of his work with Nisei dancers in Southern California. But here, this attention also represents the passing on of his legacy, which has, with some prominent exceptions, substantially persisted in the bodies of generations of female students. So too do the activities considered in this chapter demonstrate that in this period, Ito's influence most fully expanded out of the world of formal concert dance into structures of quotidian movement carried out by women in their daily lives, a legacy that is untraceable, but imaginable all the same.

As Ito taught young women new repertoires with which to embody the nation's reconstruction, he also imparted the necessity of fantasy as a way to project themselves into their own desired performances of self. Throughout this book, I have offered fantasy as a methodology to engage the past, and as a framework for understanding how Ito performed himself into a sense

Being Watched   217

of continuity across the ruptures and dislocations of his career. As I have argued, these fantasies, these performances of self, helped to bind Ito to the social worlds in which he lived, and it is to this sense of social relationality in particular that this chapter attends. Here, Ito shows that fantasy is a deeply self-conscious practice of relationality, in which the experiences of watching and being watched help constitute the self as meaningfully in the world.

Etiquette continues with Makiko's story in the next chapter, which presents her version of the meeting with S—Sensei, through the device of her personal diary, which she has left on S—Sensei's desk to attest to her commitment to becoming a dancer and a true artist:

> With that, "Come in," I had the feeling not of one Japanese person visiting another, but rather that I was hailed as a cosmopolitan. In that instant of insight, I fell into confusion. My appearance, my belongings, manner, suddenly I couldn't help feeling it was all shabby, and overwhelmed with misery. This was the first time I'd had such an experience. To knock at the door of someone you're visiting, in elementary school, at my girls' school, and in the factory even, I've always done that, it's an everyday occurrence. But with that greeting, "Come in," in English, I became totally flustered.[3]

The casual greeting, "Come in," precipitates a crisis for Makiko, as the foreign language in which it is uttered interpellates her not as a Japanese person, but as a cosmopolitan. Yet Makiko does not feel herself to be cosmopolitan; instead, she is self-conscious about the "shabbiness" of her "outfit, personal effects, and manner," all of which become markers of her Japaneseness, given away by her incessant bowing. As the diary continues:

> When I left the theater, the words "Come in" would not leave my head. . . . As I darted between the foreign cars crisscrossing each other amid soldiers and civilians—there flowed the colors of every nation of the world. It was truly a deluge of internationalism. Up to that moment I had thought it ordinary that Japan was welcoming foreigners. But suddenly, I became aware that the present situation is much more than that. Instead, it is that Japan is being called by all the various people of the world.[4]

Makiko recognizes S—Sensei's "Come in" as Japan's cue to reenter the world. The problem, as she has just discovered, is that her body, bearing, and behavior are unequipped to do so. A new corporeal vocabulary would be necessary, or, as Ito would have it, a new etiquette, to guide Japanese in inhabiting their new society.

It is significant that in the narrative of S—Sensei and Makiko, Ito has Makiko submit her journal to S—Sensei. Indeed, she is writing with the knowledge that she will hand it over to be read. This is a public performance masquerading as private confessional, and it is a deeply self-conscious performance of self. This quality of self-consciousness permeates all of Ito's activities during the Occupation, a self-consciousness frequently manifested through the bodies of the young women he trained. As we will see, in photographs taken of the Erniettes (the young female corps attached to the Ernie Pyle Theatre), the dancers exhibit a self-consciousness that encompasses the tension between their enjoyment and their anxiety in working as entertainers for the former enemy. Likewise, in Ito's magazine columns, he urges readers to alter the mechanics of their walking, and to do so with a sense of intentionality that will mark their bodies as self-confident, fashionable, and ready to meet the world. And again, in images of Ito teaching models how to pose, we see self-consciousness not merely as a byproduct of the awkwardness of learning something new, but as a cultivated affect communicating awareness of one's own body, and the intention that that awareness should be legible to others. Indeed, these moments of self-consciousness mirrored the unfolding of the Occupation itself, in which both Allied personnel and the Japanese themselves went about reconstructing society through top-down directives and intentional changes in personal behavior and social life (even as all these changes masked the innumerable continuities that persisted—and were even safeguarded by SCAP). The self-consciousness exhibited in Makiko's narrative reflects a preoccupation of this period, a manifestation of the challenge facing Ito, his students, and Japanese at large: how do you remake yourself when the world is watching?

Ito's answer to this question is epitomized in another of Makiko's journal episodes. The other students have gone shopping, but she decides to return to the rehearsal room. She stands in front of the mirror, examining her body, alone, apparently for the first time, and sees herself as if she were looking at someone else's body. Suddenly, she freezes, and locks eyes in the mirror with someone who is standing in the doorway, also staring at her. It is S—Sensei, puffing a cigar. He comes to where she is standing and declares that to become a dancer, she must truly know herself. He instructs her to investigate every point of her body, to become aware of how her neck moves her head, how her shoulders slope down to her arms, how the bones of her feet

Being Watched 219

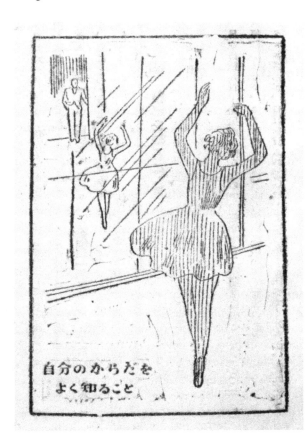

Fig. 18. *Echiketto* by Ito Michio. The Japanese reads: "Know your body well." [Jibun no karada wo yoku shiru koto]. Asian Division, Library of Congress.

hold their stance.[5] The self-consciousness of feeling oneself being watched, of needing to perform under a watchful gaze, is here literalized. The supposedly private moment of self-reflection turns out, disconcertingly, to be a public moment of being watched. And the advice Ito gives her is not to resist or subvert this gaze, but rather to embrace it, and to produce oneself, even more fully, as a scrutinized body.

Ito is, in this illustration and scenario, rather obviously correlated with S—Sensei. But he is also, without a doubt, Makiko. (Note the first initial.) This lesson, then, in which Michio teaches Makiko, and his readers, how to respond to this gaze, recapitulates his own career-long experience of being the object of innumerable scrutinizing, desirous gazes. Canny, artful responsiveness to the gaze of others was, after all, the key to so many of Ito's performances over the course of his career—from his engagement in the homo-social world of japoniste erotics in Alvin Langdon Coburn's London studio, to the embodiment of a fantasy of access through the genre of "oriental" dance in New York, and as a reflection of the various national and imperial identificatory desires that his audiences in California, Mexico, and interwar Japan had ascribed to him. Ito's awareness of the ways that gaze and desire circulate through the performance of fantasy was at the heart of what he offered to his students and the broader public during the Occupation. There, in the final two decades of his life, Ito allowed the focus of this gaze to shift, away from himself and onto the performances carried out by young Japanese women. The lessons he imparted to these women were both the promises of modern dance as a vehicle of self-expression and individual freedom, and also the techniques of sustaining oneself through fantasy, a performance of self while being watched.

Staging a "New" Japan at the Ernie Pyle

At the corner of a wide thoroughfare in Tokyo's Yurakucho district stood the Ernie Pyle Theatre, its name conspicuously advertised in thick, suspended letters at the top of its façade. Built in 1934 as the Tokyo Takarazuka Theatre, it was requisitioned by American Occupation forces in December 1945 as the epicenter of entertainment for Allied forces stationed across the Pacific. Though its staff and performers were mostly Japanese, its audience was almost exclusively restricted to Allied servicemen, Occupation personnel, and their families. With its emblazoned new name and off-limits facilities, the building served as a daily reminder of Japan's defeat. Yet the Ernie Pyle Theatre was more than a monument of resentment; it also became a potent sign of longing for the potential freedom and prosperity that peace and the Occupation promised. Ito's work there, as choreographer, director, and producer, was central to the creation of its allure.

Not just for Ito but for many who passed through the building, the Ernie Pyle was a formative site of technical training and cultural experience, that multiplied as they moved on to work in theaters and other institutions. For instance, under Ito's tutelage, many of the Erniettes later gained fame as dancers, actors, and teachers. Similarly, the house orchestra soon became the Tokyo Philharmonic; and, as Kuwahara Noriko has documented, the venue facilitated important exchange between American and Japanese visual art-

Being Watched   221

ists, and served as an exhibition space for the first generation of Japanese artists working after the war.[6] Nor was this a one-way transfer of knowledge: in addition to the USO entertainers who eagerly absorbed snippets of Japanese performance and material culture during their tours in Japan, many of the scholars who are now considered the first generation of US specialists in Japanese theater served as censors in the Occupation or were stationed in Japan during the Korean War, during which time they honed their Japanese language skills and gained appreciation for the Japanese theatrical forms they would study later in their careers.[7]

Ito had been recommended to the Occupation authorities by a former student from his Hollywood studio, who was now a commissioned officer with the special services.[8] Engaged to direct the venue's first production, *Fantasy Japonica*, in February 1946, Ito was permanently hired a month later, responsible for conceiving, producing, choreographing, and directing stage productions, supervising dance instruction, designing costumes, and overseeing stage design.[9] Ito's years of experience in the entertainment industry in the US meant that he understood both the expectations of his GI spectators as well as the rehearsal and production practices of American theaters. Over the years of the Occupation, he had a hand in a significant number of the shows at the Ernie Pyle, ranging from plays such as *The Brigadier's Wife* and *Snow Queen Fantasy*, to pageant-style pieces such as *1776* and the yearly Christmas show, musicals and operetta such as *The Mikado*, and revues such as *Tabasco, Rhapsody in Blue*, and *Jungle Drums*.[10] Ito also brought onto the staff his brother, the scenic designer Kisaku, who was responsible for some of the most spectacular sets from the period. When the theater finally closed (reverting back to the Takarazuka company) in 1966, Ito was hailed as the "principle figure behind many of the biggest shows staged at the theater. . . . A friendly, affable man, . . . known as 'Papa' Ito to the many GI's who have known him and worked with him since his coming to the theater in 1946."[11] The article's gloss on the chumminess between Ito and the GIs is borne out in Ito's own writings; the Occupation represented for Ito a sort of remote reentry into the US, a nation whose customs had become "second nature" to him, as he explained to a journalist from the magazine *Maru* in 1948.[12] At the Ernie Pyle, Ito worked alongside Americans whose manner was deeply familiar to him; the informal friendliness of his relations there, reminding him of his life before the war, became a common theme of his magazine articles. One gets the sense that although for many Japanese, the Ernie Pyle was a painful symbol of the complicated sense of exclusion and opportunity wrought by the Occupation, for Ito, it offered a sort of return to his adopted home, while remaining in the nation of his birth.

At the Ernie Pyle, Ito was in the business of staging fantasy—theatrical productions that played to spectators' desires for spectacle, for exotic scenarios, and for dancing girls. And predominant among the theater's staged fantasies was that of Japan itself. The visions of Japan that Ito oversaw—and taught his fellow Japanese to inhabit—consistently staged the trope of Japan as a nation with both a rich cultural history and a unique capacity for cosmopolitan engagement with the rest of the world. The astute construction of "Japan" as a product to be consumed by foreigners was by the time of the Occupation a long-running practice, dating at least to the Meiji Restoration. But the very literal presence of the GI spectators at the Ernie Pyle made the stakes of this performance especially apparent. Moreover, in using these tropes to reassure their spectators of Japan's unthreatening, welcoming essence, the dancers who appeared on stage at the Ernie Pyle were performing, as Adria Imada puts it, an "imperial hospitality," a form of "imagined intimacy" proffered by cultural workers to the military presence that they had no choice but to host.[13]

Inasmuch as Ito's productions at the Ernie Pyle staged fantasies of Japan for an audience of occupying forces, these shows might also, in different and complicated ways, have offered fantasies for the performers themselves. As Michelle Carriger observes, "internalized pressures may look very like, or indeed be indistinguishable from, personal desire."[14] After years of ideological authoritarianism, death, and suffering, the opportunity to reimagine Japan, and to embody it through glamorous and fun dancing, might have provided the theater's dancing corps, the Erniettes, with the chance not only to represent, but even to become part of, Japan's new postwar vision of itself. In productions that allowed them to inhabit imaginaries not only of "old" and "new" Japan, but also of New York, Mexico, Indonesia, France, and more, the Erniettes could project themselves into different geographic fantasies, and perhaps feel those fantasies as embodied repertoires. In the movements they performed on stage, the Erniettes might have found a sense of corporeal possibility, different ways of imagining and performing themselves.

In this section, through analyses of several of Ito's Ernie Pyle productions, I reconstruct what was a surprisingly cohesive fantasy staged across many of the theater's offerings. Under Ito's direction, a Japan rich in cultural inheritance combined with a contemporary cosmopolitanism, to reestablish the nation within the international order. In communicating this vision, Ito used

Being Watched   223

movement vocabularies coded as either traditional or modern, Japanese or Western, along with similarly emblematic costumes, to corporealize Japan as uniquely able to hold together the past and the present, Asia and the West. This formulation certainly reiterated common binaries. But, in Ito's use of the same bodies—the Erniettes—to embody all these referents, these spatio-temporal poles were staged as flexible repertoires accessible to anyone. With such staging, Ito not only presented Japan as fundamentally adaptable, but also asserted dance as an exemplary practice for enabling bodies to transition from one repertoire to the next.

Ito's first production at the Ernie Pyle, *Fantasy Japonica*, offered a proto-type for the way he would go on to stage Japan throughout the Occupation. A production photograph shows an audience of Allied servicemen represent-ing various branches of the armed services; we see the backs of their heads, pomaded hair gleaming in the light, as they all gaze at the stage. Around thirty women, dressed in formal kimono, dance in two mirrored groups. Behind them is a painted backdrop representing a pastiche of Japanese landscape—rolling hills with the *kuromatsu* pine tree, a branching cherry blossom tree, a *tō* (Japanese pagoda) rising above low clouds—this is not any specific place, but rather, a collage of scenic items indexing Japan. This image evokes a nostalgic, pastoral scene of traditional Japan, a place of scenic beauty, filled with beautiful maidens. But the striping on the lanterns and stage flat—even through the photograph's sepia, it seems likely that these are red and white stripes—also suggests the US flag, a scenic framing that indicates a dramatur-gical, and even historical framing.

The next photograph is unlabeled in the archive, but my hunch is that it is from the second act of *Fantasy Japonica*. Where once there were women delicately dancing in kimonos, now they move with physical expansiveness. They wear short, pleated skirts and tops cut high to reveal bare midriff; ear-lier in the number they wore white pumps, which they have now kicked off in order to dance barefoot. The Japanese pastoral backdrop has been replaced with a glittering New York City scene. It is not visible here, but another pho-tograph shows that overhead, where lanterns once hung, there is now a row of national flags, with the US and Britain's placed prominently at the cen-ter. The women face the audience in a messy kick line. Legs are flung up, each dancer hitting however high she can reach; some point their foot, oth-ers have it flexed; some bend their standing knee, some manage to keep it straight; some of the dancers are even up on relevé to get more propulsion for their kicking leg. We see in this photograph the amateur status of these

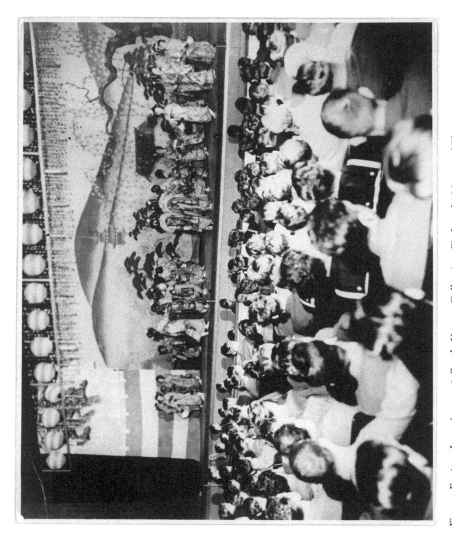

Fig. 19. *Fantasy Japonica*, 1946. Senda Koreya Collection, Tsubouchi Memorial Theatre Museum, Waseda University.

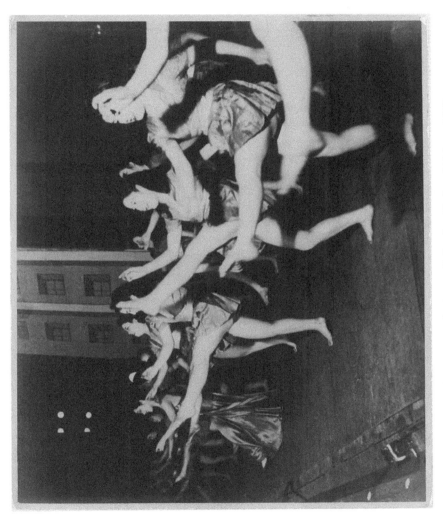

Fig. 20. *Fantasy Japonica* (?), 1946. Senda Koreya Collection, Tsubouchi Memorial Theatre Museum, Waseda University.

dancers; these are not trained professionals, but rather young women who were recently working in wartime factories or trying to sustain their starving families at home. The photograph also suggests that they are having fun; they are perhaps amused or surprised at finding themselves on a lavish stage, performing in a revue for Allied servicemen.

The implied message of *Fantasy Japonica* is fairly clear: with a bit of help (or framing) from the US, lovely but quaint Japan can cast off its traditionalism to enter the postwar world. There, with exuberant smiles and bodies moving expansively, Japan (or Japan's women) can be part of a new internationalism. Whose fantasy is this *Fantasy Japonica*? To be sure, with the Latinate "Japonica" and the scenic framing of the US's paternalistic presence, this is a white, Western, heterosexual, male fantasy of what Occupation looks like, and of what Japan represented in the white-supremacist imaginary. This is not only a geopolitical, but a sexual fantasy as well, as the rows of male spectators gazing up into the women's kicks makes clear. Such a fantasy not only recapitulated a classic colonial script, but also involved a reeducation of the GIs themselves, shifting their perception of Japan from that of Theodore Geisel's (Dr. Seuss's) propaganda film *Know Your Enemy—Japan* to one of Japan as a junior Eastern partner, compliant and assimilable to US values. In this shift of perception, the GIs, who had undergone their own trauma of war, had to reimagine themselves as well: no longer fierce soldiers in the island campaigns, they were, rather, benevolent liberators and rebuilders of a valuable society.[15]

But this is also an odd, more ambiguous fantasy for the women on stage. Though they are smiling in the second photograph, surely these women felt moments of strangeness and terror, facing an auditorium filled with the men who had, months earlier, been committed to indiscriminately killing them and their families. Indeed, though the war was over, conditions in Tokyo were devastating; extreme inflation, widespread malnutrition and starvation, and a bombed-out and burned city full of rubble meant that daily life for most Japanese was still a matter of sheer survival. *Fantasy Japonica*'s brightly lit, gayly costumed, jazzy theatrical scene must have felt like an extraordinary world, suspended from the harsh environment outside the Ernie Pyle. The fantasy staged in *Fantasy Japonica*, then, is not only Japan's supposed transition from feudal to modern (a shift that had taken place more than half a century earlier), nor Japan's reentry into a peaceful internationalism; it is also the enchantment of the theater, whereby two groups, facing each other across the footlights, were supposed to reimagine each other as part of their new present and future. Here, sexual desire, and

Being Watched

a performance geared to elicit that desire, undergirds a deeper, more amorphous intimacy, as the theatrical event becomes an opportunity to engage others in new performances of the self.

Ito's subsequent productions relied on many aspects of *Fantasy Japonica*'s formulations: dance as a representation of the transition from traditional to modern; the female body as a site of national-cultural expression; and even dance as a mode of travel. As the Erniettes professionalized, these visions took on a glossier, more cohesive aspect. For instance, *Sakura Flowers* (April 1947), like *Fantasy Japonica*, presented Japan as a series of costumed dance scenes, each representing an era. Eighth-century *bugaku* shifted to Edo-period *kabuki*-style dancing, next to a ballet-styled number, and on to a nightclub-style finale. Here again, choreographic history serves as teleology of modern development. In a photograph that probably depicts the show's finale, the men from the Nara-period *gagaku* are back on stage. They are surrounded by women in long contemporary gowns, with one arm bared, tight bodices leading down to a flowing skirt with a deep slit. Their pose, with one leg stretched out in *tendu* to push through the skirt's slit, and their heads tilted out over a bare shoulder, suggests choreography typical of a revue's line of chorus girls. Another woman, wearing a vampish gown of black lace and sequins, posed in a deep lunge to the side with her torso twisted front, grounds this scene's focus as resolutely contemporary. While the men in the background remind us of Japan's past, even they, standing with arms outstretched, have adopted the physical repertoire of the modern Broadway-style show. In this number, Japan's rich cultural past is incorporated into a jazzy and seductive present, the two temporalities coexisting in a production of Japan as a site of entertainment and enticement.

While Ito's Japan-centered choreography, such as *Fantasy Japonica* and *Sakura Flowers*, used dance as a vehicle for historical narrative, it is notable that in these shows, ballet and other nonnative forms did not just *represent* the presence and incorporation of Western practices, but were *embodied modes* of that assimilation and cosmopolitanism. Where theatrical representation is sometimes understood as a symbol or analogy of historical events, here (and indeed, since his earliest days at Hellerau) Ito understood choreographic embodiment as a literal instantiation of the social-political phenomena depicted. In his Japan-centered revues at the Ernie Pyle, Ito asserted that Japan had changed, over time and over the course of its history, *because* its bodily modes of comportment had changed. Dance was thus the manifestation of, and easiest way to observe, this corporeal history.

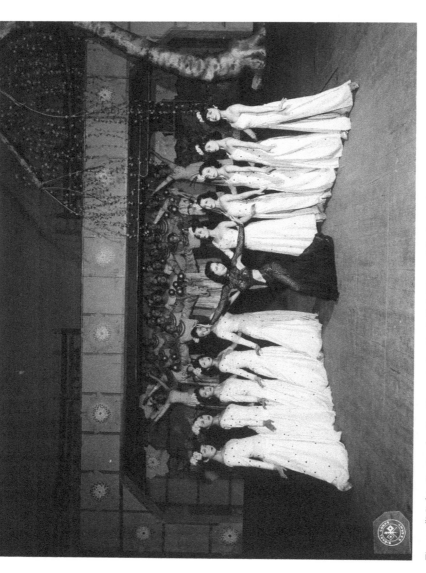

Fig. 21. "Michio Ito Production Presented at Ernie Pyle Theatre" (*Sakura Flowers*), April 25, 1947. National Archives, photographs of American Military Activities, ca. 1918–ca. 1981.

Being Watched   229

In addition to shows that staged new visions of Japan, Ito created a number of revues set in foreign locales. These productions used settings abroad to imagine a new, more cosmopolitan Japan, but did so through nostalgic evocation, using tropes that would be especially pertinent to the audience of Allied servicemen. As with the Japan-centered shows, even as these productions were aimed at the theater's Western, male spectators, they offered intriguing forms of reverie for the Japanese women performing in them, who could, perhaps, imagine themselves as figures belonging to this cosmopolitan world.

Rhapsody in Blue, presented in mid-August of 1947 and set to George Gershwin's famous composition, transported performers and spectators to the exhilarating scene of New York City. Production photos demonstrate Ito's fluency with Broadway-style choreography and jazz: torsos counterposed against hips, pressed arches, and popped hips all reveal how many different choreographic modes Ito had absorbed while in the US—and the open traffic between modern concert dance and other forms of dance modernism. We also see the incorporation of his own choreographic technique; photographs show dancers in poses where their arms are outstretched in precisely the positions from his method; and there are echoes with some of Ito's earlier solo and group pieces. The production's set consisted of a bandstand at the back of the stage, on which the orchestra played, and a backdrop across which fans the twinkling skyline of New York City. New York's metropolitan grandeur envelopes the dancers, and in the high-contrast stage lighting, the women seem to glow like the windows above them. *Rhapsody in Blue*, then, evokes the glossy, moody image of New York City, an image that for many young servicemen—whose first experience traveling might have been their military tours in the Pacific—may well have been as mediated by Hollywood movies and media representations as it was for the young women dancing as "New Yorkers" on stage. In such an iconic setting, the production's jazz-inflected choreography allowed the dancers to inhabit this imagined New York, and to feel themselves become a part of its alluring vision.

Tabasco, presented in late February of 1947, offered another exotic excursion, this time set in Mexico. A series of Latin and Latin-flavored dance numbers, strung together without any narrative to speak of, *Tabasco*, like the other revues Ito created for the Ernie Pyle, was constructed to evoke a particular atmosphere of tropical exoticism communicated through familiar choreographies and the narratives of imperial access they encoded.[16] Moving through the rhumba, the huapango, the tango, the conga, and finally the cucaracha, *Tabasco* offered the range of what Brian Herrera has called

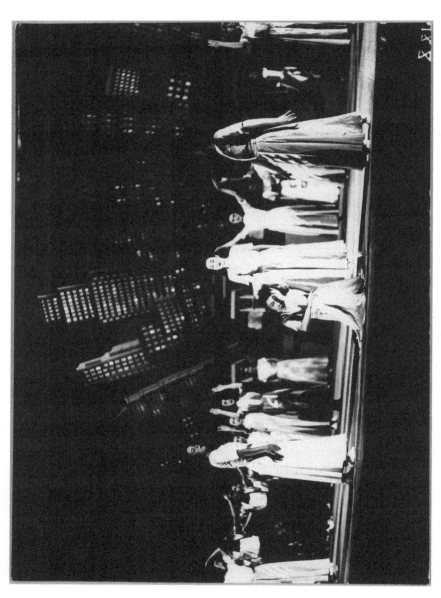

Fig. 22. *Rhapsody in Blue*, 1947. Senda Koreya Collection, Tsubouchi Memorial Theatre Museum, Waseda University.

Being Watched 231

"Latin numbers"—"the stylized mode of musical-theatrical presentation that deployed a shifting constellation of visual, musical, and linguistic cues to enact a distilled fantasy of Latin American peoples, places, and traditions, presumably for US audiences."[17] *Tabasco* invoked multiple waves of nostalgia for its audience, both for being back home in the US, where such routines were standard in Broadway and Hollywood musicals, as well as for the recent war years, when Latin-themed numbers had been a mainstay of productions sponsored by Special Services Divisions, including United Service Organization (USO) entertainments, jeep shows, and field camp theatricals. (Indeed, since the Ernie Pyle was run by the Eighth Special Services Division, the production offered GIs a sense of both nostalgia and continuity.)

Although *Tabasco* staged an established genre of American entertainment, because it was carried out by Japanese performers, the production also served to recast an overall image of Japan as an expansive site of foreign seduction. For example, one photographed scene suggests how fully Ito's production borrowed from the Latin fantasy of popular entertainment. The women, in costumes resembling Carmen Miranda's famous outfits, are in the middle of a shimmy as they direct attention to a female lead dancer who is similarly attired, though with more sequins. With their bared midriffs and flouncy skirts, the dancers perform the sensual and energetic physicality expected of the Latin number, demonstrating mastery of the stylized aggregation of the Latin idea. In doing so, however, the performers appear as a doubled ethnic exotic. Already fulfilling the fantasy of "oriental" allure, in performing *Tabasco*'s Latin numbers, the dancers also seem to embody Latin exoticism (and eroticism). *Tabasco*, then, made use of the Latin number to stage Japan as a geographically capacious site of racially ambiguous fantasy.

The overt message of productions such as *Rhapsody in Blue* and *Tabasco* was a demonstration of Japan's new cosmopolitanism—both its openness to other cultures and also, because these cultures were embodied by the Erniettes, as a sort of welcome to foreigners, who might feel "at home" through these representations. But the depiction of Japan as a place that could hold other geographic imaginaries within its realm also contained echoes of the country's recent imperial past, which, as I traced in earlier chapters, involved its own version of cosmopolitan absorption. Productions such as the 1946 *Jungle Drums*, ostensibly set in Indonesia, recalled the revue Ito had planned during the last year of the war, as well as the many performed by the Takarazuka Revue, on the very stage where the Erniettes now danced. As with so much in the Occupation, proclamations of newness intersected with continuities of Japan's only recently abandoned imperial project.

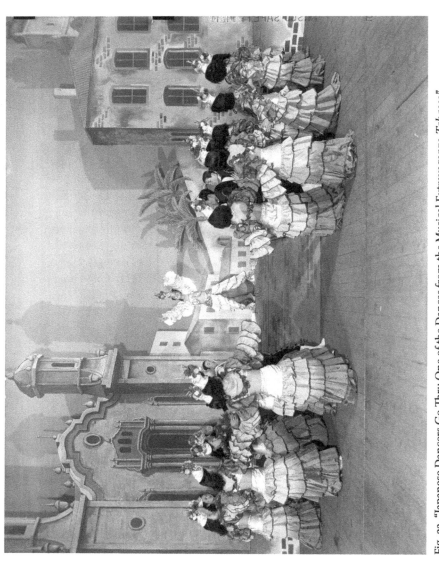

Fig. 23. "Japanese Dancers Go Thru One of the Dances from the Musical Extravaganza *Tabasco*," February 24, 1947. National Archives, photographs of American Military Activities, ca. 1918–ca. 1981.

Being Watched 233

Though the productions at the Ernie Pyle were all staged to provide a sense of pleasurable nostalgia and allure for the military spectators in the audience, Ito and the Erniettes perhaps attached other meanings to these shows. Like Ito's first experience of stage orientalism at the Imperial Theatre forty years earlier, for the Erniettes, dancing on stage in glamorous costumes and surrounded by beautifully painted sets and stage lights, the productions must have been transporting—transporting not only away from the misery of postwar Tokyo, but also *to* these far-off, dreamlike locales. Such productions offered something oddly like touristic travel, an embodied experience of possibility, a chance to imagine oneself *in* a fantasy, not simply in a dreamlike state, but as a corporeal repertoire. For Ito, too, these productions were a kind of fantasy—though no longer the kind of transporting, imaginative experiences of his early encounters with stage orientalism. Instead, these are fantasies of places Ito had lived in and visited; they are, like his postwar memoirs, projections propelled by his experiences and memories.

The fantasies Ito staged at the Ernie Pyle used the bodies of the theater's dance corps to materialize visions of Japan as culturally rich, cosmopolitan, and ready to welcome foreigners. In communicating such visions of a new Japan, Ito's choreography was effective because it was set on the gendered, raced bodies of the Erniettes, a conjunction suggestive of Anne Cheng's concept of "ornamentalism." As Cheng defines it, ornamentalism "names the peculiar processes (legally, materially, imaginatively) whereby *personhood is named or conceived through ornamental gestures*, which speak through the minute, the sartorial, the prosthetic, and the decorative."[18] That is, in Cheng's theory, ornamentalism emerges through the Asian woman's contiguity with decorative surfaces, which constitute her as a surface as well, a being at the border of objecthood and personhood. In her book, Cheng's focus is on the objects, surfaces, and bursts of light that produce her subjects at the meeting point of racial and aesthetic abstraction. But Ito's Ernie Pyle productions suggest that dance itself can serve as the ornamental prosthetic through which this kind of personhood is produced. The kick line in *Fantasy Japonica*, for instance, which in its very amateur roughness highlights the choreography as a not-entirely-seamless appendage to the body, or the shoulder shimmies in *Tabasco*, which overlay racialized indices of tropical enjoyment and female corporeality on the dancers, are both instances in which choreography acts ornamentally, to produce the dancers as subjects "whose personhood is animated, rather than eviscerated, by aesthetic congealment."[19] Though the Occupation aimed to produce democratic liberal subjects in the model of

Enlightenment ideals, Cheng's theory suggests a more complicated type of personhood was produced here. Choreographic ornamentalism might have been a way for these dancers to exist between the contradictory poles of their performances at the Ernie Pyle: the unavoidable objectification and abjection of presenting oneself as a racialized, gendered body for others' spectatorial consumption, alongside the possibility that these dance movements, shifting in geographic and generic registers, might offer a kind of prosthetic escape. In this reading, the Erniettes are not transparent liberal subjects; they are, rather, self-conscious performers of the imbrication of person and material goods on which the Occupation's claims were ultimately premised.

The Backstage on Stage

The Ernie Pyle has been thought of as off-limits to Japanese, a potent sign of exclusion in their own capitol. It is true that, with a few exceptions, Japanese spectators were not admitted to the theater. However, an extraordinary number of Japanese worked at the institution, in addition to the Erniettes. The building contained two live performance theaters, a film-screening room, a library, five restaurants, rehearsal rooms, offices for the theater's staff, and a billiards room—all of which were staffed by local Japanese workers. Due to the Occupation's policy of "blocked yen," which mandated that the reparations paid by Japan could not be spent outside of the country, the facility had a huge budget for both material and personnel. The scale of the venue meant that several thousand Japanese passed in and out of the Ernie Pyle. One document listing musicians alone includes over 800 names; another, enumerating the categories of backstage personnel (typists, boilermen, elevator operators, and so on), estimates that 178 people were required to keep the facility running on a daily basis. All of these workers were involved in producing the fantasies of a "new" Japan that materialized on the theater's stages. This work contained an odd kind of self-consciousness, one that I suggest pervaded the Occupation as a whole, and the task of rebuilding Japan under it.

At the Ernie Pyle, then, the backstage as much as the onstage was an active place of reimagining what it might mean to be Japanese in the postwar era. Considering the backstage draws attention to the hopes and attachments that Japanese workers at the Ernie Pyle invested into their activities at the theater as they created its onstage fantasies. This investment does not mean that they did not also critique it, feel cynical about it, or reject the meanings

Being Watched   235

that their superiors and the Occupation authorities assigned to the production. On the contrary, the backstage offers a way of leaving room for Japanese subjects to have conflicting feelings about the Occupation, or to assign multiple meanings to their endeavors to reconstruct themselves and their nation after the war.

A photograph of a rehearsal of *Rhapsody in Blue* might serve as a stand-in for the myriad activities carried out by workers in the building. Ito, dancing among a group of six women, is perhaps going over the choreography, checking spacing on the theater's stage, or marking the steps for lighting cues. The dancers hold an open fourth position, with torsos counterposed against hips and arms extended out, hands flipped up at the wrists. They are in costume, so this is probably a dress rehearsal. But I also take this moment as a rehearsal for the many fantasies that the production—and working at the Ernie Pyle—may have activated. For one, in addition to rehearsing the choreography, the dancers might corporeally imagine the urbanity and abundance that the production evoked and that working at the theater also provided. This was not mere illusion; working as an Erniette meant access to resources that others could only dream of: former Erniettes interviewed by Saitō Ren recalled the thrill of getting to wear the short culotte skirts that had been banned for many years, and being served hamburger at the rehearsal hall.[20] So too, the photograph might suggest Ito's own desire to remain relevant, as he marks the choreography in his casual shorts and T-shirt. Together, the group gestures toward a set of desires that remain mostly unexpressed, as they carry out the hard work of theater-making.

My reading of the backstage in this photograph, and my insistence on the multiplicity of desires it might contain, might suggest the established dyads of *soto* and *uchi* (outside and inside), *omote* and *ura* (front and behind), and *tatemae* and *honne* (public face and inner feeling). These are paired concepts that for many thinkers, building on the original work of sociologist Doi Takeo, articulate the particularity of Japanese self-conception, and how an individual relates herself to the world around her.[21] In fact, anthropologist Nancy Rosenberger has articulated *tatemae* and *honne* through the metaphor of the front-stage and backstage, which she productively multiplies into countless stages and backstages, illuminated at varying levels of consciousness and intentionality.[22] Under these paradigms, the formal performances that the Erniettes gave for Allied personnel, all smiles and welcoming choreography, would be *tatemae*, while their inner feelings about the Occupation would be *honne*; a photograph such as this one, in its almost-performance-readiness, might be read as

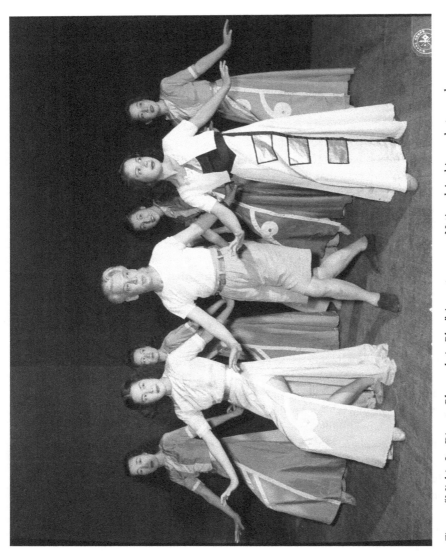

Fig. 24. "Michio Ito Directs *Rhapsody in Blue*," August 12, 1947. National Archives, photographs of American Military Activities, ca. 1918–ca. 1981.

Being Watched 237

a kind of middle state. But I am interested in the self-consciousness, not just of the performance, or of the onstage, but of the backstage as well. This is a self-awareness of being watched while going about a putatively nonperforming job, that is perhaps better evoked by the *kuroko*, the black-garbed stagehands of many forms of traditional Japanese theater who do their work in full view of the audience, within the performance's diegetic space, even as they remain to some extent "unseen." The backstage, then, is a way of thinking about Japanese subjects, at the Ernie Pyle and around the country, who were in many respects unseen, even as they were intensely watched, and deeply self-conscious of this attention. Under this odd form of scrutiny, they began to construct their own fantasies for a postwar life. While these endeavors frequently supported the grand production of "democratization and demilitarization" envisioned by SCAP, they were also part of longer lives and private meanings.

If it is useful to think about the Occupation as a kind of backstage onstage, then this peculiar self-consciousness was in no small part due to the fact that in the immediate postwar period, the Occupier's gaze was everywhere. Sometimes, this was experienced quite literally, as in the photograph of the GI spectators enjoying *Fantasy Japonica*, but more frequently this was evident in the many ways the Occupation authorities tracked their unfolding agenda, through the daily lives of Japanese throughout the country. Indeed, most of the evidence analyzed in this chapter is the result of SCAP's vast apparatus: all printed material in Japan was subject to censorship, and it is for this reason that thousands of publications—including the women's magazines for which Ito wrote numerous articles, which I will analyze in the next section—were saved, and ultimately transported to the University of Maryland to form the Gordon W. Prange Collection.[23] Likewise, the photographs were mostly taken by the US Signal Corps Photographers, whose innumerable images documented the unfolding of the Occupation in both its formal and informal moments.

In most of the photographs of Ito and the Erniettes, the subjects are looking away from the camera, as if the camera has caught them in the middle of an absorbing activity—rehearsing a dance number, socializing with each other, introducing GIs to some aspect of Japanese culture. This was probably an intentional framing, given that the Signal Corps Photographers' assignment was to unobtrusively record the effects of the Occupation on the reorganization of Japanese social and political life. The frequency of subjects looking away might also be deflection; these cameras were a form of surveillance. But to look away from the camera is not to be unaware of it, or even to ignore it.

Indeed, as the postmodern dancer/artist Yvonne Rainer insisted in a conversation about the famous averting of the dancer's gaze from that of the audience in her piece *Trio A*, avoiding eye contact is not ignoring the audience.[24] On the contrary, it is a tensely aware form of spectatorial engagement. We see in photographs of the Occupation what Carrie Lambert-Beatty describes as the "peculiar tension . . . between the body being, and being watched."[25] I want to suggest that as much as the Occupation was, for Japanese citizens, about remaking their society and themselves, in both disjunction and continuity with their wartime lives, the Occupation was also about being watched, while going about the work of being, and becoming themselves.

Being watched is a porous, kinesthetic state of being that produces a heightened self-consciousness in the act of working to appear natural. And this "peculiar tension" between being and being watched is central to understanding the working of fantasy in the Occupation. For if Japanese during this period could be said to be exploring and enacting all kinds of fantasies—of political and social freedom, of the different corporeal habits that suited those freedoms, of the various ways of reimagining what it might mean to be Japanese—then the fact that all this fantasizing, and the work of trying to inhabit these fantasies, was done while being watched, made these fantasies seem at once more real and more elusive. To have someone watch while you enact your fantasy makes it seem more real, in that spectators serve as a kind of witness, but also more illusive, because they make you aware that this might be "just" a performance, the acting out of a fantasy, without the making it so. It was this artful work of becoming oneself while being watched that Makiko discovered in the rehearsal studio, when she became aware of S—Sensei standing behind her, and that Ito taught to his dancers, students, and readers during the Occupation.

In one striking backstage photograph, the camera's subjects do meet its gaze. Ito is in a practice hall, leaning against an upright piano, his back to the camera. He is watching as a line of women, in tap character shoes and short rehearsal skirts, walk toward us, their arms swinging back and forth at a 90-degree angle. The women seem to be practicing a train formation, with their arms representing train axles, and their feet swiping the floor to create the "choo choo choo choo" sound of a train. Seen from the side, as it would be in performance, the effect is of human bodies embodying the mechanistic through precision and uniformity (and it offers yet another example of choreographic ornamentalism). But here in this rehearsal shot, we do not yet see the corporealized train; instead, our attention is on the three women whose faces can be clearly seen. The

Being Watched 239

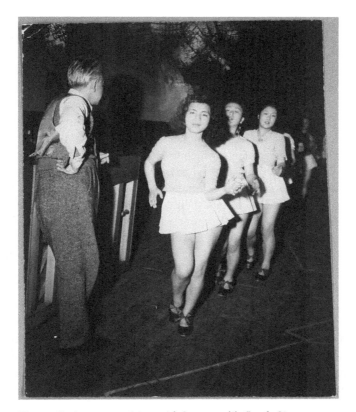

Fig. 25. Erniettes practicing with Ito, 1947 (?). Senda Koreya Collection, Tsubouchi Memorial Theatre Museum, Waseda University.

woman at the front of the line looks directly at the camera, and yet does not entirely engage it. She wears an expression of relaxed concentration, with perhaps some pride, and perhaps a hint of challenge too. This is not the face she will wear in performance, all smiles and sparkling eyes. It is assuredly still a performance, however, and a knowing arrangement of her body and face for the camera, even as she is engaged in the semiprivate work of rehearsal. Unlike Makiko, who thought herself alone, this dancer knows that the Occupation, even in its private moments, involves a sort of public awareness. It is this image, of doing the work of performing herself, while being watched, that illuminates the strange self-consciousness that was part of the Occupation's daily unfolding.

Walking into Fantasy

The photograph of the line of Erniettes contains an unavoidable theatricality. It also shows something quite mundane: women walking. Alongside his work at the Ernie Pyle, Ito expanded his choreographic pedagogy to the general public, and his prime focus was on walking as a movement practice that could provide a foundation for the remaking of individuals, and even Japanese society at large. Ito disseminated his walking tutorials in numerous articles in women's magazines, which as a prime vehicle for the reeducation of Japan's women, had returned to glossy, full-color printing long before most publications.[26] His books, such as *Etiquette*, similarly offered lessons in comportment, building on the established genre of women's edification guides that proliferated in Meiji to help women acquire the markers of middle-class status after the dismantling of the Tokugawa status system.[27]

In these tutorials, Ito offered walking—that mundane, almost unconscious activity—as the foundation for Japanese people to remake themselves after the war. As I trace in this section, in Ito's formulation, walking was not simply a practice of social engagement, but a performative mode of manifesting oneself as a liberal subject. Like the Occupation as a whole, Ito's lessons were complicated by underlying questions about who the "ideal" liberal subject is—and whether Japanese women could naturally embody such subjects. Not surprisingly, Ito also understood walking as the first step in dancing, and he positioned dancers as the people most capable of executing this corporeal renovation. Walking thus offered Ito both a concrete way to position his expertise as broadly relevant, and the chance to insist that dance—as it had been at Hellerau—was the foundational practice for remaking individuals, and society at large.

Walking is an activity that can be both mundane and virtuosic, both fundamentally unremarkable and deeply theatrical. For many people, though not all, walking is the most basic mode for moving through the world, encountering others. Walking, then, is simultaneously a form of self-mobilization and of self-presentation. Though walking might be transhistorical, in Kant, Hobbes, and other Enlightenment theorists, walking takes on significance as the preeminent manifestation of bourgeois liberal individualism, as Andrew Hewitt has traced.[28] Likewise, as Hagar Kotef delineates, as a form of mobility, walking allows individuals to take and express their freedom (they can walk anywhere); at the same time, by choosing not to go absolutely anywhere (escaping), but instead, by walking within bounds (of the state, of political

Being Watched 241

and social norms), individuals demonstrate that they are in control of themselves, and thus, the ideal "free" subjects.[29] The fantasy of this self-making embodiment is not only that it allows walkers to realize themselves as self-possessed individuals, but that their state of self-possessed freedom is manifest, evident in their gait and carriage to anyone they encounter along the way. Thus, as Hewitt observes, lessons in comportment in general, and walking in particular, make "the very condition of man ('walking on his own two feet') an aesthetic gesture, a mode of representation."[30] In these ways, walking is an embodied practice of self-making and of self-legitimation as a social subject.

Not surprisingly, Ito's model student Makiko is also interested in walking. In another section of *Etiquette*, she recounts a momentous day in the rehearsal room:

> When rehearsal had finished, S—Sensei was about to leave the room when a foreigner walked toward him briskly. Since the middle of practice, this blond, beautiful person had been standing in a corner of the rehearsal room. The woman was talking rapidly, saying who knows what, and suddenly stretched out her hand and shook Sensei's hand. Then they continued their conversation for a while, and with sensei leading the way, the woman's figure disappeared from the rehearsal room.
>
> For these moments, not more than two minutes, I drank in that woman's every single move as if possessed. It wasn't just me, there was total and utter silence as everyone in the rehearsal room observed her.
>
> What an incredible woman![31]

The next time Makiko and the other students see S—Sensei, they ask who this stunning woman is, and learn she is one of S—Sensei's students, just arrived from Hollywood. Makiko feels like she has solved a piece of the mystery: "The way one could feel the whole movements of her body, that was just as you'd expect from someone trained in dancing!"[32] Inspired to emulate the woman's way of moving, they take turns guessing at the foundations of her elegant movement: "Lack of bashfulness?" "Having confidence?" "A wealthy lifestyle?" Ito surprises them with the simplicity of the secret: walking. "Sure enough," thinks Makiko, "perhaps that is it; it was her way of walking that first fascinated us."[33]

Makiko's enthralling encounter with this blond American woman fixates on the way the woman talks, shakes hands, engages with their teacher, and most importantly, walks. Walking figures in this anecdote as a self-making, revelatory behavior; this woman's walking, above all else, is what manifests her as a confident, beautiful, self-possessed individual. Ito's vision of walking is thus in line with the "epistemology of walking" that Hewitt traces through Western theorizations of liberal subjectivity. Indeed, here, walking is such a force for enacting a legible self-possession that the woman is not only in control of herself, but has "possessed" (*tsukareru*) Makiko as well. We might read this as suggesting that if one is not in full possession of oneself, one is at risk of being possessed by others—through desire, not necessarily to *have* the other, but to *be* her, a desire so overwhelming as to cause one to lose oneself. In this moment of loss of self in the encounter with another's self-possession, we see one of the ways in which the Occupation at times produced conditions of racial mimesis and abjection that, as Karen Shimakawa has delineated, have been understood both as a part of Asian American subjectivity and as constitutive of legal and cultural Americanness.[34] Shimakawa's paradigm applies to this scene precisely because of the aspects of imperial racialization that structured the US-led Occupation, in ways that resembled US racial logic "at home." At the moment when Makiko gazes on the blond American woman as an object of desire, she is also painfully reminded of the fantasy-status of assimilation—always to be pursued, always left incomplete.

But as much as Ito's lessons may have aligned with Occupation authorities' program to remake Japan through a process of partial "Americanization," I think Ito was actually after a different kind of fantasy: Japaneseness. "Japan," as an unstable but nearly always desirable image, was the cornerstone of Ito's career and production of himself. He sought, in his walking tutorials, to delineate a mode of bodily presentation that, certainly, would suit the era's ideological calls for democratization and Westernization, but that would nevertheless specifically fit Japan and the construction of a new vision of "Japan-ness," one that could continue to fuel the many fantasies that relied on this shifting national imaginary.

Ito's instructions, though they resemble much of the discourse pressed on Japanese women during the Occupation, are also striking for their insistence that dance—that is, modern dance—was the key to a new kind of embodiment, and thus a new kind of social attitude. As we saw, Makiko is no longer mystified by the elegant woman once she understands that this striking figure is a dancer. "*Sasuga*," Makiko thinks—"Just as you'd expect." Ito's insistence on dance as a mode of physical renovation might well be understood as an intervention in one of the central discourses of the Occupation era: *nikutai*. Literally "meat body," the word connotes the physical body, its flesh. As Douglas

Being Watched

Slaymaker explains, the concept of *nikutai* registered on several semantic levels at once: it highlighted the immediate corporeal needs (starvation, injury) that occupied so much attention; it operated in contrast to the nonphysical or spiritual; and it emphatically differed from the ideology of *kokutai* (the body politic or national body—see chapter 4) that had been a dominant paradigm during the war.[35] Across all these registers, Japanese society was permeated with "the widespread notion that the fleshly body provided the gateway to liberation and authentic subjectivity."[36] This notion was, as the omnipresent figure of the *panpan* girl—the Occupation era's streetwalker—suggests, frequently imagined via a female figure.[37] But, as Michael Bourdaghs, among others, has noted, there was also strong pushback against this fleshly glorification, from critics such as Maruyama Masao and artists such as Kurosawa Akira, who instead argued for an embrace of rationality and spirituality. Ito offered a different approach to this new culture of the body. For while he emphatically believed that the physical body could provide access to liberation and subjectivity, such expressiveness could not be achieved through total corporeal release and abandonment. Rather, as his own education at Hellerau had required, corporeal liberty and the artistic remaking of the self would involve intense, precise bodily practice. For Ito, then, the body was not something to be feared, but neither could it be allowed undisciplined free rein. Instead, the body was a tool that required intentional training and a belief in its signifying capabilities, and dance was the surest way to experience this new bodily regime.

At their most fundamental, Ito's lessons in walking were lessons in dancing. In *Etiquette*, Ito advanced a distinction between inattentive walking and walking with intentionality. When one walks without thinking about it, according to Ito, the heel comes down first, followed by the toe. By contrast, when one walks with intentionality, the toe precedes the heel. As Ito writes, "Toe—Heel, toe—heel. In other words, the same as walking in dance."[38] Ito goes on to explain that if one walks with heels first, one cannot quickly come to a stop, but if one walks with toes first, one can immediately and smoothly stop as needed. That is, if one walks with toes first, as a dancer does, one is always ready. Dance—and walking as a dancerly movement—is therefore a practice of corporeal readiness.[39] The dancer, in Ito's characterization, is a person who can quickly read the world and respond to it. The dancer, then, is very much the embodiment of an ideal of cosmopolitan openness that aligned with the Occupation's stated aims of reform.

Ito's focus on walking as the behavior through which Japanese women could retrain themselves for the new postwar era involved not simply a corporeal mimesis, but an absorption—through embodied practice—of the ideologies of liberal individualism and free consumerism that the Occupation aimed to inculcate. For example, in the June 1946 issue of *Style*, in an article titled "How to Walk Beautifully," Ito offered the following lesson: the body should form a triangle; the shoulders should be aligned as a level base, with the rest of the body narrowing to the triangle's point at the feet.[40] To achieve this triangular shape, one must walk along a single line, one foot placed in front of the other. The outcome of walking in this way, Ito suggested, would be a wholesale remaking of the body, and thus of the self: by broadening out her shoulders, for instance, a woman would necessarily open herself to the world. Likewise, by walking with one foot in front of the other along a single line, the torso rotates from one side to the other; consequently, the woman by default greets others with a sense of expansive self-possession. Walking thus becomes the key to corporeal renovation. As a repetitive activity necessary to daily life, it can retrain the body into a different posture, and, as a result of that posture, a different attitude and a different way of interacting with the world.

Although Ito's lesson implicitly connects particular modes of comportment with particular societies—that is, being confident and open to the world is framed as common to a Western, or American, attitude—Ito does not end in a confirmation of cultural essentialism. According to Ito, it is the kimono that encourages a slumped, rectangular posture, in which women move with small, quick steps from the knees, following two lines with their feet, instead of one. As he argues, this is a posture that is appropriate for the kimono, but unsuitable for Western fashions. Walking and clothing, then, go hand in hand, and a change in fashion requires a change in bodily comportment. Ito thus creates a sense of naturalistic fallacy—but also of mutability: the Japanese woman is not destined to walk in a timid, retiring way, but has simply been shaped by her clothing. Once she casts off her kimono in favor of the modern suit, her body will naturally fall into a different shape, and as she moves, her body will naturally take on the confidence and self-possession that, Ito argues, is inherent to the mode of walking he teaches.

It is worth noting that, like much in the Occupation, while Ito's mode of walking was announced as "new," Western fashions and the walking that supposedly suited those styles had been part of many Japanese women's repertoire for decades. What was significant, however, was what this corporeal renovation could be taken to mean: a rejection of the period of authoritari-

Being Watched 245

anism and restricted gender roles, a reappearance (and update) of the Taisho era's modern girl, and an embrace of international trends. This shift was alluring precisely because it remained out of reach for so many women, even after the war. The wartime *monpe* (loose work trousers) that had been required by the state were still common; women otherwise wore adapted military surplus that had made its way from the occupying troops to domestic markets, or secondhand clothing donated by American churches.[41] In the early postwar years, then, Ito's lessons were as much a set of sketches for a corporeal fantasy as they were concrete physical tutorials.

Ito's lessons in walking asserted that the individual emerges as a free, liberal subject through quotidian movement. In this, he echoed the Enlightenment philosophers who also took walking as a figuration of modern personhood, because, as such a fundamental, "natural" form of movement, it has the power to naturalize whatever social and political meanings are ascribed to it. It is thus that free, liberal subjecthood comes to appear as a natural state, rather than as a politically constructed and contingent position, available only to some humans and not others. And it is as such a naturalized but revelatory activity that walking serves as an example of Ju Yon Kim's theorization of the "racial mundane." As Kim argues, within US racial logic, the mundane often serves as the site of racialization, when seemingly familiar behaviors are received as foreign.[42] The mundane becomes both a way of measuring distance from the unmarked racial norm of whiteness, and a potential method of "reprogramming" the foreign into the familiar or assimilated. Ito's lessons in walking highlighted how such a simple activity could simultaneously serve as a site of racialization, but also of assimilation via the intentional changes in posture and gait that he prescribed. And under the conditions of the Occupation, these mundane changes were attributed the power to change the status of Japan on the world stage.

But the tension inherent in what, exactly, the mundane reveals about race is also its source of ambiguity. As Kim writes, the mundane "is enacted *by* the body, but may or may not be *of* the body."[43] If women did adopt this new mode of walking, and to whatever degree, we might think of it as just this kind of theatrical performance, where we can never precisely identify the boundary between actor and role, between naturalized embodiment and citational enactment. Ito's instructions in walking held in tension the promise and problem of the mundane: as tutorials that could transform behavior, they held the promise of offering assimilation—if not into whiteness, then into the purportedly universal category of the individual liberal subject, imagined by

Enlightenment thinkers and very much espoused by Occupation authorities. At the same time, if it were something learnable rather than innate, then it was possible for it to be a "mere" performance. This is a dynamic that has haunted Western Euro-America's relationship with Japan since its whirlwind process of modernization/Westernization during the Meiji era.[44] The racial mundane thus throws into question the supposed performativity of walking and its promise to manifest the walker as a free political subject, even as it nevertheless offers a form of intentional engagement with the body, and the tantalizing possibility of remaking the self.

• • •

The ways in which Ito's tutorials might have produced knowledge and prompted movement are untraceable. Some students, perhaps, simply sat and were content to imagine themselves carrying out this movement. Some, I imagine, practiced Ito's tutorials in the privacy of their own homes, or on an empty street where they hoped no one would see them. And some, I like to think, boldly tried out these postures on the busiest thoroughfares and in the sensorium of newly reopened department stores. In all of these possibilities, Ito's magazine articles offered the promise of potentiality and the pleasure of reimagining oneself. Crucially, this was a reimagining rooted in the body, and in a kinesthetic awareness of oneself as a body. Ito's lessons in walking, then, suggest that fantasy is more than, or not only, an act of imagination taking place within one's mind. Fantasy can also be the acts of imagination that take place within the body, not as a reflection or acting-out of mental-psychological-emotional states, but as corporeal expressivity. The body itself can fantasize, in the stretching out of limbs in unexpected directions, in the pivoting of the torso in a more expansive manner, in the arching of the neck and swiveling of the head to encompass a new gaze.

And perhaps a few of the women who read Ito's tutorials showed up at the audition for Ito's three-month actor and model training course; the first recruitment session in 1953 received 1,500 applications, from which Ito and his colleagues chose 88. Ito turned to the fashion industry as the Occupation closed; it was a resource-rich industry, in which his lifetime of physical training and teaching experience could be offered as a foundation on which to develop Japan as a center of high fashion. In 1951 and 1952, he served as a judge for the Tina Leser competition for Japanese designers, an event sponsored by the American sportswear designer best known for her use of Hawaiian textiles and her introduction of sarong- and dhoti-inspired "at home" clothes. In

Being Watched 247

1953, Ito began work with the newly founded Sumire Model Group, one of the earliest organizations specializing in fashion floor shows. Over the following years, Ito directed and served as fashion show advisor for foreign designers such as Christian Dior and Howard Greer, as well as for Japanese companies such as the textile firm Toyobo and for various iterations of the Miss Universe pageant.[45] Fashion modeling, though perhaps an unexpected turn in his career, is an almost obvious outcome of his postwar interest in instructing women in modes of walking and bodily comportment through the principles of modern dance. The fashion runway, after all, lies somewhere between the explicit theatricality of the proscenium stage and the apparent ordinariness of everyday walking, and (high) fashion is, among other things, the aestheticization of the mundane necessity of wearing clothing.[46] The end of the Occupation overlapped with the start of the Korean War. The US's ability to declare the Occupation successfully concluded was in no small degree based on the sense that Japan had been successfully reconstructed as a capitalist nation, and could be relied on as an anticommunist base in the Pacific. In this register, Ito's interest in the world of fashion not only reiterates his always-present desire to seek out well-funded projects, but, as an industry particularly tuned to capitalist production and consumption, it marks Ito's understanding of the political milieu of 1950s Japan.

A photograph from 1954 shows Ito, seated at a table at the end of a rehearsal hall, evaluating potential students for his course. A woman, #38, dressed in a swimsuit and white pumps, with glinting earrings and a watch, moves toward us, away from the table. She is exhibiting her walk for the judges, and in the process, exhibiting her ability to display clothing, to present herself as a consumer subject who might inspire other consumer subjects; she is exhibiting her ability to make the body look natural even as it performs in a highly theatrical manner. This is walking, as Ito taught it, and even, in her poise, her self-consciousness, her aestheticized presentation of self, this is walking as the Enlightenment theorists might have meant it. That is, this woman's mode of walking is intended as a legible, self-making gesture. And yet, perhaps because of the slightly downward cast of her face, with its impassive expression, or perhaps because of the way this scene so explicitly stages female display for the male gaze, it is hard to take this photograph as evidence that the Occupation produced female "freedom"—even as it, assuredly, does represent certain kinds of freedom.

SanSan Kwan has offered the figure of the flâneuse as a feminist rejoinder to the flâneur, that male walker of the city who takes in the urban space

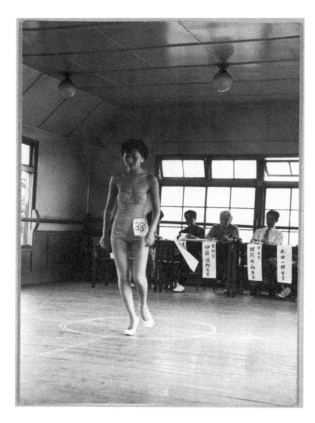

Fig. 26. Ito pro model first-round auditions, August 1954, at the Kakinokizaka Institute, Jack K. Ohi. Senda Koreya Collection, Tsubouchi Memorial Theatre Museum, Waseda University.

through his gaze and physical occupation of its spaces. Kwan writes, "While the flâneur relies on his sense of sight as a kind of mastering, objectifying gaze, the flâneuse instead gathers her information through the body.... The flâneuse is, for me, an ideal dance researcher—kinesthetically aware, self-reflectively analytic."[47] Kwan takes the figure of the flâneuse as a model for her own walks through Chinese urban spaces, offering a methodology of producing knowledge and a sense of embeddedness through visceral experience. Bounded by the studio's walls, the woman in this photograph does not appear as this kind of flâneuse. But it is possible to imagine her kinesthetic experience of this space, and how her kinesthetic awareness constructs a deep knowledge of the possibilities—and limitations—that this room holds.

She must hear the taps of her heels on the wood floor, the kind of personal sound that seems to fill space with its volume. The fresh air coming

through the open windows mingles with cigarette smoke; it must also produce goosebumps on her skin, making her even more aware of her skin's
bareness, in contrast to the fully clothed judges sitting behind her. Kinesthesia, the sensing of other bodies and the production of a knowledge of space
through that co-sensing of presence, is often understood as an empathetic
form of relationality—one that Kwan cautions us about. Indeed, though this
woman surely, overwhelmingly senses the presence of the other people in
the room, this is not a kinesthesia of empathy, of feeling with each other.
Rather, in sensing the bodies around her, and the tense, unequal relationship
between herself and them, she assembles knowledge of her own position, of
the opportunities that this measured walk through the studio seems to promise, as well as its limitations. I imagine that she can feel them behind her, she
can feel the space in the room open up as she moves farther away, and as this
space grows, she can feel her own body, small and discrete in the open space
of the studio.

This is a woman who assuredly has made walking into a fulfillment of
Hewitt's gloss, "an aesthetic gesture, a mode of representation," but she has
also, in the process, rendered herself into a kind of aesthetic object. The
promise of walking as a performative manifestation of liberal subjectivity
here collides with the material conditions of being a gendered, raced body,
and returns us to Anne Cheng's ornamentalism. Modeling extends my earlier comments on choreographic ornamentalism, because it involves a curious form of embodiment, where the model is supposed to disappear into
the impersonality of a mannequin, and yet retain something of liveness and
of individuality, to allow the potential consumer to impose herself on the
model and into the clothing she wears. Modeling is, then, a mode of self-
presentation as self-objectification, and a kind of abstraction of the self, a
"disappearance into appearance."[48] Moreover, if modeling can be taken as a
certain form of dance, then this photograph makes clear that there is nothing
inherently liberatory in dance; it neither distracts from the fleshly body nor
offers some kind of insight or interiority.

But if this woman's walk is an instance of ornamentalism, it is also an
instance of fantasy—and not simply because modeling is intended to sell consumers some kind of fantasy, or because her dream of becoming a glamorous
model is, perhaps, illusory. Rather, it is fantasy in the sense that I have tried
to offer in this book: a self-conscious performance of self that allows an individual to survive, and to construct a sense of continuity across life's ruptures.
After growing up under the war and then the Occupation, for this young

woman, the very circumstance of auditioning to be a model must have felt improbable. For her, it is perhaps this walk—both mundane and aesthetic—that allows her to continue to make herself, in the body she's always had.

Ito, like the Enlightenment philosophers and like so many of his modern dance peers, wanted to believe in the honesty of corporeal expression, in some kind of fundamental truthfulness to be found in dance. His obsession with comportment, and with etiquette, during the Occupation and the final decades of his career was a manifestation of his desire for the body to work as an unmediated register of the self. In a chapter of *Etiquette* titled "Form and Spirit" (*kata to kokoro*), he writes:

> The rules of etiquette [are intended] to express in outward form the idea of inner respect.
>
> Speaking solely from this point of view, [the rules of etiquette share a] path with artistic expression. The artist especially must not intentionally debase or deceive himself. He dearly wishes to re-extend his true feelings accurately to the world of beauty and to the world of ideas. I wish for the rules of etiquette to be such workings of the heart.
>
> Originally, in what was called etiquette, the externally appearing form, accepted by numerous people, became a kind of agreement. And of course, most people quickly learn the form of that promise, but in that condition lose their inner feeling. . . .[49]

This passage is, in many ways, a reworking of old Confucian principles, repackaged as a new prescription for corporeal sincerity appropriate for the new era. But in his insistence that movement not be conventionalized, or emptied of meaning, we see the persistence of Ito's own fantasy, of dance as a form of self-realization.

If Ito's fantasy of his choreography was of dance as honest self-expression, it was nevertheless, and especially as he taught it to young Japanese and Japanese American women, in Japan and in the US, a repertoire of persistence. In another photograph, Ito coaches a woman who stands on a dais before a group of thirty of her peers. With her right hand resting on her hip, the left arm reaches down and away from her body in a gentle point. Her feet are arranged in a seemingly casual third position—ladylike, but ready to move. The women behind her hold similar poses, though most of them have their left arm bent up in a suspended gesture of indication. In these poses, we might trace residues of the Delsarte system, some of which Ito certainly

Being Watched

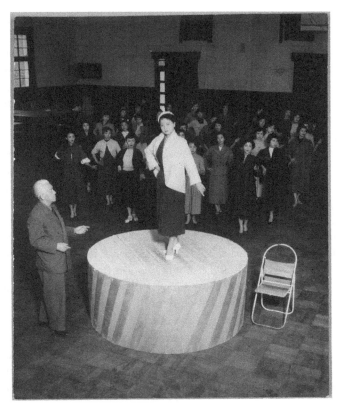

Fig. 27. "Sumire Models First-Generation Training." Senda Koreya Collection, Tsubouchi Memorial Theatre Museum, Waseda University.

absorbed in Germany and the US, and which had also been incorporated into physical education regimens in Japan.[50] As Hewitt writes, Delsarte's system of gestural expression had been so popular with the bourgeoisie in Europe and the US because his gestures appeared to "naturally" represent, in the language of the body, a person's inner state.[51] These women's poses, then, in all their stiff formality, might be read as both a manifestation of the bourgeois leisure class that fashion modeling often aims to evoke (and the Occupation's promise of that economic vision), and also of Ito's dream that movement be honest and meaningful.

But this photograph also reminds us that while fantasy may appear to be something deeply private, it is, in fact, always about the individual in relation to others, and the spectatorial awareness that engenders that relationality. In addition to the interpretations of walking already considered here, Marié Abe provides one more, in her study of *chindon-ya*. It is this paradigm that perhaps offers ground between the ideology of dance as honest manifestation of the self, and the congealment of selfhood within objectification. *Chindon-ya* are troupes of street musicians who advertise for a local business or sponsor by parading through the city. As Abe argues, key to the *chindon-ya*'s magnetism is the practice of walking—*horyū*—in which questions of pace, of footwork, of length of stride become not only the foundation for the troupe's artistic appeal (and capacity to walk for hours), but also the basis for the performers' ability to create connection among themselves and the many listeners they encounter along the way. Abe shares details from a *horyū* workshop she attended in which Hayashi Kōjirō, the leader of the prominent troupe Chindon Tsūshinsha, advised participants to "be conscious of people's gazes. . . . No one should feel ignored. On the street, too, you need to make them aware that you're watching them, even with your back and with your butt. Express, through your whole body, that you're being seen, and that you're seeing them."[52] The lesson is humorous; the fuller quotation includes an analogy with a nightclub hostess, whose performance of attentiveness has clear parallels with Ito's various students. But what is instructive here is the notion of walking as a way of moving the body into relationality with those around you, through the self-consciousness that movement can engender.

For Ito, too, I think watching and being watched were not merely ocular but corporeal practices of fantasy-making as self-performance. And it was in this practice of self-conscious seeing that Ito taught his students to form—both materially and imaginatively—a possible postwar world. During the Occupation and its aftermath, Ito taught dance as a way to reimagine the self, in service of reimagining a postwar Japan. From the Erniettes on stage, whose ebullient dancing vivified the fantasy of postwar prosperity, to his walking tutorials, which imagined mundane self-presentation as the foundation of the self-possessed liberal subject, as well as in his modeling lessons, in which the kinesthetic sense of being watched—so often a source of profound alienation—could also be made into a form of relationality, Ito wove his own fantasies into a greater historical fabric. Perhaps his abiding desire to achieve historical significance was, in the end, what allowed his many lessons, and his own example, to be remembered in bodily traces that persist today.

Conclusion

Ito died of a brain hemorrhage in 1961, in the midst of preparing for the 1964 Tokyo Olympics. His death brought to a close his choreographic and theatrical inventions, his utopic opportunism, and, seemingly, the fantasies that propelled him through his life. But fantasies sometimes live on beyond those who initiated them. As I have explored, Ito's fantasies took many different shapes: invented anecdotes, unrealized projects, socio-political affiliations, and dance-making itself—and all of these were central to Ito's performance of self, and the fantasies that sustained him. Across two World Wars, and experiences of racialization, internment, and imperialism, these fantasies persisted, even as they shifted and transformed to accommodate each historical moment. For instance, the fantasy of Ito as an object of desire bound up in both Western and Japanese orientalism, that was so resonant in London and New York, transformed to Ito as cultural diplomat in California, as he aged and as the relationship between Japan and the US deteriorated. Likewise, the fantasies of "Japan" to which he was so closely tied shifted across his career, as a mounting accrual of associations. The pervasive notion of Japan as a land of aesthetic supremacy, for example, did not disappear as Japan's imperialist visions took hold, but rather, became a layer upon which Ito, like many others, could imagine Japan's imperialism as a force of cultural Pan-Asianism. Again, after the war, even as these fantasies were repudiated, they became the ground for a vision of Japan as a peaceful, cosmopolitan, modern nation. Across all these fantasies, Ito's desire to be at the center remained. However, his belief in art as a force by which he could mediate between cultures and nations, though he never relinquished it, was profoundly diminished by his experiences during the war. Although his death might seem like the stopping point for a narrative of Ito's career, his story (like the ones he loved to tell) doesn't quite end there. Ito's legacy—the ways his dance practice and story have influenced subsequent generations—stretches on, as do his fantasies.

In dance history, it is useful to think of a person's dance descendants—the lineage of dancers who carry on a choreographer's method and repertoire in their bodies, constituting a chain of corporeal transmission. Ito's primary dance descendants are concentrated in Japan and the US. The effort to reconstitute Ito's body of work after his death involved oceanic crossings and combining different threads in a way that very much resembled the patterns of Ito's own life.

In 1977, one of Ito's dancers in Southern California, Helen Caldwell, pieced together an early biography of him, using materials she had from her own collection, Toyo Miyatake's photographs, and the stories she recalled Ito telling in the 1930s. This book represented an assertion of Ito's place in American modern dance, providing readers with a wealth of photographs, appendices of Ito's works, and Caldwell's own reports of the sensorial and imagistic associations that she learned for many of Ito's dances. Meanwhile, in Japan, Ito's protégé Maki Ryūko had taken on leadership of the studio at the time of his death, and she continued to teach his technique and his dances to new students. Imura Kyoko, another of Ito's final students, oversaw the Michio Ito Alumni Association, which she has run, along with her student Komine Kumiko. As the designated living repository of Ito's works, Maki trained many dancers, including Satoru Shimazaki, who in the late 1970s traveled to the US to study American forms of modern dance. In New York, Shimazaki offered master classes in Ito's technique, and mounted several concerts that presented both his own and Ito's choreography, thereby offering a vivid (re-)introduction of Ito to the public.[1] While in the US, Shimazaki also taught at Washington University in St. Louis for a few years, and there, he met Mary-Jean Cowell, who became a crucial partner in establishing Ito's legacy. Cowell, who trained as both a dancer and as a PhD in Japanese literature, learned Ito's technique and pieces from his repertoire from Shimazaki, and in 1994, wrote with Shimazaki "East and West in the Work of Michio Ito," which began to critically engage with Ito's career from a scholarly perspective.[2] Through subsequent articles, ongoing workshops in his technique, and numerous lectures in the US and Japan, Cowell has continued to establish Ito's importance to dance history. Her forthcoming biography, written for a wide audience, ensures that his story will reach those beyond the circles of dancers and scholars who have already been engaged by him.

The narrative above is one thread of Ito's legacy, that begins in Japan with his death, and crosses back over to the US. Another thread begins with Ito's Japanese American students in Los Angeles in the 1930s, through the period of their own incarceration at WRA centers during the war, and after, as they

Conclusion   255

pieced together their lives and in many cases became important figures for the reconstitution of the Los Angeles Little Tokyo community. In 1988, a young Korean American student in the dance program at the University of New Mexico walked the halls with his hair cut in a bob; a professor there, Dr. Judith Bennahum, was struck by the resemblance and told him he should do some research on Ito.[3] And so Dana Tai Soon Burgess found Helen Caldwell's biography and became determined to learn some of Ito's repertoire and carry on his legacy as an Asian American choreographer. After graduation, Burgess moved to Washington, DC, where he became connected to Lily Arikawa Okura, one of Ito's Los Angeles dancers, and to Michiko Yoshimura Kitsmiller, who had trained with Ito in Japan; he soon also connected with Shimazaki. These three different living repositories of Ito's method taught to Burgess and his dance company Ito's technique and some of his repertoire. Burgess continues to perform these pieces and to advocate, in his dancing, his writing, and his outreach from his position as the Smithsonian's choreographer-in-residence, for the artistic and sociopolitical significance of his own work as an Asian American choreographer, and of the larger field of Asian American dance-making.

In Burgess's story, we see a version of how Ito, both during his life and afterward, has served as an anchor for others to articulate aspects of their own self-becoming. For Burgess, Ito represents a figure for the fantasy of social justice and Asian American belonging—and, as has been the case throughout this book, by "fantasy" I do not mean an illusion or utopian hope, but rather a focal point for the affiliative identities that bind an individual to the world in which they live. We see this in Burgess's writings on Ito—for example, in his discussion of performing *Pizzicati*: "Whenever I perform *Pizzicati*, I experience a feeling akin to entering battle. [. . .] I am able to dance choreography that represents how I look and feel, that portrays me as strong and that was created by a like-minded artist who also shared my deep sense of 'otherness.'"[4] Burgess's articulation of what dancing *Pizzicati* means to him is suggestive of how, even in his afterlife, Ito is a figure through whom others can articulate their deepest, sustaining desires. As I asserted in the introduction, fantasy is different from escapism, because fantasy is grounded in a fundamental belief in its possibility. This, I think, is why Ito has become such a key fantasy for subsequent generations of Asian American dancers. His career, in real ways, set the conditions for a different set of possibilities to be realized.

Like Burgess, Bonnie Oda Homsey is a dancer (and now director of the Los Angeles Dance Foundation and cofounder of its American Repertory Dance

Company [ARDC]) who found in Ito a missing piece of history.[5] Trained at Julliard and then having worked as a principal dancer in Martha Graham's company, when she finally encountered Ito's story from Karoun Tootikian, the director of the Ruth St. Denis Foundation, Homsey wondered how Ito had been missing from her education. This absence prompted her to reconstruct six of Ito's dances for the ARDC, and to direct a documentary about his life, *Michio Ito, Pioneering Dancer-Choreographer*.[6] Meanwhile, interdisciplinary performance artist Denise Uyehara, whose great-aunt danced with Ito in Los Angeles and then later became a nightclub dancer, has taken Ito as a figuration of the exoticization of Asian and Asian diasporic people in America in her collaboration with Indonesian dancer Sri Susilowati, *Pageantry*.[7] For many dancers, then, especially those who identify as Japanese American or Asian American, Ito has become a resonant figure who stands as a kind of ancestor, a troubled and troublesome forerunner, an historic inspiration, and a foil for their own negotiations of working as artists in the US.

In addition to those dancers who trace direct choreographic lineages from Ito, many who studied with him or with his students have incorporated aspects of Ito's practice into other threads of modern and contemporary dance. Pulling on these threads leads us to other moments and major figures in dance history—Luigi, Pauline Koner, Waldeen, Lester Horton, Alvin Ailey. Ito's traces run through many repertoires.

If Ito's dance descendants have sustained Ito's repertoire in their bodies, his familial descendants have been central to these endeavors of reconstruction and to assisting scholars, choreographers, and artists to engage with Ito's life. For example, when Homsey sought to reconstruct pieces from Ito's repertoire, the work of setting the pieces on the ARDC dancers was done by Taeko Furushō, Ito's niece (and daughter of Michio's eldest sister, Yoshiko, and her husband Furushō Motō, the army general who had looked after Ito when he first arrived in Germany). Likewise, music for the film was provided by Teiji Ito, son of Michio's brother Yūji and his wife, Teiko. Above all, Ito's granddaughter, Michele Ito, has been a resource, a keeper of records, and in many respects, a guardian of Ito's legacy. As she observed of her work creating the Michio Ito Foundation: "I thought it was important for somebody to have a little control over what was being handed down to new dancers. That was really the crux of why the foundation exists, to save the dances, the surviving dances, and to make sure that they get handed down, as best as they could."[8]

Across the work of these many descendants, there now exists a body of reconstructed pieces from Ito's repertoire that work alongside the written

Conclusion

documents in his archive to provide points of access to his choreography and career. These re-performances, or reenactments, in particular, can be understood as one more nuance of my use of the term "fantasy." As André Lepecki has argued, dance reenactments can be understood as performances that "unlock, release, and actualize a work's many (virtual) com- and incompossibilities, which the originating instantiation of the work kept in reserve, virtually."[9] Dance reenactments are opportunities to explore—and for spectators to see materialized—the multiple desires that a dance can contain, not all of which are given expression in its earlier showings, even by its "originator." Ito's dances act as fantasies for his many descendants precisely because they hold room for the expression of possibilities that Ito himself may have only limned, and of new possibilities that these dancers hold for themselves.

Across the stories, images, and dances of Ito's life, fantasy was, for Ito, a way of performing himself as an object of desire—for himself and others—through constant oscillations of watching, and being watched, and watching himself being watched. As I have offered at various moments, for many theorists building on the work of Laplanche and Pontalis (including myself), fantasy has been crucially defined as a scene of desire that the fantasizer projects themself into, and effectively spectates, as the possibilities allowed for in this scene unfold. This projection is almost always understood as ocular, and indeed, my own use of "watching" follows that figuration. But the watching I am thinking of, the deep self-consciousness of feeling oneself in a theatrical setting, is corporeal. It is this sense of kinesthetic "watching" or awareness that I have articulated as the body itself fantasizing. By performing himself as an object of desire, above all, *for himself,* Ito sustained a sense of his own meaningfulness, a desire that became persistence, and perhaps, his very ability to survive.

Ito's fantasies, especially the unrealized artistic projects and utopian political affiliations, also tell us something about how his larger world worked. It is a cornerstone of theater, dance, and performance studies that bodies not only hold memories, collective and individual, but they can also manifest history itself, in gestural movement, in surrogated affect, in the ways they are read by others. I have sought to argue in this book that Ito's fantasies are similar vessels of historical events. His plan for the Philippines "independence" mass pageant, for instance, is extraordinary only for how representative it actually was, of Japanese artists' involvement in the imperial war effort, of the dream of Pan-Asianism, of Japanese imperialism's appeal to numerous individuals' personal aspirations, and of the belief that art could simultaneously chart history—and make it. Ito's fantasies are important because across a lifetime that encompassed two world wars, virulent forms of racialization, and the violently shifting borders of nations and empires, they suggest how innumerable individuals charted lives in some intimate mix of survival and personal desire.

At a remove from that historic period, the echoes of Ito's fantasies that surface most readily are those most obviously connected to empowering histories of modern dance, of community formation, of aesthetic and choreographic innovation. But Ito's fantasies were formed within, and by, the circumstances of his world: his utopic fantasies of embodied diplomacy emerge alongside the fantasy of a Japanese imperial cosmopolitanism; and his fantasies of a new corporeality, for Nisei girls and for postwar Japanese women, emerge alongside fantasies of US hegemony in the Pacific. That is, as much as Ito's fantasies sustained *him*, they also, in ways both mundane and spectacular, sustained fantasies of imperialism, racialization, and nationalism. Fantasy, after all, is licentious; its apparent—and sustaining—flights are ultimately what bind each of us to this very world. Fantasy entangles—Ito with his world, and us, perhaps, with him.

NOTES

Introduction

1. Waseda University, Tsubouchi Memorial Theatre Museum, Senda Koreya Archive, J24 #6, 7.

2. Oguma Eiji, *A Genealogy of "Japanese" Self-Images*, trans. David Askew (Melbourne: Trans Pacific Press, 2002), 3–15.

3. See William LaFleur, "A Turning in Taishō: Asia and Europe in the Early Writings of Watsuji Tetsurō," in *Culture and Identity: Japanese Intellectuals during the Interwar Years*, ed. Thomas J. Rimer (Princeton: Princeton University Press, 1990); Stefan Tanaka, "Imaging History: Inscribing Belief in the Nation," *Journal of Asian Studies* 53, no. 1 (Feb. 1994).

4. Okakura Kakuzō, *Ideals of the East: With Special Reference to the Art of Japan* (London: J. Murray, 1903, reprint, Tokyo: Charles E. Tuttle, 1970), 7–8.

5. Sandra Collins, *The 1940 Tokyo Games: The Missing Olympics* (New York: Routledge, 2007), 126.

6. Fujita Fujio, *Itō Michio, sekai wo mau* [Itō Michio, dancing through the world] (Tokyo: Musashino Shobō, 1992), 293.

7. Helen Caldwell, *Michio Ito: The Dancer and His Dances* (Berkeley: University of California Press, 1977); Mary-Jean Cowell and Satoru Shimazaki, "East and West in the Work of Michio Ito," *Dance Research Journal* 26, no. 2 (Autumn 1994); Carrie J. Preston, *Learning to Kneel: Noh, Modernism, and Journeys in Teaching* (New York: Columbia University Press, 2016); Kevin Riordan, "Performance in the Wartime Archive: Michio Ito at the Alien Enemy Hearing Board," *American Studies* 55/56, no. 4/1 (2017); Yutian Wong, "Artistic Utopias: Michio Ito and the Trope of the International," in *Worlding Dance*, ed. Susan Leigh Foster (New York: Palgrave Macmillan, 2009); Carol Fisher Sorgenfrei, "Strategic Unweaving: Itō Michio and the Diasporic Dancing Body," in *Politics of Interweaving Performance Cultures: Beyond Postcolonialism*, ed. Erika Fischer-Lichte, Torsten Jost, and Saskya Iris Jain (London: Routledge, 2014); Takeishi Midori, *Japanese Elements in Michio Ito's Early Period: 1915–1924: Meetings of East and West in the Collaborative Works*, ed. David Pacun (Tokyo: Gendai tosho, 2006); Yagishita Emi, "Itō Michio no amerika ni okeru buyō katsudō: rosanzerusu de no katsudō wo chūshin ni" [Itō Michio's dance activities in America: focusing on his activities in Los Angeles], *Waseda RILAS Journal* 4 (October 2016).

8. Jacqueline Rose, *States of Fantasy* (Oxford: Oxford University Press, 1996), 3.

9. Quoted in and translated by Mitchell Greenberg, *Baroque Bodies: Psychoanalysis and the Culture of French Absolutism* (Ithaca: Cornell University Press, 2001), 108, fn 96.

259

10. Rose, *States of Fantasy*, 3.

11. Rose, *States of Fantasy*, 21.

12. Neferti Tadiar, *Fantasy-Production: Sexual Economies and Other Philippine Conse-quences for the New World Order* (Chicago: University of Chicago Press, 2004), 30, 9.

13. Leslie Bow, *Racist Love: Asian Abstraction and the Pleasures of Fantasy* (Durham: Duke University Press, 2022), 15.

14. Lauren Berlant, *The Anatomy of National Fantasy: Hawthorne, Utopia, and Every-day Life* (Chicago: University of Chicago Press, 1991); Anne Anlin Cheng, *The Melancholy of Race: Psychoanalysis, Assimilation, and Hidden Grief* (Oxford: Oxford University Press, 2000); David L. Eng, *Racial Castration: Managing Masculinity in Asian America* (Durham: Duke University Press, 2001); Karen Shimakawa, *National Abjection: The Asian American Body Onstage* (Durham: Duke University Press, 2002); Juliana Chang, *Inhuman Citizen-ship: Traumatic Enjoyment and Asian American Literature* (Minneapolis: University of Minnesota Press, 2012).

15. Greg Clancey, *Earthquake Nation: The Cultural Politics of Japanese Seismicity, 1868–1930* (Berkeley: University of California Press, 2006), 186–202.

16. Senda Koreya, "Atogaki: yume to genjitsu" [Afterword: dream and reality], in the Japanese version of Helen Caldwell's biography: *Itō Michio: Hito to geijutsu*, trans. Nak-agawa Enosuke (Tokyo: Hayakawa Shobō, 1985), 161–64.

17. Ishibashi remained in France, served in the French air force during World War I, and returned to Japan after being injured in a crash. He and Ito remained friends for the rest of their lives.

18. Marcia Siegel and Peggy Phelan both advanced formative arguments about the fun-damental nature of dance and performance as disappearance. Since then, a rich discourse around this presumption of ephemerality has developed, complicating what Anna Pakes has characterized as a "binary ontology that parcels the world into either concrete physical objects or transient events" (6). Marcia Siegel, *At the Vanishing Point: A Critic Looks at Dance* (New York: Saturday Review Press, 1973); Peggy Phelan, *Unmarked: The Politics of Performance* (London: Routledge, 1993); André Lepecki, "Inscribing Dance," in *Of the Presence of the Body: Essays on Dance and Performance Theory*, ed. André Lepecki (Mid-dletown: CT: Wesleyan University Press, 2004); Anthea Kraut, *Choreographing Copyright: Race, Gender, and Intellectual Property Rights in American Dance* (New York: Oxford Uni-versity Press, 2016); Anna Pakes, *Choreography Invisible: The Disappearing Work of Dance* (New York: Oxford University Press, 2020).

19. Ju Yon Kim, *The Racial Mundane: Asian American Performance and the Embodied Everyday* (New York: New York University Press, 2015), 7.

20. Shane Vogel, *The Scene of Harlem Cabaret: Race, Sexuality, Performance* (Chicago: University of Chicago Press, 2009), 176.

21. Vogel, *Harlem Cabaret*, 179.

22. Susan Manning, *Ecstasy and the Demon: The Dances of Mary Wigman* (Minneapo-lis: University of Minnesota Press, 1993), 11.

23. Pannill Camp, "The Poetics of Performance Nonevents," *Journal of Dramatic Theory and Criticism* 32, no. 2 (2018): 148.

24. VK Preston, "Baroque Relations: Performing Silver and Gold in Daniel Rabel's *Bal-*

lets of the Americas," in *The Oxford Handbook of Reenactment,* ed. Mark Franko (New York: Oxford University Press, 2017), 302.

25. Tavia Nyong'o, *Afro-Fabulations: The Queer Drama of Black Life* (New York: New York University Press, 2019), 7. See also Saidiya Hartman, *Wayward Lives, Beautiful Experiments: Intimate Histories of Social Upheaval* (New York: Norton, 2019).

26. Amy Stanley, *Stranger in the Shogun's City: A Japanese Woman and Her World* (New York: Scribner, 2020).

27. Aaron C. Thomas, "Infelicities," *Journal of Dramatic Theory and Criticism* 35, no. 2 (Spring 2021).

28. Many thanks to Holly Poe Durbin and Marcy Froehlich for their expert reading of Ito's costume in this photograph.

29. My thanks to Matthew Isaac Cohen for his identification of the costume pieces in this photograph.

30. Yutian Wong, "Toward a New Asian American Dance Theory: Locating the Dancing Asian American Body," *Discourses in Dance* 1, no. 1 (2002): 72.

31. Senda Koreya, "Atogaki," 160.

32. Naoki Sakai, "Subject and Substratum: On Japanese Imperial Nationalism," *Cultural Studies* 14, nos. 3–4 (2000); John Namjun Kim, "On the Brink of Universality: German Cosmopolitanism in Japanese Imperialism," *Positions: East Asia Cultures Critique* 17, no. 1 (Spring 2009).

33. Stefan Tanaka, *Japan's Orient: Rendering Pasts into History* (Berkeley: University of California Press, 1993).

34. Wan-yao Chou, "The *Kōminka* Movement in Taiwan and Korea: Comparisons and Interpretations," in *The Japanese Wartime Empire, 1931–1945,* eds. Peter Duus, Ramon H. Myers, and Mark R. Peattie (Princeton: Princeton University Press, 1996).

35. Eiichiro Azuma, *In Search of Our Frontier: Japanese America and Settler Colonialism in the Construction of Japan's Borderless Empire* (Oakland: University of California Press, 2019).

36. Mitziko Sawada, *Tokyo Life, New York Dreams: Urban Japanese Visions of America, 1890–1924* (Berkeley: University of California Press, 1996).

37. T. Fujitani, *Race for Empire: Koreans as Japanese and Japanese as Americans during World War II* (Berkeley: University of California Press, 2011), 29.

38. Azuma, *In Search of Our Frontier.*

39. Josephine Nock-Hee Park, *Apparitions of Asia: Modernist Form and Asian American Poetics* (Oxford: Oxford University Press, 2008), 19.

40. Shirley Hune, "Asian American Studies and Asian Studies: Boundaries and Borderlands of Ethnic Studies and Area Studies," in *Color-Line to Borderlands: The Matrix of American Ethnic Studies,* ed. Johnnella Butler (Seattle: University of Washington Press, 2001); Eiichiro Azuma, "Pioneers of Overseas Japanese Development: Japanese American History and the Making of Expansionist Orthodoxy in Imperial Japan," *Journal of Asian Studies* 67, no. 4 (Nov. 2002); Augusto Espiritu, "Inter-Imperial Relations, the Pacific, and Asian American History," *Pacific Historical Review* 83, no. 2 (May 2014).

41. Christine Yano, "Global Asias: Improvisations on a Theme (a.k.a Chindon-ya Riffs)," *Journal of Asian Studies* 80, no. 4 (Nov. 2021): 859.

262 Notes to Pages 31–42

42. Sara Ahmed, *Queer Phenomenology: Orientations, Objects, Others* (Durham: Duke University Press, 2006), 114.

43. Arata Isozaki, *Japan-ness in Architecture*, trans. Sabu Kohso (Cambridge, MA: MIT Press, 2006).

44. Kandice Chuh, *Imagine Otherwise: On Asian Americanist Critique* (Durham: Duke University Press, 2003), 8.

45. Chuh, *Imagine Otherwise*, 8.

46. Many thanks to Joshua Chambers-Letson for his help thinking through this point.

Chapter One

1. Yamada Kōsaku, "Michio Itō no purofairu," foreword to *Utsukushiku naru kyōshitsu* [A classroom for beauty] (Tokyo: Hōbunkan, 1956), 3.

Ito published four books in Japan: *Amerika* [America] (Tokyo: Hata Shoten, 1940); *Amerika to nihon* [America and Japan] (Tokyo: Yakumo Shoten, 1946, 1949); *Josei hando-bukku, echiketto* [A handbook for women, etiquette] (Tokyo: Rōdōbunkasha, 1947); and *Utsukushiku naru kyōshitsu* [A classroom for beauty] (Tokyo: Hōbunkan, 1956).

2. Shane Vogel, *The Scene of Harlem Cabaret: Race, Sexuality, Performance* (Chicago: University of Chicago Press, 2009), 176.

3. Itō, *Amerika to nihon*, 35.

4. Itō, *Amerika to nihon*, 35

5. Itō, *Amerika to nihon*, 35.

6. Itō, *Amerika to nihon*, 36.

7. Itō, *Utsukushiku naru kyōshitsu*, 14. Itō, *Amerika to nihon*, 38–39.

8. Itō, *Amerika to nihon*, 40–41.

9. David Ewick and Dorsey Kleitz, *Michio Ito's Reminiscences of Ezra Pound, W. B. Yeats, and Other Matters: A Translation and Critical Edition of a Seminal Document in Modernist Aesthetics* (Lewiston, NY: Mellen, 2018), 18.

10. Or perhaps Reimann; we have only the kana, which Ito gives as レイマン; she has not been more precisely identified.

11. Itō, *Amerika to nihon*, 43.

12. On the self-inventing nature of autobiography, see, for example: Timothy Dow Adams, *Telling Lies in Modern American Autobiography* (Chapel Hill: University of North Carolina Press, 1990); Paul John Eakin, *Fictions in Autobiography: Studies in the Art of Self-Invention* (Princeton: Princeton University Press, 1995); and Kimberly Mack, *Fictional Blues: Narrative Self-Invention from Bessie Smith to Jack White* (Amherst: University of Massachusetts Press, 2020).

13. Susanna Fessler, *Musashino in Tuscany: Japanese Overseas Travel Literature, 1860–1912* (Ann Arbor: Center for Japanese Studies, University of Michigan Press, 2004); Joshua A. Fogel, *The Literature of Travel in the Japanese Rediscovery of China, 1862–1945* (Stanford: Stanford University Press, 1996).

14. Christopher Bush, *Ideographic Modernism: China, Writing, Medium* (Oxford: Oxford University Press, 2010), 19, 34.

15. Fogel, *Literature of Travel*, xv.

16. Lisa Lowe, *Critical Terrains: French and British Orientalisms* (Ithaca, NY: Cornell University Press, 1991, 2018), 53.

Notes to Pages 42–53

17. Rana Kabbani, *Europe's Myths of Orient: Devise and Rule* (London: Palgrave Macmillan, 1986), 73.

18. The innovator of the method is known as Émile Jaques-Dalcroze, though he was born Émile Jaques and added the Dalcroze while in Algeria. I follow standard usage and use the shortened phrase "the Dalcroze method" or "Dalcrozian rhythms" when discussing the technique as distinct from its inventor.

19. Julia Walker, *Performance and Modernity: Enacting Change on the Globalizing Stage* (New York: Cambridge University Press, 2022), 111.

20. Selma Landen Odom, "Wigman at Hellerau," *Ballet Review* 14, no. 2 (Summer 1986): 46.

21. There are video clips of Carrie Preston performing both sequences, as well as reconstructions of *Tone Poem II* and *Pizzicati* performed by Dana Tai Soon Burgess Dance Company on the website accompanying Preston's book on modernism and noh. "Ito Michio's Hawk's Tours in Modern Dance and Theater," Clips 5–10, accessed August 22, 2023, https://sites.bu.edu/learningtokneel/home/ito-michios-hawk-tours-in-modern-dance-and-theater/. There is also a series of film stills of Helen Caldwell moving through the sequences in her book: *Michio Ito: The Dancer and His Dances* (Berkeley: University of California Press, 1977), 143–53.

22. Mary-Jean Cowell and Satoru Shimazaki, "East and West in the Work of Michio Ito," *Dance Research Journal* 26, no. 2 (Autumn 1994): 15.

23. Conversation with the author, August 18, 2023.

24. *Michio Ito Workshop*, filmed by George Lamboy, workshop conducted by Satoru Shimazaki, May 11, 1980. New York Public Library for the Performing Arts.

25. Interview with Pauline Koner, 1975. New York Public Library for the Performing Arts, MGZTL 4–355.

26. Interview with Beatrice Seckler, 1974, transcript. New York Public Library for the Performing Arts, MGZTC 3–2196, 8.

27. Carrie J. Preston, *Learning to Kneel: Noh, Modernism, and Journeys in Teaching* (New York: Columbia University Press, 2016), 106.

28. "Michio Ito, Japanese Dancer, to Give Three Recitals in New York," *Musical Courier*, November 3, 1927, 40.

29. Didem Ekici, "'The Laboratory of a New Humanity': The Concept of Type, Life Reform, and Modern Architecture in Hellerau Garden City, 1900–1914" (PhD diss., University of Michigan, 2008), 72–73.

30. Michael J. Cowan, *Cult of the Will: Nervousness and German Modernity* (University Park: Pennsylvania State University Press, 2008). See also Stephen Kern, *The Culture of Time and Space, 1880–1918* (Cambridge, MA: Harvard University Press, 1983).

31. Walker, *Performance and Modernity*, 109.

32. Walker, *Performance and Modernity*, 122.

33. Various accounts suggest that Ito must have met Wigman in Hellerau, and that he played a fury in the *Orpheus* production. Given the timing of his arrival, both of these are incorrect.

34. Homi Bhabha, "'Race,' Time and the Revision of Modernity," *Oxford Literary Review* 13, no. 1/2 (1991): 205.

264 Notes to Pages 53–64

35. Lisa Lowe, *Intimacies of Four Continents* (Durham: Duke University Press, 2015), 189, fn 24.

36. Tessa Morris-Suzuki, "Becoming Japanese: Imperial Expansion and Identity Crises in the Early Twentieth Century," in *Japan's Competing Modernities: Issues in Culture and Democracy, 1900–1930*, ed. Sharon A. Minichiello (Honolulu: University of Hawai'i Press, 1998), 161, 175.

37. Harry Harootunian, *Overcome by Modernity: History, Culture, and Community in Interwar Japan* (Princeton: Princeton University Press, 2000), xvi.

38. Itō, *Amerika to nihon*, 144.

39. Anne Anlin Cheng, *The Melancholy of Race: Psychoanalysis, Assimilation, and Hidden Grief* (Oxford: Oxford University Press, 2001), xi.

40. Émile Jaques-Dalcroze, "Remarks on Arrhythmy," trans. F. Rothwell, *Music & Letters* 14, no. 2 (April 1933): 142–43.

41. Itō, *Amerika to nihon*, 145.

42. Itō, *Amerika to nihon*, 147–48, 149.

43. Itō, *Amerika*, 141–42. Note that Ito gives himself three years at the institute in this narrative, yet another expression of his desire, if not of chronology.

44. Quoted in Senda Koreya, "Atogaki: yume to genjitsu" [Afterword: dream and reality] in the Japanese version of Helen Caldwell's biography: *Itō Michio: Hito to geijutsu* [Michio Ito: the dancer and his dances], trans. Nakagawa Enosuke (Tokyo: Hayakawa Shobō, 1985), 178.

45. Robin Bernstein, *Racial Innocence: Performing American Childhood from Slavery to Civil Rights* (New York: New York University Press, 2011), 71.

46. On the proximity of Japanese people and objects, see, among many: Christopher Bush, "The Ethnicity of Things in America's Lacquered Age," *Representations* 99, no. 1 (Summer 2007); Josephine Lee, *The Japan of Pure Invention: Gilbert and Sullivan's The Mikado* (Minneapolis: University of Minnesota Press, 2010).

47. Michelle Liu Carriger, *Theatricality of the Closet: Fashion, Performance, and Subjectivity between Victorian Britain and Meiji Japan* (Evanston: Northwestern University Press, 2023), 74.

48. Selma Landen Odom, "Choreographing *Orpheus*: Hellerau 1913 and Warwick 1991," in *Dance Reconstructed: A Conference on Modern Dance Art, Past, Present, Future* (Rutgers University, New Brunswick, NJ: October 16 and 17, 1992): 128–29.

49. Quoted in Senda, "Atogaki," 183.

Chapter Two

1. For instance, Carol Sorgenfrei reads the image as suggesting a militaristic superiority of the Japanese body. Carol Fisher Sorgenfrei, "Strategic Unweaving: Itō Michio and the Diasporic Dancing Body," in *Politics of Interweaving Performance Cultures: Beyond Postcolonialism*, eds. Erika Fischer-Lichte, Torsten Jost, and Saskya Iris Jain (Florence, KY: Taylor & Francis, 2014).

2. Arabella Stanger, *Dancing on Violent Ground: Utopia as Dispossession in Euro-American Theater Dance* (Evanston: Northwestern University Press, 2021), 98.

3. For representative readings of these dancers' use of energy, see Vera Maletic, *Body,*

Notes to Pages 64–70

Space, Expression: The Development of Rudolf Laban's Movement and Dance Concepts (Berlin: Mouton de Gruyter, 1987); Carrie J. Preston, *Modernism's Mythic Pose: Gender, Genre, Solo Performance* (Oxford: Oxford University Press, 2011), 144–90; and Stanger, *Dancing on Violent Ground*, 64–76, 89–112.

4. Many thanks to Rosemary Candelario for articulating this.

5. Ezra Pound and Ernest Fenollosa, *The Classic Noh Theater of Japan* (1917; repr. New York: New Directions, 1959), 153.

6. "In the Spotlight," *American Dancer*, June 1929, 25.

7. Helen Caldwell, *Michio Ito: The Dancer and His Dances* (Berkeley: University of California Press, 1977), 4.

8. When Yamada returned to Japan he helped to organize the first expressionist art show, of Der Sturm group, at the Hibiya Art Museum, March 14–28, 1914.

9. For instance, Yamada taught and helped design the curriculum at the Bunka Gakuin school for girls in the 1920s. Hirasawa Nobuyasu, "Shoki bunkagakuin ni okeru buyō kyōiku jissen—Yamada Kōsaku ni yoru" [Implementation of dance education at the early Bunka Gakuin: experiments in Yamada Kōsaku's "dance-poem"], *Gakujutsu Kenkyū Kiyō, Kanoya Taiiku Daigaku* 34 (March 2006).

10. David Pacun, "Nationalism and Musical Style in Interwar 'Yōgaku': A Reappraisal," *Asian Music* 43, no. 2 (July 2012); David Pacun, "'Thus We Cultivate Our Own World, and Thus We Share It with Others': Kósçak Yamada's Visit to the United States in 1918–1919," *American Music* 24, no. 1 (April 2006).

11. "Asakusa Opera" was a music hall phenomenon that emerged in 1917 and was named for its location—the Asakusa district of Tokyo. With Western-style scenery and costumes, Italian operas were loosely translated and truncated into popular Japanese forms. With the 1923 Kantō earthquake, this form abruptly vanished, but left a generation of trained performers, and a lasting mark on how Japanese theater workers approached the localization of Western forms. Charles Exley, "Popular Musical Star Tokuko Takagi and Vaudeville Modernism in the Taishō Asakusa Opera," *Japanese Language and Literature* 51, no. 1 (April 2017).

12. Quoted in Kataoka Yasuko, "Ishii Baku—Buyōshi to tenkai" [Ishii Baku: the development of the dance poem], *Buyōgaku* 13, no. 1 (1989): 49.

13. Yamada Kōsaku, "Buyō to watashi" [Dance and myself] (1922), in *Yamada Kōsaku Collected Works, Vol. 1*, eds. Gotō Nobuko, Dan Ikuma, and Tōyama Kazuyuki (Tokyo: Iwanami Shoten, 2001), 11.

14. Nohara Yasuko, "Yamada Kōsaku no Sukuriabin juyō" [Yamada Kōsaku's reception of Scriabin], *Musashino ongaku daigaku kenkyū kiyō* no. 51 (2019).

15. Yamada Kōsaku, "Buyōshi to buyōgeki" [Dance-poem and dance-drama] (1916), in *Yamada Kōsaku Collected Works, Vol. 1*, 218.

16. Yamada, "Buyōshi to buyōgeki," 218.

17. Ito later choreographed his own dance to Yamada's "Oto no nagare."

18. On Isadora Duncan's dancing to poetry recitation, see Ann Daly, *Done into Dance: Isadora Duncan in America* (Middletown, CT: Wesleyan University Press, 2002).

19. Yamada, "Buyōshi to buyōgeki," 218.

20. Quoted in Ishii Kan, *Buyō shijin Ishii Baku* (Tokyo: Miraisha, 1994), 111.

266　Notes to Pages 70–76

21. Ishii Kan, *Buyō shijin*, 113.

22. Funeyama Takashi, "Yamada Kōsaku no buyōshi—Taisho modanizumu no yume to zasetsu" [Yamada Kōsaku's dance-poem: Taisho modernism's dreams and failures], *Ongaku Geijutsu* 44, no. 2 (Feb. 1986).

23. For instance, Mary Fleischer, *Embodied Texts: Symbolist Playwright-Dancer Collaborations* (Amsterdam: Rodopi, 2007).

24. Yamada Kōsaku, "Tsuide ni kaete" [In place of a preface], in *Yamada Kōsaku Collected Works*, Vol. 1, 7.

25. Yamada Kōsaku, "Michio Itō no purofairu," in Itō Michio, *Utsukushiku naru kyōshitsu* [A classroom for beauty] (Tokyo: Hōbunkan, 1956), 1.

26. Ezra Pound, "Sword-Dance and Spear-Dance: Texts of the Poems Used with Michio Itow's Dances. By Ezra Pound, from Notes of Masirni Utchiyama," *Future* 1, no. 2 (Dec. 1916), in *Ezra Pound's Poetry and Prose*, Vol. 2, eds. Lea Baechler, A. Walton Litz, and James Longenbach (New York: Garland, 1991), 182.

27. H. T. Parker, "Roshanara and Ito," December 5, 1917, in *Motion Arrested: The Dance Reviews of H. T. Parker*, ed. Olive Holmes (Middletown, CT: Wesleyan University Press, 1982), 258–59.

28. Harriette Underhill, "Michio Itow," *New York Tribune*, August 19, 1917, C2.

29. Quoted in Kataoka, "Ishii Baku," 49.

30. Elizabeth Cullingford, *Yeats, Ireland, and Fascism* (London: Macmillan, 1981), 72. See also James W. Flannery, *W. B. Yeats and the Idea of a Theatre* (Toronto: Macmillan, 1976); Karen Dorn, *Players and Painted Stage: The Theatre of W. B. Yeats* (Sussex: Harvester Press, 1984).

31. Joseph Lennon, "W. B. Yeats's Celtic Orient," *Irish Orientalism: A Literary and Intellectual History* (Syracuse: Syracuse University Press, 2004).

32. As Eric Hayot, Josephine Park, and others have shown, Pound's "China" is not merely invented, but more crucially, the relationship between Pound, China, and modernist literary production has shaped notions of representation, authenticity, and universalism in English literature and critical discourse ever since. Eric Hayot, *Chinese Dreams: Pound, Brecht, Tel Quel* (Ann Arbor: University of Michigan Press, 2004); Josephine Nock-Hee Park, *Apparitions of Asia: Modernist Form and Asian American Poetics* (Oxford: Oxford University Press, 2008).

33. See footnotes 36, 43, 46, 49, 53, and 54.

34. Itō Michio, "Sekai ni odoru" [Dancing through the world], *Geijutsu Shinchō*, July 1955, 216–27.

35. Ezra Pound, "How I Began," *T.P.'s Weekly*, June 6, 1913, 707.

36. David Ewick, "Strange Attractors: Ezra Pound and the Invention of Japan, II," *Essays and Studies in British and American Literature*, Tokyo Woman's Christian University, 64 (2018).

As Carrie Preston observes of the wide-ranging influence of this idea: "Pound invoked a spirit of unity that helped him solve the problems he was facing in his own poetic writing, and it appeared for him in other plays. He passed on the idea of noh's unity to Euro-American poets, especially Yeats and T. S. Eliot, and it is now a commonplace that modernist and contemporary poetry, in the absence of classical form, regular meter, and rhyme,

Notes to Pages 76–81

is organized by recurring images that build on one another until the trope resolves itself in a revelation or unified impression." Carrie J. Preston, *Learning to Kneel: Noh, Modernism, and Journeys in Teaching* (New York: Columbia University Press, 2016), 45.

37. As Carrie Preston models in her book, we should rightly call the publication resulting from this process "the Fenollosa-Hirata-Pound" translations, given Hirata's central contribution. *Learning to Kneel*, 36.

38. The standard story has Pound seeking out Ito at the Café Royal sometime in June 1915, and subsequently introducing him to Yeats. But, as David Ewick has traced, Yeats was present at Ito's first drawing-room performance at Lady Ottoline Morrell's in late 1914. Pound, it seems, separately saw Ito perform at the Coliseum shortly before he found him at Café Royal. David Ewick, "Notes Toward a Cultural History of Japanese Modernism in Modernist Europe, 1910–1920, with Special Reference to Kōri Torahiko," *Hemingway Review of Japan* no. 13 (June 2012): 21.

39. For more on Kume, and especially Kōri and his relation to Pound, see Ewick, "Notes Toward a Cultural History," 21–22. On Kōri's own fascinating, if short, career as a playwright, see Yoko Chiba, "Kori Torahiko and Edith Craig: A Japanese Playwright in London and Toronto," *Comparative Drama* 30, no. 4 (Winter 1996–97).

40. Preston, *Learning to Kneel*, 74–76.

41. Itō Michio, *Utsukushiku naru kyōshitsu*, 28

42. Ezra Pound, "Vorticism," *Fortnightly Review* 96 (September 1, 1914): 471.

43. Midori Takeishi, *Japanese Elements in Michio Ito's Early Period: 1915–1924: Meetings of East and West in the Collaborative Works*, ed. David Pacun (Tokyo: Gendai tosho, 2006), 27. Andrew Houwen, *Ezra Pound's Japan* (London: Bloomsbury Academic, 2021), 148.

44. Preston, *Learning to Kneel*, 118, 120.

45. Ezra Pound, "Sword-Dance and Spear-Dance," 182.

46. Andrew Houwen, "Ezra Pound's Early Cantos and His Translation of *Takasago*," *Review of English Studies* 65 (2013); Ewick, "Strange Attractors."

47. Ezra Pound, "Vorticism," 466.

48. Ezra Pound, "Vorticism," 464–65, 469.

49. Christopher Bush, "I Am All for the Triangle: The Geopolitical Aesthetic of Pound's Japan," in *Ezra Pound in the Present: Essays on Pound's Contemporaneity*, eds. Josephine Park and Paul Stasi (New York: Bloomsbury, 2016); Diego Pellecchia, "Ezra Pound and the Politics of Noh Film," *Philological Quarterly* 92, no. 4 (Fall 2013).

50. Bush, "I Am All for the Triangle," 85.

51. Bush, "I Am All for the Triangle," 93.

52. Ernest Fenollosa and Ezra Pound, *The Chinese Written Character as a Medium of Poetry*, cited in Bush, "I Am All for the Triangle," 95.

53. David Ewick, "The Instigations of Ezra Pound by Ernest Fenollosa I: The Chinese Written Character, Atlantic Crossings, Texts Mislaid, and the Machinations of a Divinely-Inspired Char Woman," *Essays and Studies*, Tokyo Christian Women's University 66, no. 1 (2015).

54. Hakutani Yoshinobu, "Ezra Pound, Yone Noguchi, and Imagism," *Modern Philology* 90, no. 1 (Aug. 1992).

268 Notes to Pages 81–90

55. Sato Hiroaki, "Yone Noguchi: Accomplishments and Roles," *Journal of American and Canadian Studies*, Sophia University (March 31, 1996): 114.

56. Houwen, *Ezra Pound's Japan*, 196.

57. Internment trial. National Archives and Records Administration, at Riverside. Record Group 85, District 16, Enemy Alien Case Files, 1941–1948. Folder Title 15942/633-Michio Ito, Box 27.

58. Pellecchia, "Ezra Pound and the Politics of Noh Film," 508–9.

59. For a clear view of the print itself, see https://artgallery.yale.edu/collections/objects /24872. Many thanks to Satoko Shimazaki for identifying this piece.

60. Gerald Groemer, *Street Performers and Society in Urban Japan, 1600–1900* (New York: Routledge, 2016), 79–85.

61. Christopher Reed, *Bachelor Japanists: Japanese Aesthetics and Western Masculinities* (New York: Columbia University Press, 2017), 5. See also, John Walter de Gruchy, *Orienting Arthur Waley: Japonism, Orientalism, and the Creation of Japanese Literature in English* (Honolulu: University of Hawai'i Press, 2003).

62. Grace Elisabeth Lavery, *Quaint, Exquisite: Victorian Aesthetics and the Idea of Japan* (Princeton: Princeton University Press, 2019), 24.

63. Amy Sueyoshi, *Queer Compulsions: Race, Nation, and Sexuality in the Affairs of Yone Noguchi* (Honolulu: University of Hawai'i Press, 2021).

64. Tara Rodman, "A Modernist Audience: The Kawakami Troupe, Matsuki Bunkio, and Boston Japonisme," *Theatre Journal* 65, no. 4 (Dec 2013).

65. Itō Michio, "Camp Livingston Notebook," J21, Senda Koreya Files, Tsubouchi Memorial Theatre Museum, Waseda University.

66. J. Keith Vincent, *Two-timing Modernity: Homosocial Narrative in Modern Japanese Fiction* (Cambridge, MA: Harvard University Asia Center, 2012), 42.

67. Emmanuel Cooper, *The Sexual Perspective: Homosexuality and Art in the Last 100 Years in the West* (New York: Routledge, 1994), 117. On the Bloomsbury/*At the Hawk's Well* queer relations, see Preston, *Learning to Kneel*, 111–14.

68. Richard Taylor, *The Drama of W. B. Yeats: Irish Myth and the Japanese Nō* (New Haven: Yale University Press, 1976); Masaru Sekine and Christopher Murray, *Yeats and the Noh: A Comparative Study* (Savage, MD: Barnes and Noble, 1990).

69. Angus Fletcher, "Ezra Pound's Egypt and the Origin of the *Cantos*," *Twentieth-Century Literature* 48, no.1 (Spring 2002); Claire Nally, *Envisioning Ireland: W. B. Yeats' Occult Nationalism* (Oxford: Peter Lang, 2010), 186.

70. Ewick notes that this residence, at 20 Cavendish Square, was actually owned by the wife of Prime Minister Asquith, and leased by Lady Cunard. Ewick, "Notes toward a Cultural History," 20.

71. Curtis Bradford, *Yeats at Work* (Carbondale: Southern Illinois University Press, 1965), 180.

72. Helen Caldwell, *Michio Ito*, 45.

73. Itō Michio, "Omoide wo kataru" [Reminiscences] *Hikaku bunka* 2, no. 1 (1956): 76.

74. Ezra Pound, *The Pisan Cantos*, ed. Richard Sieburth (New York: New Direction Books, 1948, 2003), 47.

Notes to Pages 91–99 269

Chapter Three

1. For instance, in Japan, Komori Toshi (1936) and Miya Misako (1933) both choreographed tangos.

2. William Hosley, *The Japan Idea* (Hartford, CT: Wadsworth Atheneum 1990); Jan Walsh Hokenson, *Japan, France, and East-West Aesthetics: French Literature, 1867–2000* (Madison, NJ: Fairleigh Dickinson University Press, 2004); for an expansive bibliography of materials on japonisme, see David Ewick's *Japonisme, Orientalism, Modernism: A Bibliography of Japan in English Language Verse of the Early 20ᵗʰ Century*, last modified August 2012, themargins.net

3. Charlotte Eubanks and Jonathan Abel, "Of Asian Boxes . . ." *Verge: Studies in Global Asias* 1, no. 2, Collecting Asias (Fall 2015): vii.

4. Stefan Tanaka, *Japan's Orient: Rendering Pasts into History* (Berkeley: University of California Press, 1995).

5. Marta Robertson, "Floating Worlds: Japanese and American Transcultural Encounters in Dance," *Conference Proceedings* (Congress on Research in Dance, 2014).

6. Susan Stewart, *On Longing: Narratives of the Miniature, the Gigantic, the Souvenir, the Collection* (Durham: Duke University Press, 1993), 132–69.

7. Clayton Hamilton, "Japanese Art Comes to Life in the Dance," *Vogue*, April 15, 1917, 60.

8. See Mari Yoshihara, *Embracing the East: White Women and American Orientalism* (Oxford: Oxford University Press, 2002); Josephine Lee, *The Japan of Pure Invention: Gilbert and Sullivan's* The Mikado (Minneapolis: University of Minnesota Press, 2010); Tara Rodman, "A Modernist Audience: The Kawakami Troupe, Matsuki Bunkio, and Boston Japonisme," *Theatre Journal* 65, no. 4 (December 2013).

9. Christopher Bush, "The Ethnicity of Things in America's Lacquered Age," *Representations* 99, no. 1 (Summer 2007); Christopher Reed, *Bachelor Japanists: Japanese Aesthetics and Western Masculinities* (New York: Columbia University Press, 2017); Grace Lavery, *Quaint, Exquisite: Victorian Aesthetics and the Idea of Japan* (Princeton: Princeton University Press, 2019).

10. Clayton Hamilton, "Japanese Art Comes to Life."

11. Rosemary Candelario, *Flowers Cracking Concrete: Eiko & Koma's Asian / American Choreographies* (Middletown, CT: Wesleyan University Press, 2016), 92; Barbara E. Thornbury, *America's Japan and Japan's Performing Arts: Cultural Mobility and Exchange in New York, 1952–2011* (Ann Arbor: University of Michigan Press, 2013).

12. Carrie J. Preston, *Learning to Kneel: Noh, Modernism, and Journeys in Teaching* (New York: Columbia University Press, 2016); Midori Takeishi, *Japanese Elements in Michio Ito's Early Period: 1915–1924: Meetings of East and West in the Collaborative Works*, ed. David Pacun (Tokyo: Gendai tosho, 2006).

13. Chizuru Sugiyama, "Shizukesa wo aisuru kokoro wo kate ni: Komori Toshi" [Nourishing a heart that loves tranquility], in *Nihon no gendai buyō no paioniā*, ed. Kataoka Yasuko (Tokyo: Maruzen and New National Theatre Tokyo, 2015).

14. Program, "Modern and Classic Japanese Pantomimes and Dances," April 6, 1918, Neighborhood Playhouse, Jerome Robbins Dance Division, New York Public Library for the Performing Arts.

270 Notes to Pages 99–109

15. Takeishi, *Japanese Elements*, 51.

16. "Programmes for the Week," *New York Tribune*, April 4, 1918.

17. Takeishi, *Japanese Elements*, 55.

18. Mitziko Sawada, *Tokyo Life, New York Dreams: Urban Japanese Visions of America, 1890–1924* (Berkeley: University of California Press, 1996).

19. Eiichiro Azuma, *Between Two Empires: Race, History, and Transnationalism in Japanese America* (Oxford: Oxford University Press, 2005). For further discussion, see chapters 4 and 5.

20. "Beijin no mita nōgeki 'tamura' beikoku gekidan no rikai" [Understanding the noh performance of "Tamura" by an American theater troupe], *Nyū Yōku Shimpō*, February 16, 1921, 3.

21. "Hagoromo wo jouen" [Performing Hagoromo], *Nyū Yōku Shimpō*, January 13, 1923, 3.

22. "Shibai sonohi sonohi" [Theater, day by day], *Nyū Yōku Shimpō*, June 21, 1922, 3.

23. "Beikokugekikai ni sakanna nihon shumi ga bokkou" [Japanese pastimes suddenly thrive in American theater], *Nichibei Shinbun*, February 15, 1917, 2.

24. "Pin Wiru geki ni nihonfujin ga iriyou" [Japanese women needed for the Pin Wheel show], *Nyū Yōku Shimpō*, June 24, 1922, 3.

25. "The Dance: Tamiris' Art," *New York Times*, February 5, 1928, 111.

26. Advertisement, Michio Itow School, *Vogue*, November 1920, 30.

27. Harriette Underhill, "Michio Itow," *New York Tribune*, August 19, 1917, C2.

28. Jane Desmond, "Dancing Out the Difference: Cultural Imperialism and Ruth St. Denis' 'Radha' of 1906," *Signs* 17, no. 1 (1991); Amy Koritz, "Dancing the Orient for England: Maud Allan's 'The Vision of Salome,'" *Theatre Journal* 46, no. 1 (March 1994); Yutian Wong, *Choreographing Asian America* (Middletown, CT: Wesleyan University Press, 2010); Priya Srinivasan, *Sweating Saris: Indian Dance as Transnational Labor* (Philadelphia: Temple University Press, 2011); SanSan Kwan, "Performing a Geography of Asian America: The Chop Suey Circuit," *The Drama Review: TDR* 55 (2011).

29. "Seen on the Stage," *Vogue*, September 1, 1917, 152.

30. Roshanara was an Englishwoman who was born and raised in Calcutta, where she learned the "Hindu dances" that made up her dance expertise. Ratan Devi (née Alice Richardson) was an Englishwoman who specialized in East Indian vocal music and was married to the renowned Indian art critic and historian of religion, Ananada K. Coomaraswamy.

31. See, among others, Yoshihara, *Embracing the East*; Eubanks and Abel, "Of Asian Boxes . . ."

32. Thomas Richards, *The Imperial Archive: Knowledge and the Fantasy of Empire* (London: Verso, 1993), 6.

33. Michelle Liu Carriger, *Theatricality of the Closet: Fashion, Performance, and Subjectivity between Victorian Britain and Meiji Japan* (Evanston: Northwestern University Press, 2023), 162.

34. Tanaka, *Japan's Orient*.

35. Kushida Kiyomi, "Yōbu sōsō-ki no kaitakusha to tōyō buyōka Teiko Itō no 'kyōdo' to 'minzoku' wo meguru gensetsu" [Discourses of "Ethnicity" and "The Homeland" surrounding Teiko Itō, East Asian dance artist and pioneer of early 20th century Western

dance], *Jissen joshi daigaku bungakubu kiyō dai* 64 (2022); and "Itō Yūji ga buro-dowei- ni motarashita 'tōyō': 1930 nendaigohan no nihon/ajia ni okeru minzoku geinō no chōsa" [Itō Yūji brought the "Orient" to Broadway: investigating folk performance of Japan/Asia in the 1930s], *Jissen joshi daigaku bungakubu kiyō dai* 65 (2023).

36. Janet Poole, *When the Future Disappears: The Modernist Imagination in Late Colonial Korea* (New York: Columbia University Press, 2015); Nayoung Aimee Kwon, *Intimate Empire: Collaboration and Colonial Modernity in Korea and Japan* (Durham: Duke University Press, 2015).

37. Kwon, *Intimate Empire*, 8.

38. Alma Talley, "The Story of Roshanara," *Dance Magazine*, November 1926, 11–13, 51.

39. Ruth St. Denis, "Oriental Dancing," *Dance Magazine*, December 1928, 16–17, 60, 62.

40. Laura Ann Stoler, *Carnal Knowledge and Imperial Power: Race and the Intimate in Colonial Rule* (Berkeley: University of California Press, 2002).

41. Tara Rodman, "Altered Belonging: The Transnational Modern Dance of Itō Michio" (PhD diss., Northwestern University, 2017).

42. Bush, "Ethnicity of Things," 81.

43. Brooks MacNamara, "'Something Glorious': Greenwich Village and the Theater," in *Greenwich Village: Culture and Counterculture*, eds. Rick Beard and Leslie Cohen Berlowitz (New Brunswick, NJ: Rutgers University Press, 1993), 313. On Greenwich Village, see also Christine Stansell, *American Moderns: Bohemian New York and the Creation of a New Century* (Princeton: Princeton University Press, 2000).

As Amy Sueyoshi's work on the "wide-open town" of San Francisco in the early 20th century reminds us, the ability to enjoy sexual freedom with impunity was an unevenly distributed privilege predominantly accorded to white people. And, as Shane Vogel has shown, Harlem residents of New York of the same period were differently policed than their primarily white counterparts in the Village. Amy Sueyoshi, *Discriminating Sex: White Leisure and the Making of the American "Oriental"* (Urbana: University of Illinois Press, 2018); Shane Vogel, *The Scene of Harlem Cabaret* (Chicago: University of Chicago Press, 2009).

44. On Ito's work in *Emperor Jones*, see Preston, *Learning to Kneel*, 137–40.

45. Percy Hammond, "The New Play: Mr. Hitchcock's 'Pin Wheel' Is, at Least, a Sober and Erudite Dancing Festival," *New York Tribune*, June 16, 1922, 10.

46. "New Theatrical Offerings," *New York Tribune*, June 11, 1922, D1.

47. The following year, Ito filed for bankruptcy due to *Pinwheel*, listing liabilities of $10,415.71 and no assets. "Itow's Bankruptcy," *Variety*, March 22, 1923, 13.

48. Hammond, "The New Play," 10.

49. Gordon Whyte, "Pin Wheel Revue," *Billboard*, August 12, 1922, 34.

50. See George Chauncey, *Gay New York: Gender, Urban Culture, and the Making of the Gay Male World, 1890–1940* (New York: Basic Books, 1994).

51. Hammond, "The New Play," 10.

52. "Inside Stuff," *Variety*, June 16, 1922, 14.

53. "Broadway Reviews," *Variety*, June 23, 1922, 15.

54. "'Pin Wheel Revue' at the Carroll Is Big Dance Revel," *New York Clipper*, June 21, 1922, 20.

272   Notes to Pages 113–22

55. "Broadway Reviews," *Variety*, June 23, 1922, 15. Such slit-legged costuming and bare feet were, in fact, fairly common in modern concert dance recitals as well (where it was a frequent point of lecherous commentary).

56. Robert C. Benchley, "Drama: An Evening with Terpsichore," *Life*, August 17, 1922, 18.

57. "'Pinwheel Revel' Odd," *New York Times*, June 16, 1922, 25.

58. Benchley, "Drama."

59. John Martin, "The Dance—Japanese Art," *New York Times*, March 9, 1930, 124.

60. M. E. H., "Through Our Own Opera Glasses," *Baltimore Sun*, August 12, 1917, SN2.

61. Lisa Lowe, *Immigrant Acts: On Asian American Cultural Politics* (Durham: Duke University Press, 1996); David Eng, *Racial Castration: Managing Masculinity in Asian America* (Durham: Duke University Press, 2001); Susan Koshy, *Sexual Naturalization: Asian Americans and Miscegenation* (Stanford: Stanford University Press, 2004); C. Winter Han, *Geisha of a Different Kind: Race and Sexuality in Gaysian America* (New York: NYU Press, 2015); and, on a critical counteranalysis that argues against "remasculinization" in favor of "a politics of bottomhood that opposes racism and heteronormativity without scapegoating femininity" (14), see Nguyen Tan Hoang, *A View from the Bottom: Asian American Masculinity and Sexual Representation* (Durham: Duke University Press, 2014).

62. Hamilton, "Japanese Art Comes to Life," *Vogue*, April 15, 1917, 60, 142.

63. Eng, *Racial Castration*.

64. Yutian Wong, "Artistic Utopias: Michio Ito and the Trope of the International," *Worlding Dance*, ed. Susan Leigh Foster (New York: Palgrave Macmillan, 2009), 157.

65. "The Artist and the Hostess as Collaborators," *Vogue*, July 15, 1917, 70.

66. Anne McClintock, *Imperial Leather: Race, Gender and Sexuality in the Colonial Contest* (New York: Routledge, 1995), 184.

67. Leslie Bow, "Fetish," in *The Routledge Companion to Asian American and Pacific Islander Literature*, ed. Rachel C. Lee (New York: Routledge, 2014), 128.

68. Leslie Bow, *Racist Love: Asian Abstraction and the Pleasures of Fantasy* (Durham: Duke University Press, 2022), 157.

69. Mary C. Panzer, "The Essential Tact of Nickolas Muray," in *The Covarrubias Circle: Nickolas Muray's Collection of Twentieth-century Mexican Art*, ed. Kurt Heintzelman (Austin: University of Texas Press, 2004).

70. Anne Anlin Cheng, *The Melancholy of Race: Psychoanalysis, Assimilation, and Hidden Grief* (Oxford: Oxford University Press, 2000), 53.

71. Rey Chow, "Fateful Attachments: On Collecting, Fidelity, and Lao She," *Critical Inquiry* 28, no. 1 (Autumn 2001).

72. Itō Michio, *Amerika*, 225–27.

73. Itō Michio, "Kurui heru Nijinsuki" [The Mad Nijinsky], *Geijutsu Shinchō*, July, 1950, 96.

74. Quoted in Penny Farfan, *Performing Queer Modernism* (New York: Oxford University Press, 2017), 41–42.

75. Joshua Takano Chambers-Letson, *A Race So Different: Performance and Law in Asian America* (New York: New York University Press, 2013), 8–9.

76. Itō, "Kurui heru Nijinsuki," 97.

Notes to Pages 122–29 273

77. Itō, "Kurui heru Nijinsuki," 99.

78. Kevin Kopelson, *The Queer Afterlife of Vaslav Nijinsky* (Stanford: Stanford University Press, 1997).

79. J. Keith Vincent, *Two-Timing Modernity: Homosocial Narrative in Modern Japanese Fiction* (Cambridge, MA: Harvard University Asia Center, distributed by Harvard University Press, 2012).

Chapter Four

1. "Michio Ito to Direct Dance, 'Prince Igor' at the Bowl," *Rafu Shimpo*, English section, August 15, 1930, 8.

2. Naima Prevots, *Dancing in the Sun: Hollywood Choreographers, 1915–1937* (Ann Arbor, MI: UMI Research Press, 1987); Mary-Jean Cowell, "Michio Ito in Hollywood: Modes and Ironies of Ethnicity," *Dance Chronicle* 24, no. 3 (2001). See also Yagishita Emi, "Itō Michio no amerika ni okeru buyō katsudō: rosanzerusu de no katsudō wo chūshin ni" [Itō Michio's dance activities in America: focusing on his activities in Los Angeles], *Waseda RILAS Journal* 4 (October 2016).

3. Mary-Jean Cowell, "Michio Ito in Hollywood," 280.

4. "Forms Dance Symphony," *Los Angeles Times*, April 28, 1929, C12.

5. *American Dance Festival Presents Pauline Koner: Speaking of Dance*, directed by Douglas Rosenberg (1998; Oregon, WI: American Dance Festival Video, 2006).

6. For example, Mary Watkins, "Michio Ito Ends Season Here with Old Numbers," *New York Herald Tribune*, March 19, 1928, 13.

7. See Susan Manning, *Modern Dance, Negro Dance: Race in Motion* (Minneapolis: University of Minnesota Press, 2004).

8. Mike Davis, *City of Quartz: Excavating the Future in Los Angeles* (London: Verso, 1990).

9. Eiichiro Azuma, *Between Two Empires: Race, History, and Transnationalism in Japanese America* (New York: Oxford University Press, 2005), 47.

10. "Colorful Lil' Tokyo Projected for L.A.," *Nichibei Shinbun*, August 6, 1935, 1.

11. "Michio Ito's Tentative Plan for the Reconstruction of East First Street: The Little Tokyo in Los Angeles," 1. B2F15, CEMA Archive, University of California, Santa Barbara.

12. Scott Kurashige, *The Shifting Grounds of Race: Black and Japanese Americans in the Making of Multiethnic Los Angeles* (Princeton: Princeton University Press, 2008), 40–43.

13. Ito knew more about this than might be supposed: his father, Tamekichi, was an architect famous for inventing a new earthquake-resistant design for homes following the devastating 1891 Nōbi earthquake. Greg Clancey, *Earthquake Nation: The Cultural Politics of Japanese Seismicity, 1868–1930* (Berkeley: University of California Press, 2006), 186–202.

14. Charlotte Brooks, *Alien Neighbors, Foreign Friends: Asian Americans, Housing, and the Transformation of Urban California* (Chicago: University of Chicago Press, 2009), 82.

15. "Michio Ito's Tentative Plan," 1.

16. "Michio Ito's Tentative Plan," 2

17. "Michio Ito's Tentative Plan," 3.

18. "Michio Ito's Tentative Plan," 3.

274   Notes to Pages 131–36

19. "Kangei teikoku renshū kantai" [Welcoming the Imperial Naval exercises], *Rafu Shimpo*, August 23, 1929, Special Section, 8.

20. The founding and expansive study here is Yuji Ichioka, *The Issei: The World of the First Generation Japanese Immigrants, 1885–1924* (New York: Collier Macmillan, 1988).

21. Wong, "Artistic Utopias," 158.

22. Eiichiro Azuma, *In Search of Our Frontier: Japanese America and Settler Colonialism in the Construction of Japan's Borderless Empire* (Oakland: University of California Press, 2019).

23. Eiichiro Azuma, *Between Two Empires: Race, History, and Transnationalism* (New York: Oxford University Press, 2005), 12–14.

24. Andrew Leong, *Roots of the Issei: Exploring Early Japanese American Newspapers* (Stanford: Hoover Institution Press, 2018). On the historiographic implications of these now-pervasive terms, and the histories they may occlude, see Eiichiro Azuma, "The Making of a Japanese American Race, and Why Are There No 'Immigrants' in Postwar Nikkei History and Community? The Problems of Generation, Region, and Citizenship in Japanese America," in *TransPacific Japanese American Studies: Conversations on Race and Racializations*, eds. Yasuko Takezawa and Gary Y. Okihiro (Honolulu: University of Hawai'i Press, 2016).

25. Kojima Shigeru, "Who Are Nikkeijin?" trans. Mina Otsuka. *Discover Nikkei*, April 17, 2017. http://www.discovernikkei.org/en/journal/2017/4/21/nikkei-wa-dare-no-koto

26. Valerie J. Matsumoto, *City Girls: The Nisei Social World in Los Angeles, 1920–1950* (Oxford: Oxford University Press, 2014), 60.

27. Lon Kurashige, *Japanese American Celebration and Conflict: A History of Ethnic Identity and Festival, 1934–1990* (Berkeley: University of California Press, 2002).

28. Eiichiro Azuma, *Between Two Empires*, 191.

29. Matsumoto, *City Girls*, 19.

30. Given Little Tokyo's location on the border of one of LA's red-light districts, and the ongoing history of equating Asian women with prostitutes, the suggestiveness inherent in bodily display was a source of real anxiety.

31. A. M., "Art in Movement," *Los Angeles Times*, June 23, 1929, 16.

32. A. M., "Art in Movement."

33. Ito had his main studio in Hollywood, and at times operated other studios in the region; he also taught at the Edith Jane Studio, and at USC.

34. On Ito's film career, see Mary-Jean Cowell, "Michio Ito in Hollywood."

35. "Argus Bowl Closes Successful Series," *Rafu Shimpo*, September 6, 1929, English Section, 1.

36. Muriel Babcock, "Rhythmics of Far East Delight Eye," *Los Angeles Times*, August 15, 1929, A11.

37. Zarina (Jane Zimmerman), following in the footsteps of La Meri, was an "oriental dance" specialist. In the late '30s, as the genre shifted to what is known as "ethnic dance," she began to study in Asia, traveling to India, Thailand, Cambodia, Java, Bali, and Japan, and authored a book on those forms: Xenia Zarina, *Classic Dances of the Orient* (New York: Crown Publishers, 1967). See also Matthew Isaac Cohen, "Dancing the Subject of 'Java': International Modernism and Traditional Performance, 1899–1952," *Indonesia and the Malay World* 35, no. 101 (2007).

Notes to Pages 137–46

38. Isabel Morse Jones, "Ito Spiritually Inspired," *Los Angeles Times*, June 2, 1929, C13.

39. See Naima Prevots, *Dancing in the Sun; American Pageantry: A Movement for Art and Democracy* (Ann Arbor: UMI Research Press, 1990); Catherine Parsons Smith, "Founding the Hollywood Bowl," *American Music* 11, no. 2 (Summer 1993); also, *Making Music in Los Angeles: Transforming the Popular* (Berkeley: University of California Press, 2007); Sarah Schrank, *Art and the City: Civic Imagination and Cultural Authority in Los Angeles* (Philadelphia: University of Pennsylvania Press, 2009).

40. Lewis Barrington, "Community Dancing," *American Dancer*, July 1929, 16.

41. Lewis Barrington, "Community Dancing Regains Popularity," *American Dancer*, January 1930, 16.

42. Barrington, "Community Dancing Regains Popularity," 31.

43. "Beginners' Dance Class Will Open on Wednesday Evening," *Rafu Shimpo*, July 29, 1929, English Section, 3.

44. "Michio Ito Is Pleased with Results of Japanese Class," *Rafu Shimpo*, August 5, 1929, English Section, 3.

45. "Dance Class Taken to See Vera Fokine," *Rafu Shimpo*, August 19, 1929, English Section, 3.

46. "Many Michio Dancers to Dance on Rose Bowl Program," *Rafu Shimpo*, September 16, 1929, English Section, 3.

47. "Prince Igor Awaited for Bowl," *Rafu Shimpo*, August 4, 1930, English Section, 1.

48. "Ballet Wins Bowl Honors," *Los Angeles Times*, August 18, 1930, A7.

49. "Ballet Wins Bowl Honors."

50. "Ito Enthralls Huge Crowd," *Rafu Shimpo*, August 18, 1930, English Section, 1.

51. T. Fujitani, *Race for Empire: Koreans as Japanese and Japanese as Americans during World War II* (Berkeley: University of California Press, 2011).

52. Stanger, *Dancing on Violent Ground*, 17.

53. Wong, "Artistic Utopias," 160.

54. Juliana Chang, *Inhuman Citizenship: Traumatic Enjoyment and Asian American Literature* (Minneapolis: University of Minnesota Press, 2012) 25, 59.

55. Kandice Chuh, *Imagine Otherwise: On Asian Americanist Critique* (Durham: Duke University Press, 2003), 9.

56. Lisa Lowe, *Immigrant Acts: On Asian American Cultural Politics* (Durham: Duke University Press, 1996), 2.

57. For more on the problem of dancing selfhood in ("oriental") modern dance, see my essay, "Ito Michio, 'Oriental Dance,' and the Surfaces of Japanese American Modern Dance," in *Border Crossings: Exile and American Modern Dance*, eds. Ninotchka D. Bennahum and Rena M. Heinrich (New York: The New York Public Library for the Performing Arts, Lincoln Center / Santa Barbara: Museum of Art, Design & Architecture, UC Santa Barbara, 2024).

58. Charles W. Mills, *The Racial Contract* (Ithaca: Cornell University Press, 1997); Joshua Takano Chambers-Letson, *A Race So Different: Performance and Law in Asian America* (New York: New York University Press, 2013).

59. Lauren Berlant, *Cruel Optimism* (Durham: Duke University Press, 2011).

60. Jacqueline Rose, *States of Fantasy* (Oxford: Oxford University Press, 1996), 21.

61. Isabel Morse Jones, "Kipling's Famous Phrase Disproved by Michio Ito," *Los Angeles Times*, August 20, 1933, A2.

62. Oguma Eiji, *A Genealogy of "Japanese" Self-Images*, trans. David Askew (Melbourne: Trans Pacific Press, 2002); Tessa Morris-Suzuki, "Becoming Japanese: Imperial Expansion and Identity Crises in the Early Twentieth Century," in *Japan's Competing Modernities: Issues in Culture and Democracy 1900–1930*, ed. Sharon A. Minichiello (Honolulu: University of Hawai'i Press, 1998).

63. Douglas Slaymaker, *The Body in Postwar Fiction: Japanese Fiction after the War* (New York: Routledge, 2004). See chapter 7 for more on *nikutai* during the Allied Occupation.

64. Bert Winther-Tamaki, *Maximum Embodiment: Yōga, the Western Painting of Japan, 1912–1955* (Honolulu: University of Hawai'i Press, 2012), 20–21. See also Noriko Horiguchi's important work on *kokutai* in mid-twentieth-century literature: *Women Adrift: The Literature of Japan's Imperial Body* (Minneapolis: University of Minnesota Press, 2011).

65. "Itō shi no buyōgeijutsu sen to ugoki to hyōgen, kono utsukushisa ni kōkotsu" [Ecstatic beauty in the lines, movement, and expression of Itō's dance art], *Rafu Shimpo*, June 9, 1929, 3.

66. Carol Sorgenfrei, "Strategic Unweaving: Ito Michio and the Diasporic Dancing Body," in *The Politics of Interweaving Performance Cultures: Beyond Postcolonialism*, eds. Erika Fischer-Lichte, Torsten Jost, and Saskya Iris Jain (London: Routledge, 2014).

67. T. Fujitani, *Race for Empire*, 125–40, 256–71.

68. "East Is East, American Divorcee Now Agrees," *New York Tribune*, April 3, 1936, 16.

69. Bill Ong Hing, *Making and Remaking Asian America Through Immigration Policy, 1850–1990* (Stanford: Stanford University Press, 1993), 45.

70. Martha Gardener, *The Qualities of a Citizen: Women, Immigration, and Citizenship, 1870–1965* (Princeton: Princeton University Press, 2005); Yuki Oda, "Family Unity in U.S. Immigration Policy, 1921–1978" (PhD diss., Columbia University, 2014), 109–24.

71. "Ballets to Be Presented at Hollywood Bowl Tonight," *Los Angeles Times*, August 19, 1937, A8. "Hidemaro Konoye Conducts Hollywood Bowl Program," *Los Angeles Times*, August 20, 1937, 15. "Nisei Girls Dance in Ito's Ballet at Bowl Tonight," *Rafu Shimpo*, August 19, 1937, English Section, 8.

72. For an interpretation arguing that the white dancer's body sticks out, see Carol Sorgenfrei's essay, "Strategic Unweaving."

73. Hollywood Bowl Program, *Dancing Under the Stars*, August 17, 1937, 34.

74. Boris Morros, "Wise Nipponese," *Los Angeles Times*, July 13, 1937, B6. The *Rafu Shimpo*, hoping for more of a story, was rebuffed, and reported that Konoe was "Mum on Far East Strife." *Rafu Shimpo*, August 16, 1937, English Section, 6.

75. Zoë Alexis Lang, *The Legacy of Johann Strauss* (Cambridge: Cambridge University Press, 2014), 86, 140.

76. Mitchell Greenberg, *Baroque Bodies: Psychoanalysis and the Culture of French Absolutism* (Ithaca: Cornell University Press, 2001), 107–8.

Chapter Five

1. Eiichiro Azuma, *In Search of Our Frontier: Japanese America and Settler Colonialism in the Construction of Japan's Borderless Empire* (Oakland: University of California Press, 2019), 125.

Notes to Pages 162–72

2. Azuma, *In Search of Our Frontier*, 6.

3. Teemu Ruskola, "Canton Is Not Boston: The Invention of American Imperial Sovereignty," *American Quarterly* 57, no. 3 (Sep. 2005): 860.

4. See Tavia Nyong'o, *The Amalgamation Waltz: Race, Performance, and the Ruses of Memory* (Minneapolis: University of Minnesota Press, 2009).

5. Ushiyama Mitsuru, "Itō Michio Buyōdan wo miru" [Seeing the Itō Michio Dance Group], *Asahi Shimbun*, April 24, 1931, 8.

6. Ushiyama Mitsuru, "Aruhentina no buyō" [Argentina's dance], *Asahi Shimbun*, January 28, 1929, 5; "Sakarofu no buyō wo miru" [Seeing the Sakaroffs dance], *Asahi Shinbun*, January 29, 1931, 5.

7. Ushiyama, "Itō Michio buyōdan wo miru."

8. Ushiyama, "Itō Michio buyōdan wo miru."

9. See, for instance, "Buyōchū no Itō fujin kōin de kaijō tachimachi daikonran" [Mrs. Itō arrested during middle of dance, performance hall thrown into great confusion], *Yomiuri Shimbun*, May 6, 1931, 7; "Dansu shintorishimari keishichō de chikaku tsukuru" [New controls on dance will soon be made by the chief superintendent], *Asahi Shimbun*, May 7, 1931, 2.

10. "Mei Torishimari" [The Great Crackdown], *Asahi Shimbun*, May 8, 1931, 3.

11. Tessa Morris-Suzuki, "Debating Racial Science in Wartime Japan," *Osiris* 13 (1998); Jennifer Robertson, "Blood Talks: Eugenic Modernity and the Creation of New Japanese," *History and Anthropology* 13, no. 3 (2002).

12. Eika Tai, "Intermarriage and Imperial Subject Formation in Colonial Taiwan: Shoji Soichi's Chin-Fujin," *Inter-Asia Cultural Studies* 15, no. 4 (2014).

13. Morris-Suzuki, "Debating Racial Science," 361.

14. Morris-Suzuki, "Debating Racial Science," 363.

15. Fujita Fujio, *Itō Michio, sekai wo mau* [Itō Michio, dancing through the world] (Tokyo: Musashino Shobō, 1992), 141.

16. Daisuke Miyao, *Sessue Hayakawa: Silent Cinema and Transnational Stardom* (Durham: Duke University Press, 2007), 38–44; 107–10.

17. Michiko Tanaka, "Seki Sano and Popular Political and Social Theatre in Latin America," *Latin American Theatre Review* 27, no. 2 (Spring 1994): 55.

18. Fujita, *Itō Michio*, 145.

19. Fujita, *Itō Michio*, 159.

20. Ellie Guerrero, *Dance and the Arts in Mexico, 1920–1950: The Cosmic Generation* (Cham, Switzerland: Palgrave Macmillan, 2018), 122–26; Mitchell K. Snow, *A Revolution in Movement: Dancers, Painters, and the Image of Modern Mexico* (Gainesville: University Press of Florida, 2021), 165–69.

21. Jose Luis Reynoso, "Choreographing Modern Mexico: Anna Pavlova in Mexico City (1919)," *Modernist Cultures* 9, no. 1 (2014); *Dancing Mestizo Modernisms: Choreographing Postcolonial and Postrevolutionary Mexico* (New York: Oxford University Press, 2023).

22. Jerry García, *Looking Like the Enemy: Japanese Mexicans, the Mexican State, and US Hegemony, 1897–1945* (Tucson: University of Arizona Press, 2014), 95–98.

23. Daniel M. Masterson with Sayaka Funada-Classen, *The Japanese in Latin America* (Urbana: University of Illinois Press, 2004), 28.

24. "Nihon wo reisan suru Itō Michio-shi no inshō" [Glorifying Japan, impressions of

278   Notes to Pages 173–77

Itō Michio], *Mehiko Shinpō*, June 6, 1934. Waseda University, Tsubouchi Memorial Theatre Museum, Senda Koreya Archive, J11 Scrapbook #5. All the Japanese- and Spanish-language articles from Mexican newspapers cited in this section are in a scrapbook at the above archive.

25. "Itō shi no buyō ni gaikōdan no shōtai" [The diplomatic corps's invitation to see Itō dance], no paper title, no date.

26. "Itō shi no buyō wo miru" [Seeing Mr. Itō dance], no paper title, no date.

27. For example, "Itō shi no buyō ni gaikōdan no shōtai."

28. "Itō shi no buyō wo miru."

29. "Itō shi no buyō ni tsuite" [About Mr. Itō's dancing], no paper title, no date.

30. Eiichiro Azuma, *Between Two Empires: Race, History, and Transnationalism in Japanese America* (Oxford: Oxford University Press, 2005), 38.

31. García, *Looking like the Enemy*, 84–85.

32. "Shōsū yūshi no moyōshita Itō shi kangei zadangō" [Theatre discussion and welcome with a few of Ito's supporters], *Mehiko Shinpō*, June 9, 1934.

33. "Seinen shokun!! Itō shi to kataru yūbe" [Come, young people!! An evening with Mr. Itō], no paper title, no date.

34. "Yoki ijō no seika wo osameru, honsha shusai Itō shi zadankai" [Better results than expected, roundtable discussion with Mr. Itō sponsored by the head office], *Mehiko Shinpō*, June 13, 1934.

35. "Shōsuu yūshi no mōshita Itō-shi kangei zadankai" [A gathering hosted by a few enthusiasts: welcome discussion for Mr. Itō], no paper title, no date.

36. The journalist here uses "zaigai dōhō" rather than "kaigai dōhō," which became the standard formulation by 1940. On the discourse of "overseas brethren," Azuma, *In Search of Our Frontier*, 230–50; Kenneth J. Ruoff, *Imperial Japan at Its Zenith: The Wartime Celebration of the Empire's 2,600th Anniversary* (Ithaca: Cornell University Press, 2010), 171–74; and Sidney Xu Li, *The Making of Japanese Settler Colonialism* (New York: Columbia University Press, 2019), 229–31.

37. As Tsuyoshi Namigata traces, the term "avant-garde" (*zen'ei*) entered Japanese in the 1920s, from French surrealist film discourse, containing as well the word's earlier military connotations. Tsuyoshi Namigata, *Ekkyō no avangyarudo* (Tokyo: NTT Shuppan, 2005).

38. "Pasado mañana debutara Michio Ito, el eximio bailarin Japones, en el Teatro Hidalgo" [The day after tomorrow, the Japanese dancer Ito Michio will make his debut at the Hidalgo Theatre], *Jueves de Excelsior*, May 31, 1934.

39. "Exicto de Michio Ito" [Michio Ito's success], *El Universal*, June 14, 1934.

40. "Escenarios: Michio Ito en el Hidalgo" [Scenarios: Michio Ito at the Hidalgo], *El Mundo*, June 4, 1934.

41. "Michio Ito y su Cuadro de Solistas En El Teatro Hidalgo" [Michio Ito and his ensemble of soloists at the Hidalgo Theater], no paper title, no date.

42. On this divide, see Susan Manning, *Modern Dance, Negro Dance: Race in Motion* (Minneapolis: University of Minnesota Press, 2004), 118.

43. Carlos Gonzalez Peña, "Michio Ito y sus Bailarinas" [Michio Ito and his ballerinas], no paper title, June 24, 1934. Thanks to José Eduardo Valadés for discussion on this commentary. The original quotation in Spanish is: "El nombre es exótico. Michio Ito. Dícesele japonés. La verdad es que viéndole bailair nos convencemos de que no tiene los ojos sufi-

Notes to Pages 177–86

cientemente oblicuos como para garantizar la procedencia. Ignoro si en el Japón la oblicuidad no sea general, sino parchial tano sólo. De todas maneras . . . ¿No será un nipón algo mestizo?"

44. Ellen Samuels, *Fantasies of Identification: Disability, Gender, Race* (New York: New York University Press, 2014).

45. Gonzalez Peña, "Michio Ito y sus Bailarinas."

46. Robert McKee Irwin, *Mexican Masculinities* (Minneapolis: University of Minnesota Press, 2003), 117.

47. Diana Taylor, *The Archive and the Repertoire: Performing Cultural Memory in the Americas* (Durham: Duke University Press, 2003), 93–96.

48. No article title, *Universal Grafico*, June 16, 1934.

49. "La Personalidad Artistica de Michio Ito" [The artistic personality of Michio Ito], no paper title, July 5, 1934.

50. "Miryoku aru gunbu 'Purinsu Igōru' Nichigeki bare—hyō" [Impressive group dance "Prince Igor" at the Nichigeki Ballet], *Asahi Shimbun*, November 3, 1939, 8.

51. "Hibonna shuwan enshutsu ni shimeshita Itō risaitaru hyō" [Rare abilities shown in the performance of the Itō recital], *Asahi Shimbun*, December 5, 1939, 8.

52. "Hibonna shuwan."

53. "Shingeki ni shinseimen" [A new phase for shingeki], *Asahi Shimbun*, December 20, 1939, 8.

54. See Ruoff, *Imperial Japan at Its Zenith*.

55. "'Daibutsu Kaigen' jūkōmi aru fūzoku byōsha" ["Daibutsu Kaigen" profound depiction of customs], *Asahi Shinbun*, February 6, 1940, 6.

56. As Eiichiro Azuma traces in the discourse around the development of farming techniques suitable for Manchurian settlements, although the most effective and widely adopted techniques all came from the US—brought by remigrated Issei who had first established themselves as farmers there—by the mid-1930s discussions of American influence had become unacceptable. Azuma, *In Search of Our Frontier*, 171–78.

57. Senda Koreya, *Mō hitotsu no shingekishi* [One more history of shingeki] (Tokyo: Chikuma Shōbō, 1975), 445.

58. "Michio Ito Brings White Peacocks as Gift to President," *Shin Sekai Asahi*, June 18, 1940, 1.

59. "Michio Ito Brings White Peacocks."

60. "Exhibit A," Department of Justice Alien Enemy Hearing Board, National Archives and Records Administration, at Riverside, Record Group 85, District 16, Enemy Alien Case Files, Folder 15942/633—Michio Ito, Box 27.

Chapter Six

1. Itō Michio, *Amerika to nihon* [America and Japan] (Tokyo: Yakumo Shoten, 1946, 1948), 259.

2. Itō, *Amerika to nihon*, 268.

3. Itō, *Amerika to nihon*, 270.

4. Fujita Fujio, *Itō Michio, sekai wo mau* [Itō Michio, dancing through the world] (Tokyo: Musashino Shobō, 1992), 110.

5. Mary F. Watkins, "The Dancers," *New York Herald Tribune*, May 6, 1928, F9.

6. Kevin Riordan, "Performance in the Wartime Archive: Michio Ito at the Alien Enemy Hearing Board," *American Studies* 55/56, no. 4 (2017).

7. On the afterlives and haunting memories of the Asia-Pacific War, see Jessica Nakamura, *Transgenerational Remembrance: Performance and the Asia-Pacific War in Contemporary Japan* (Evanston: Northwestern University Press, 2020).

8. Yutian Wong, "Artistic Utopias: Michio Ito and the Trope of the International," in *Worlding Dance*, ed. Susan Leigh Foster (New York: Palgrave Macmillan, 2009).

9. Carol Sorgenfrei, "Strategic Unweaving: Itō Michio and the Diasporic Dancing Body," in *The Politics of Interweaving Performance Cultures: Beyond Postcolonialism*, eds. Erika Fischer-Lichte, Torsten Jost, and Saskya Iris Jain (New York: Routledge, 2014).

10. The word "internment" is commonly, but inaccurately, used to refer to the broad phenomenon of the imprisonment of Japanese nationals and Japanese Americans during the Pacific War. In fact, the vast majority of prisoners, who were held under Roosevelt's Executive Order 9066, were imprisoned at the ten camps administered by the War Relocation Authority, which were called "relocation centers," and their experience is properly referred to as "incarceration." (While these centers were being constructed, these prisoners were held at temporary "assembly centers.") Ito, however, *was* interned; he underwent a "trial," at which he was "convicted" and ordered to be interned, and then was imprisoned at four of the "internment camps" administered by the Justice Department. These were used to imprison German, Italian, and Japanese "enemy aliens" who were considered dangerous. See Tetsuden Kashima, *Judgment without Trial: Japanese American Imprisonment during World War II* (Seattle: University of Washington Press, 2003), 8–9.

11. Gail Okawa, "Putting Their Lives on the Line: Personal Narrative as Political Discourse among Japanese Petitioners in American World War II Internment," *College English* 74, no. 1 (September 2011): 52.

12. On the precisely choreographed and spectacular performance of the first forty-eight hours of these arrests, see the chapter "Spectacularizing Japanese American Suspects" in Emily Roxworthy's *The Spectacle of Japanese American Trauma: Racial Performativity and World War II* (Honolulu: University of Hawai'i Press, 2008).

13. National Archives and Records Administration at Kansas City, Record Group 566, Records of the U.S. Citizenship and Immigration Services, Alien Case Files, 1944–2003, Alien Case File A5783768, Michio Ito.

14. National Archives and Records Administration at Kansas City.

15. "Exhibit 'A,'" Department of Justice Alien Enemy Hearing Board, National Archives and Records Administration, National Archives at Riverside. Record Group 85, Records of the Immigration and Naturalization Services, District 16. Alien Enemy Case Files, 1941–1948, Folder 15942/633 Michio Ito, Box 27.

16. Sakomizu was to become the chief secretary to Kantarō Suzuki, the final prime minister of the war. During this time, Sakomizu determined that Japan did not have the resources to continue fighting the war for much longer. In this, he and Ito agreed, and perhaps even discussed after Ito's repatriation.

17. Yuji Tosaka, "The Discourse of Anti-Americanism and Hollywood Movies: Film Import Controls in Japan, 1937–1941," *Journal of American–East Asian Relations* 12, no. 1/2 (Spring-Summer 2003).

Notes to Pages 191–97

18. Cemil Aydin, *The Politics of Anti-Westernism in Asia* (New York: Columbia University Press, 2007), 172–73.

19. "Memorandum for Major Lemuel B. Schofield," November 18, 1941, Alien Case Files, National Archives at Kansas City.

20. "Memorandum," November 27, 1941, Alien Case Files, National Archives at Kansas City.

21. "Memorandum for Mr. L. M. C. Smith," November 4, 1941, Alien Case Files, National Archives at Kansas City.

22. Paul J. Clark, "Those Other Camps: An Oral History Analysis of Japanese Alien Enemy Internment During World War II" (master's thesis, California State University, Fullerton, 1980).

23. Carol Bulger Van Valkenburg, "An Alien Place: The Fort Missoula, Montana, Detention Camp, 1941–1944" (master's thesis, University of Montana, 1988).

24. We might compare Ito's wartime notebooks to those of the Japanese writer Nagai Kafu, who consistently wrote withering criticism of Japan's military regime in his diary (published in 1947 under the title *Risai Nichiroku, A Daily Account of the Calamity*). During most of the Fifteen Years War, Nagai was publicly silent, unwilling to publish writing that accorded with the government's propaganda demands. Instead, he wrote in his diary in the voice of his literary alter ego, the Danchōtei. Though Nagai hid this and other manuscripts in a Boston bag that he kept with him throughout the war, *Risai Nichiroki* is written with a sense of future readership—whether or not Nagai himself survived. David C. Earhart, "Nagai Kafu's Wartime Diary: The Enormity of Nothing," *Japan Quarterly* 41, no. 4 (Oct 1994).

25. Internment Notebook, Tsubouchi Memorial Theatre Museum, Waseda University, Senda Koreya Archive, J21.

26. Satō Yoshiaki, *J-Pop Shinkaron: "Yosahoi bushi" kara "automatic" e* (Tokyo: Heibonsha Shinsho, 1999), 52–58. In a *yosahoi bushi*, usually the first word of each verse echoes the sound of the number being counted. So in the first verse, *hitotsu* (one) should then be followed by a line that begins with the sound "hi." Here, I have opted for a translation emphasizing meaning rather than trying to find aural equivalents of the song's wordplay. Many thanks to Kushida Kiyomi for working through this song with me, and to Asako Katsura for her thoughtful suggestions.

27. The *shūyō* of "self-improvement" in this line has the same pronunciation as a different *shūyō*, meaning "custody" or "internment," as used in the word *shūyōjo*—internment or concentration camp. We might read this line, then, as containing a sardonic pun on the long-term self-improvement possible under long-term imprisonment. Many thanks to Andrew Leong for this reading.

28. The corporeal emphasis also finds echoes in the references to the body in lines 5 and 8.

29. J21 Internment Notebook.

30. J21 Internment Notebook.

31. J21 Internment Notebook.

32. J21 Internment Notebook.

33. J21 Internment Notebook.

282   Notes to Pages 198–203

34. Taki Ryōichi, "Tōyō ni okeru būyō ni tsuite," *Tōyō ongaku kenkyū* 2 (1937).

35. Eri Hotta, *Pan-Asianism and Japan's War, 1931–1945* (New York: Palgrave Macmillan, 2007); *Pan-Asianism in Modern Japanese History: Colonialism, Regionalism and Borders*. eds. Sven Saaler and J. Victor Koschmann (London: Routledge, 2007).

36. Jawaharlal Nehru, *Glimpses of World History* (Bombay: Asia Publishing House, 1934, 1962), 413–14.

37. Sven Saaler, "Pan-Asianism in Modern Japanese History: Overcoming the Nation, Creating a Region, Forging an Empire," in *Pan-Asianism in Modern Japanese History*; Cemil Aydin, "Japan's Pan-Asianism and the Legitimacy of Imperial World Order, 1931–1945," *Asia-Pacific Journal: Japan Focus* 6, no. 3 (March 2008).

38. Louise Young, *Japan's Total Empire: Manchuria and the Culture of Wartime Imperialism* (Berkeley: University of California Press, 1998), 239.

39. This included Hong Kong, French Indochine (Vietnam, Cambodia, Laos), British New Guinea, the Philippines, Malaya, and Brunei.

40. There is a large and growing literature on these topics. Here, I cite only a few representative English-language sources that I have not listed elsewhere. John Dower, *War Without Mercy: Race and Power in the Pacific War* (New York: Pantheon Books, 1993); Mark Peattie, *Nan'yō: The Rise and Fall of the Japanese in Micronesia, 1885–1945* (Honolulu: University of Hawai'i Press, 1992, 1998); Elizabeth W. Son, *Embodied Reckonings: "Comfort Women," Performance, and Transpacific Redress* (Ann Arbor: University of Michigan Press, 2018).

41. Ishii Kan, *Ishii Baku—buyōshijin* [Ishii Baku: dance-poet] (Tokyo: Miraisha, 1994), 265.

42. War Notebook, Tsubouchi Memorial Theatre Museum, Waseda University, Senda Koreya Archive, J30 #2, p. 20.

43. On the "three human bullets" mass media boom in the early 1930s that established this trope, see Louise Young, *Japan's Total Empire*, 77–78.

44. R. James Brandon, *Kabuki's Forgotten War, 1931–1945* (Honolulu: University of Hawai'i Press, 2009); Samuel Leiter, "Wartime Colonial and Traditional Theatre," in *A History of Japanese Theatre*, ed. Jonah Salz (Cambridge: Cambridge University Press, 2016); Benjamin Uchiyama, *Japan's Carnival War: Mass Culture on the Home Front, 1937–1945* (Cambridge: Cambridge University Press, 2019).

45. Jennifer Robertson, "Ethnicity and Gender in the Wartime Japanese Revue Theatre," in *War and Militarism in Modern Japan: Issues of History and Identity*, ed. Guy Podoler (Folkestone, UK: Global Oriental, 2009).

46. When performers entertained military troops, their work frequently was categorized under the term *imon*, or "comfort." In Japanese, *imon* is distinct from the "comfort" of *ian*, which is used for the system of sexual slavery known as "comfort women." *Imon* has the sense of (female-provided) reassurance, and so, while *imon* is used for concepts such as theatrical support troupes, or care packages (*imon-dan* and *imon-bukuro*), it is important to emphasize how these different notions of "comfort" were all part of the same integrated system.

47. J. Thomas Rimer, *Toward a Modern Japanese Theatre: Kishida Kunio* (Princeton: Princeton University Press, 1974).

Notes to Pages 203–10

48. Guohe Zheng, "From War Responsibility to the Red Purge," in *Rising from the Flames: The Rebirth of Theater in Occupied Japan, 1945–1952*, ed. Samuel Leiter (Lanham, MD: Lexington Books, 2009).

49. Hoshino Yukiyo, "Use of Dance to Spread Propaganda during the Sino-Japanese War," *Athens Journal of History* 2, no. 3 (July 2016): 195.

50. See, for instance, Faye Yuan Kleeman, *In Transit: The Formation of the Colonial East Asian Cultural Sphere* (Honolulu: University of Hawai'i Press, 2014); Emily Wilcox, "Crossing Over: Choe-Seung-hui's Pan-Asianism in Revolutionary Times," *Journal of Society for Dance Documentation and History of South Korea* 51 (December 2018).

51. Nayoung Aimee Kwon, *Intimate Empire: Collaboration and Colonial Modernity in Korea and Japan* (Durham: Duke University Press, 2015), 8, 15.

52. On Japanese cultural activities in occupied Southeast Asia, see Leiter, "Wartime Colonial and Traditional Theatre"; Kleeman, *In Transit*, 251–66; Sang Mi Park, "Wartime Japan's Theater Movement," *WIAS Research Bulletin* 1 (2009); Yoshida Yukihiko, "National Dance under the Rising Sun, Mainly from National Dance, Buyō Geijutsu and the Activities of Takaya Eguchi," *International Journal of Eastern Sports and Physical Education* 7, no. 1 (October 2009); Matthew Isaac Cohen, *Inventing the Performing Arts: Modernity and Tradition in Colonial Indonesia* (Honolulu: University of Hawai'i Press, 2016).

53. Motoe Terami-Wada, "The Japanese Propaganda Corps in the Philippines: Laying the Foundation," in *Japanese Cultural Policies in Southeast Asia during World War 2*, ed. Grant K. Goodman (New York: St. Martin's Press, 1991).

54. Mark Ethan, "The Perils of Co-Prosperity: Takeda Rintarō, Occupied Southeast Asia, and the Seductions of Postcolonial Empire," *American Historical Review* 119, no. 4 (2014).

55. Numerous artists were sent on "comfort tours" to provide entertainment and assuage the homesickness of Japanese troops; they also performed for local populations across the empire.

56. John D. Swain, "Senda Koreya and the *Tenkō* Paradigm," in *Modern Japanese Theatre and Performance*, eds. David Jortner, Keiko McDonald, and Kevin J. Wetmore Jr. (Lanham, MD: Lexington Books, 2006).

57. Fujita Fujio, ed. *Daitōa butai geijutsu kenkyūjo kankei shiryō* [Greater East Asia Stage Arts Research Institute related documents] (Tokyo: Fujishuppan, 1993), 12.

58. For more on Watsuji Tetsurō and Ito's interest in this concept, see this book's introduction.

59. Document #7, Fujita, *Greater East Asia*.

60. Document #7, Fujita, *Greater East Asia*.

61. Document #7, Fujita, *Greater East Asia*.

62. See, for instance, Kim Brandt, "Objects of Desire: Japanese Collectors and Colonial Korea," *Positions* 8, no. 3 (Winter 2000).

63. Senda, *Mō hitotsu no shingekishi* [One more history of shingeki], (Tokyo: Chikuma Shōbō, 1975), 476.

64. The historian Hatano Sumio has argued that Japan's granting of "independence" in the Philippines and Burma was precisely in accordance with Senda's third hypothesis—that government officials surrounding Shigemitsu Mamoru—who was appointed foreign

284 Notes to Pages 210–21

minister in April 1943—began preparing for defeat and the war crime trials that would accompany it by effecting policies that would contribute to Japan's defense on the grounds of Asian liberation. Saaler, "Pan-Asianism in Modern Japanese History," 14.

65. Itō Michio, "Amerika no kokuminsei to geinō," *Engekikai* 2, no. 11 (November 1944): 10–12. R. James R. Brandon also discusses this article, and its appearance along with six other articles condemning American culture—all commissioned by the Bureau of Information, in *Kabuki's Forgotten War*, 289–93.

66. On *Miikusabune*, see Higashiya Sakurako, "Shinsakunō 'Miikusabune' no tamondai" [The various problems of the new piece 'Miikusabune'], *Japanese Literature Bulletin*, Showa Women's University 28 (2017); Satō Kazumichi, "Senjika no nogaku: 'Chūrei' 'Miikusabune' wo chūshin ni" [Wartime theatre: focusing on 'The Faithful' 'Miikusabune'], *Theatre Studies: Journal of the Japanese Society for Theatre Research* (November 2017). The play's author is given as Sako shōi (Second lieutenant Sako). It has not been determined who this is—nor whether it was an individual or a group—and for what exact security reasons their identity was kept hidden.

67. Senda, *Mō hitotsu no shingekishi*, 481–82.

68. Jennifer Robertson, *Takarazuka: Sexual Politics and Popular Culture in Modern Japan* (Berkeley: University of California Press, 1998), 115–20.

Chapter Seven

1. Itō Michio, *Josei handobukku, Echiketto* [Women's handbook: etiquette] (Tokyo: Rōdōbunkasha, 1947). Library of Congress, Asian Reading Room, 5.

2. Mark McLelland, *Love, Sex, and Democracy in Japan during the American Occupation* (New York: Palgrave Macmillan, 2012).

3. Itō, *Echiketto*, 9.

4. Itō, *Echiketto*, 10.

5. Itō, *Echiketto*, 13–14.

6. Kuwahara Noriko, "Ānīpairu gekijō wo meguru bijutsukatachi" [Concerning artists at the Ernie Pyle Theatre], *Seitoku Daigaku Kenkyū Kiyō* 18 (2007).

7. See, for example: Marlene J. Mayo, "To Be or Not to Be: *Kabuki* and Cultural Politics in Occupied Japan," in *War, Occupations, and Creativity: Japan and East Asia, 1920–1960*, eds. Marlene J. Mayo and Thomas J. Rimer (Honolulu: University of Hawai'i Press, 1999); James R. Brandon, "Myth and Reality: A Story of *Kabuki* during American Censorship, 1945–1949," *Asian Theatre Journal* 23, no. 1 (Spring 2006); Samuel L. Leiter, "The Good Censors: Evading the Threat to Postwar Kabuki," in *Rising from the Flames: The Rebirth of Theater in Occupied Japan, 1945–1952*, ed. Samuel Leiter (Lanham, MD: Lexington Books, 2009).

8. Itō Michio, "Ānīpairu Gekijō no koto: watashi no shigoto" [About the Ernie Pyle Theatre: my work], *Nihon Engeki*, October 1947, 41–42. The Gordon W. Prange Collection, Publications and Unpublished Materials from the Allied Occupation of Japan within the East Asian Collection, McKeldin Library, University of Maryland, College Park.

9. Tsubouchi Memorial Theatre Museum, Waseda University. Senda Korea Archive, J23 #8.

10. On Ito's postwar productions of *The Mikado* in Japan, see my essay "A More Humane

Notes to Pages 221–40

Mikado: Re-envisioning the Nation through Occupation-Era Productions of *The Mikado* in Japan," *Theatre Research International* 40, no. 3 (October 2015). On *Jungle Drum*, see Kushida Kiyomi, "Ānī Pairu gekijō no sutēji shō" [The Ernie Pyle Theatre's stage shows], *Jissen joshi daigaku bungakubu kiyō dai* 35 (2021).

11. George H. Lambert, "End of an Era: Far East's Largest Service Club Closes," *The Brigadier*, January 25, 1966, 5. Tsubouchi Memorial Theatre Museum, Waseda University. Senda Koreya Archive, J23 #14.

12. Shimada Toshio, "Ānīpairu gekijō Itō Michio hōmonki" [Ernie Pyle Theatre: notes from visiting Itō Michio], *Maru*, May 1948: 25–29. Gordon W. Prange Collection, University of Maryland.

13. Adria Imada, *Aloha America: Hula Circuits through the U.S. Empire* (Durham: Duke University Press, 2021), 217, 222.

14. Michelle Liu Carriger, *Theatricality of the Closet: Fashion, Performance, and Subjectivity between Victorian Britain and Meiji Japan* (Evanston: Northwestern University Press), 169.

15. This reimagining mirrored simultaneous efforts within the US to retrain the domestic public to think favorably of Japan, as Naoko Shibusawa has shown. *America's Geisha Ally: Reimagining the Japanese Enemy* (Cambridge, MA: Harvard University Press, 2006).

16. Tabasco Scenario, Tsubouchi Memorial Theatre Museum, Waseda University. Senda Koreya Archive, J23–1.

17. Brian Herrera, *Latin Numbers: Playing Latino in Twentieth-Century U.S. Popular Performance* (Ann Arbor: University of Michigan Press, 2015), 20.

18. Anne Anlin Cheng, *Ornamentalism* (New York: Oxford University Press, 2019), 18.

19. Anne Anlin Cheng, "Ornamentalism: A Feminist Theory for the Yellow Woman," *Critical Inquiry* 44 (Spring 2018): 415.

20. Saitō Ren, *Anī Pairu Gekijō, GI wo ian shita rebyū gāru* [Ernie Pyle Theatre: the revue girls who entertained GIs] (Tokyo: Bronze Shinsha, 1998), 75.

21. Takeo Doi, *The Anatomy of Self: The Individual Versus Society* (Tokyo: Kodansha USA Publishing, 1985). See also Carriger, *Theatricality of the Closet*, 168–69.

22. Nancy Rosenberger, *Gambling with Virtue: Japanese Women and the Search for Self in a Changing Nation* (Honolulu: University of Hawai'i Press, 2001), 29–31.

23. In addition to the titles in fn 7, see, for example, Marlene Mayo, "Civil Censorship and Media Control in Early Occupied Japan," in *Americans as Proconsuls: United States Military Government in Germany and Japan, 1944–1952*, ed. Robert Wolfe (Carbondale: Southern Illinois University Press, 1984); Sara Christine Snyder, "Odyssey of an Archives: What the History of the Gordon W. Prange Collection of Japanese Materials Teaches Us about Libraries, Censorship, and Keeping the Past Alive" (master's thesis, University of Maryland, 2007).

24. Carrie Lambert-Beatty, *Being Watched: Yvonne Rainer and the 1960s* (Cambridge, MA: MIT Press, 2008), 7.

25. Lambert-Beatty, *Being Watched*, 6.

26. Malia McAndrew, "Beauty, Soft Power, and the Politics of Womanhood During the U.S. Occupation of Japan, 1945–1952," *Journal of Women's History* 26, no. 4 (Winter 2014): 90.

27. Rebecca Corbett, *Cultivating Femininity: Women and Tea Culture in Edo and Meiji Japan* (Honolulu: University of Hawai'i Press, 2018).

28. Andrew Hewitt, *Social Choreography: Ideology as Performance in Dance and Everyday Movement* (Durham: Duke University Press, 2005), 80. Other important reflections on walking include Susan Leigh Foster, "Walking and Other Choreographic Tactics: Danced Inventions of Theatricality and Performativity," *SubStance* 31, no. 2/3 (2002); André Lepecki, *Exhausting Dance: Performance and the Politics of Movement* (New York: Routledge, 2006).

29. Hagar Kotef, *Movement and the Ordering of Freedom: On Liberal Governances of Mobility* (Durham: Duke University Press, 2015), 9.

30. Hewitt, *Social Choreography*, 80.

31. Itō, *Echiketto*, 45–46.

32. Itō, *Echiketto*, 48.

33. Itō, *Echiketto*, 49–50.

34. Karen Shimakawa, *National Abjection: The Asian American Body Onstage* (Durham: Duke University Press, 2002).

35. Douglas Slaymaker, *The Body in Postwar Fiction: Japanese Fiction after the War* (New York: Routledge, 2004), 8.

36. Michael Bourdaghs, *Sayonara Amerika, Sayonara Nippon: A Geopolitical Pre-History of J-Pop* (New York: Columbia University Press, 2012), 37.

37. On the *panpan* girl, see Slaymaker, *The Body in Postwar Fiction*, 40–42. See also Michael Molasky, *The American Occupation of Japan and Okinawa* (London: Routledge, 1999).

38. Itō, *Echiketto*, 50–51.

39. Danielle Goldman, *I Want to be Ready: Improvised Dance as a Practice of Freedom* (Ann Arbor: University of Michigan Press, 2010).

40. Itō Michio, "How to Walk Beautifully" [Utsukushii arukikata], *Style*, June 1946, 54–55.

41. Andrew Gordon, *Fabricating Consumers: The Sewing Machine in Modern Japan* (Oakland: University of California Press, 2021), 190.

42. Ju Yon Kim, *The Racial Mundane: Asian American Performance and the Embodied Everyday* (New York: NYU Press, 2015), 6, 15.

43. Kim, *Racial Mundane*, 3.

44. Christopher Bush, "The Ethnicity of Things in America's Lacquered Age," *Representations* 99, no. 1 (Summer 2007): 91.

45. Tsubouchi Memorial Theatre Museum, Waseda University. Senda Korea Archive, J2–1.

46. Carriger, *Theatricality of the Closet*, 4–7.

47. SanSan Kwan, *Kinesthetic City: Dance and Movement in Chinese Urban Spaces* (Oxford: Oxford University Press, 2013), 7.

48. Cheng, *Ornamentalism*, 85.

49. Itō, *Echiketto*.

50. See, for example, Katagiri Yoshio, "Naruse Jinzo to joshi taiiku: Nihon Daigakkou no 'yōgi taisō'" [Naruse Jinzo and women's physical education: 'yōgi gymnastics' at Japan Women's University], *Hikaku buyō kenkyū* 26, no. 3 (2020).

Notes to Pages 251–57

51. Hewitt, *Social Choreography*, 80.

52. Marié Abe, *Resonances of Chindon-ya: Sounding Space and Sociality in Contemporary Japan* (Middletown, CT: Wesleyan University Press, 2018), 52–53.

Conclusion

1. See, for example, clippings from the Ito file at the New York Public Library for Performing Arts: Sally Banes, "Remembering Michio Ito," *Village Voice*, May 15, 1978, 86; Susan Reiter, "Reviving and Restoring," no paper title, June 14, 1979, 7.

2. Mary-Jean Cowell and Satoru Shimazaki, "East and West in the Work of Michio Ito," *Dance Research Journal* 26, no. 2 (Autumn 1994).

3. Author's conversation with Dana Tai Soon Burgess, May 3, 2021. See also Dana Tai Soon Burgess, *Chino and the Dance of the Butterfly: A Memoir* (Albuquerque: University of New Mexico Press, 2022).

4. Dana Tai Soon Burgess, "Dance and Social Justice: Retracing the Steps of Michio Itō," in *Milestones in Dance History*, ed. Dana Tai Soon Burgess (New York: Routledge, 2023), 151.

5. Timothy Cowert, "Interview with Director Bonnie Oda Homsey," *DanceFilms.org* https://www.dancefilms.org/2013/01/23/interview-with-director-bonnie-oda-homsey/

6. *Michio Ito: Pioneering Dance-Choreographer*, directed by Bonnie Oda Homsey (Los Angeles Dance Foundation, 2013).

7. Daphne Lei, "Ruptures Within and Without: *Pageantry*—A Work in Progress by Denise Uyehara and Sri Susilowati," *Theatre Research International* 35, no. 2 (July 2010).

8. Author's conversation with Michele Ito, August 15, 2023.

9. André Lepecki, "The Body as Archive: Will to Re-Enact and the Afterlives of Dances," *Dance Research Journal* 42, no. 2 (Winter 2010): 31.

BIBLIOGRAPHY

Abe, Marié. *Resonances of Chindon-ya: Sounding Space and Sociality in Contemporary Japan*. Middletown, CT: Wesleyan University Press, 2018.

Adams, Timothy Dow. *Telling Lies in Modern American Autobiography*. Chapel Hill: University of North Carolina Press, 1990.

Ahmed, Sara. *Queer Phenomenology: Orientations, Objects, Others*. Durham: Duke University Press, 2006.

Aydin, Cemil. *The Politics of Anti-Westernism in Asia*. New York: Columbia University Press, 2007.

Aydin, Cemil. "Japan's Pan-Asianism and the Legitimacy of Imperial World Order, 1931–1945." *Asia-Pacific Journal: Japan Focus* 6, no. 3 (March 2008): 1–33.

Azuma, Eiichiro. "Pioneers of Overseas Japanese Development: Japanese American History and the Making of Expansionist Orthodoxy in Imperial Japan." *Journal of Asian Studies* 67, no. 4 (Nov. 2002): 1187–226.

Azuma, Eiichiro. *Between Two Empires: Race, History, and Transnationalism in Japanese America*. New York: Oxford University Press, 2005.

Azuma, Eiichiro. "The Making of a Japanese American Race, and Why Are There No 'Immigrants' in Postwar Nikkei History and Community? The Problems of Generation, Region, and Citizenship in Japanese America." In *TransPacific Japanese American Studies: Conversations on Race and Racializations*, edited by Yasuko Takezawa and Gary Y. Okihiro, 257–87. Honolulu: University of Hawai'i Press, 2016.

Azuma, Eiichiro. *In Search of Our Frontier: Japanese America and Settler Colonialism in the Construction of Japan's Borderless Empire*. Oakland: University of California Press, 2019.

Berlant, Lauren. *The Anatomy of National Fantasy: Hawthorne, Utopia, and Everyday Life*. Chicago: University of Chicago Press, 1991.

Berlant, Lauren. *Cruel Optimism*. Durham: Duke University Press, 2011.

Bernstein, Robin. *Racial Innocence: Performing American Childhood from Slavery to Civil Rights*. New York: New York University Press, 2011.

Bhabha, Homi. "'Race,' Time and the Revision of Modernity." *Oxford Literary Review* 13, no. 1/2 (1991): 193–219.

Bourdaghs, Michael. *Sayonara Amerika, Sayonara Nippon: A Geopolitical Pre-History of J-Pop*. New York: Columbia University Press, 2012.

Bow, Leslie. "Fetish." In *The Routledge Companion to Asian American and Pacific Islander Literature*, edited by Rachel C. Lee, 122–31. New York: Routledge, 2014.

Bow, Leslie. *Racist Love: Asian Abstraction and the Pleasures of Fantasy.* Durham: Duke University Press, 2022.

Bradford, Curtis. *Yeats at Work.* Carbondale: Southern Illinois University Press, 1965.

Brandon, James R. "Myth and Reality: A Story of *Kabuki* during American Censorship, 1945–1949." *Asian Theatre Journal* 23, no. 1 (Spring 2006): 1–110.

Brandon, James R. *Kabuki's Forgotten War, 1931–1945.* Honolulu: University of Hawai'i Press, 2009.

Brandt, Kim. "Objects of Desire: Japanese Collectors and Colonial Korea." *Positions* 8, no. 3 (Winter 2000): 711–46.

Brooks, Charlotte. *Alien Neighbors, Foreign Friends: Asian Americans, Housing, and the Transformation of Urban California.* Chicago: University of Chicago Press, 2009.

Burgess, Dana Tai Soon. *Chino and the Dance of the Butterfly: A Memoir.* Albuquerque: University of New Mexico Press, 2022.

Burgess, Dana Tai Soon. "Dance and Social Justice: Retracing the Steps of Michio Itō." In *Milestones in Dance History*, edited by Dana Tai Soon Burgess, 134–58. New York: Routledge, 2023.

Bush, Christopher. "The Ethnicity of Things in America's Lacquered Age." *Representations* 99, no. 1 (Summer 2007): 74–98.

Bush, Christopher. *Ideographic Modernism: China, Writing, Medium.* Oxford: Oxford University Press, 2010.

Bush, Christopher. "I Am All for the Triangle: The Geopolitical Aesthetic of Pound's Japan." In *Ezra Pound in the Present: Essays on Pound's Contemporaneity*, edited by Josephine Park and Paul Stasi, 75–106. New York: Bloomsbury, 2016.

Caldwell, Helen. *Michio Ito: The Dancer and His Dances.* Berkeley: University of California Press, 1977.

Camp, Pannill. "The Poetics of Performance Nonevents." *Journal of Dramatic Theory and Criticism* 32, no. 2 (2018): 141–50.

Candelario, Rosemary. *Flowers Cracking Concrete: Eiko & Koma's Asian/American Choreographies.* Middletown, CT: Wesleyan University Press, 2016.

Carriger, Michelle Liu. *Theatricality of the Closet: Fashion, Performance, and Subjectivity between Victorian Britain and Meiji Japan.* Evanston: Northwestern University Press, 2023.

Chambers-Letson, Joshua Takano. *A Race So Different: Performance and Law in Asian America.* New York: New York University Press, 2013.

Chang, Juliana. *Inhuman Citizenship: Traumatic Enjoyment and Asian American Literature.* Minneapolis: University of Minnesota Press, 2012.

Chauncey, George. *Gay New York: Gender, Urban Culture, and the Making of the Gay Male World, 1890–1940.* New York: Basic Books, 1994.

Cheng, Anne Anlin. *The Melancholy of Race: Psychoanalysis, Assimilation, and Hidden Grief.* Oxford: Oxford University Press, 2000.

Cheng, Anne Anlin. *Second Skin: Josephine Baker and the Modern Surface.* Oxford: Oxford University Press, 2010.

Cheng, Anne Anlin. "Ornamentalism: A Feminist Theory for the Yellow Woman." *Critical Inquiry* 44 (Spring 2018): 415–46.

Bibliography

Cheng, Anne Anlin. *Ornamentalism*. Oxford: Oxford University Press, 2019.

Chiba, Yoko. "Kori Torahiko and Edith Craig: A Japanese Playwright in London and Toronto." *Comparative Drama* 30, no. 4 (Winter 1996–97): 431–51.

Chou, Wan-yao. "The *Kōminka* Movement in Taiwan and Korea: Comparisons and Interpretations." In *The Japanese Wartime Empire, 1931–1945*, edited by Peter Duus, Ramon H. Myers, and Mark R. Peatti, 40–70. Princeton: Princeton University Press, 1996.

Chow, Rey. "Fateful Attachments: On Collecting, Fidelity, and Lao She." *Critical Inquiry* 28, no. 1 (Autumn 2001), Things: 286–304.

Chuh, Kandice. *Imagine Otherwise: On Asian Americanist Critique*. Durham: Duke University Press, 2003.

Clancey, Greg. *Earthquake Nation: The Cultural Politics of Japanese Seismicity, 1868–1930*. Berkeley: University of California Press, 2006.

Clark, Paul J. "Those Other Camps: An Oral History Analysis of Japanese Alien Enemy Internment During World War II." Master's thesis, California State University, Fullerton, 1980.

Cohen, Matthew Isaac. "Dancing the Subject of 'Java': International Modernism and Traditional Performance, 1899–1952." *Indonesia and the Malay World* 35, no. 101 (2007).

Cohen, Matthew Isaac. *Inventing the Performing Arts: Modernity and Tradition in Colonial Indonesia*. Honolulu: University of Hawai'i Press, 2016.

Collins, Sandra. *The 1940 Tokyo Games: The Missing Olympics*. New York: Routledge, 2007.

Cooper, Emmanuel. *The Sexual Perspective: Homosexuality and Art in the Last 100 Years in the West*. New York: Routledge, 1994.

Corbett, Rebecca. *Cultivating Femininity: Women and Tea Culture in Edo and Meiji Japan*. Honolulu: University of Hawai'i Press, 2018.

Cowan, Michael J. *Cult of the Will: Nervousness and German Modernity*. University Park: Pennsylvania State University Press, 2008.

Cowell, Mary-Jean, and Satoru Shimazaki. "East and West in the Work of Michio Ito." *Dance Research Journal* 26, no. 2 (Autumn 1994): 11–23.

Cowell, Mary-Jean. "Michio Ito in Hollywood: Modes and Ironies of Ethnicity." *Dance Chronicle* 24, no. 3 (2001): 263–305.

Cullingford, Elizabeth. *Yeats, Ireland, and Fascism*. London: Macmillan, 1981.

Daly, Ann. *Done into Dance: Isadora Duncan in America*. Middletown, CT: Wesleyan University Press, 2002.

Davis, Mike. *City of Quartz: Excavating the Future in Los Angeles*. New York: Verso, 1990.

de Gruchy, John W. *Orienting Arthur Waley: Japonism, Orientalism, and the Creation of Japanese Literature in English*. Honolulu: University of Hawai'i Press, 2003.

Desmond, Jane. "Dancing Out the Difference: Cultural Imperialism and Ruth St. Denis' 'Radha' of 1906." *Signs* 17, no. 1 (1991): 28–49.

Doi, Takeo. *The Anatomy of Self: The Individual versus Society*. Tokyo: Kodansha USA Publishing, 1985.

Dorn, Karen. *Players and Painted Stage: The Theatre of W. B. Yeats*. Sussex: Harvester Press, 1984.

Dower, John. *War without Mercy: Race and Power in the Pacific War*. New York: Pantheon Books, 1993.

Dower, John. *Embracing Defeat: Japan in the Wake of World War II.* New York: W. W. Norton and Company, 1999.

Eakin, Paul John. *Fictions in Autobiography: Studies in the Art of Self-Invention.* Princeton: Princeton University Press, 1995.

Earhart, David C. "Nagai Kafu's Wartime Diary: The Enormity of Nothing." *Japan Quarterly* 41, no. 4 (Oct. 1994): 488–504.

Ekici, Didem. "'The Laboratory of a New Humanity': The Concept of Type, Life Reform, and Modern Architecture in Hellerau Garden City, 1900–1914." PhD diss., University of Michigan, 2008.

Eng, David L. *Racial Castration: Managing Masculinity in Asian America.* Durham: Duke University Press, 2001.

Espiritu, Augusto. "Inter-Imperial Relations, the Pacific, and Asian American History." *Pacific Historical Review* 83, no. 2 (May 2014): 238–54.

Ethan, Mark. "The Perils of Co-Prosperity: Takeda Rintarō, Occupied Southeast Asia, and the Seductions of Postcolonial Empire." *American Historical Review* 119, no. 4 (2014): 1184–206.

Eubanks, Charlotte, and Jonathan Abel. "Of Asian Boxes . . ." *Verge: Studies in Global Asias* 1, no. 2, Collecting Asias (Fall 2015): vii–xv.

Ewick, David. "Notes Toward a Cultural History of Japanese Modernism in Modernist Europe, 1910–1920, with Special Reference to Kōri Torahiko." *The Hemingway Review of Japan* No. 13 (June 2012): 19–36.

Ewick David. *Japonisme, Orientalism, Modernism: A Bibliography of Japan in English Language Verse of the Early 20ᵗʰ Century.* Last modified August 2012. themargins.net

Ewick, David. "The Instigations of Ezra Pound by Ernest Fenollosa I: The Chinese Written Character, Atlantic Crossings, Texts Mislaid, and the Machinations of a Divinely-Inspired Char Woman." *Essays and Studies,* Tokyo Christian Women's University 66, no. 1 (2015): 53–72.

Ewick, David. "Strange Attractors: Ezra Pound and the Invention of Japan, II." *Essays and Studies in British and American Literature,* Tokyo Woman's Christian University 64 (2018): 1–40.

Ewick, David, and Dorsey Kleitz. *Michio Ito's Reminiscences of Ezra Pound, W. B. Yeats, and Other Matters: A Translation and Critical Edition of a Seminal Document in Modernist Aesthetics.* Lewiston, NY: Mellen, 2018.

Exley, Charles. "Popular Musical Star Tokuko Takagi and Vaudeville Modernism in the Taishō Asakusa Opera." *Japanese Language and Literature* 51, no. 1 (April 2017): 63–90.

Farfan, Penny. *Performing Queer Modernism.* New York: Oxford University Press, 2017.

Fessler, Susanna. *Musashino in Tuscany: Japanese Overseas Travel Literature, 1860–1912.* Ann Arbor: Center for Japanese Studies, University of Michigan Press, 2004.

Flannery, James W. *W. B. Yeats and the Idea of a Theatre.* Toronto: Macmillan, 1976.

Fleischer, Mary. *Embodied Texts: Symbolist Playwright-Dancer Collaborations.* Amsterdam: Rodopi, 2007.

Fletcher, Angus. "Ezra Pound's Egypt and the Origin of the *Cantos.*" *Twentieth-Century Literature* 48, no. 1 (Spring 2002): 1–21.

Bibliography

Fogel, Joshua A. *The Literature of Travel in the Japanese Rediscovery of China, 1862–1945*. Stanford: Stanford University Press, 1996.

Foster, Susan Leigh. "Walking and Other Choreographic Tactics: Danced Inventions of Theatricality and Performativity." *SubStance* 31, no. 2/3 (2002): 125–46.

Fujita Fujio. *Itō Michio, sekai wo mau* [Itō Michio, dancing through the world]. Tokyo: Musashino Shobō, 1992.

Fujita Fujio, ed. *Daitōa butai geijutsu kenkyūjo kankei shiryō* [Greater East Asia Stage Arts Research Institute related documents]. Tokyo: Fujishuppan, 1993.

Fujitani, T. *Race for Empire: Koreans as Japanese and Japanese as Americans during World War II*. Berkeley: University of California Press, 2011.

Funeyama Takashi. "Yamada Kōsaku no buyōshi—Taisho modanizumu no yume to zasetsu" [Yamada Kōsaku's dance-poem: Taisho modernism's dreams and failures]. *Ongaku Geijutsu* 44, no. 2 (Feb. 1986): 32–39.

García, Jerry. *Looking Like the Enemy: Japanese Mexicans, the Mexican State, and US Hegemony, 1897–1945*. Tucson: University of Arizona Press, 2014.

Gardener, Martha. *The Qualities of a Citizen: Women, Immigration, and Citizenship, 1870–1965*. Princeton: Princeton University Press, 2005.

Goldman, Danielle. *I Want to Be Ready: Improvised Dance as a Practice of Freedom*. Ann Arbor: University of Michigan Press, 2010.

Goodman, Grant K. ed. *Japanese Cultural Policies in Southeast Asia during World War 2*. New York: St. Martin's Press, 1991.

Gordon, Andrew. *Fabricating Consumers: The Sewing Machine in Modern Japan*. Oakland: University of California Press, 2021.

Greenberg, Mitchell. *Baroque Bodies: Psychoanalysis and the Culture of French Absolutism*. Ithaca: Cornell University Press, 2001.

Groemer, Gerald. *Street Performers and Society in Urban Japan, 1600–1900*. New York: Routledge, 2016.

Guerrero, Ellie. *Dance and the Arts in Mexico, 1920–1950: The Cosmic Generation*. Cham, Switzerland: Palgrave Macmillan, 2018.

Hakutani Yoshinobu. "Ezra Pound, Yone Noguchi, and Imagism." *Modern Philology* 90, no. 1 (August 1992): 46–69.

Han, C. Winter. *Geisha of a Different Kind: Race and Sexuality in Gaysian America*. New York: NYU Press, 2015.

Harootunian, Harry. *Overcome by Modernity: History, Culture, and Community in Interwar Japan*. Princeton: Princeton University Press, 2000.

Hartman, Saidiya. *Wayward Lives, Beautiful Experiments: Intimate Histories of Social Upheaval*. New York: W. W. Norton, 2019.

Hayot, Eric. *Chinese Dreams: Pound, Brecht, Tel Quel*. Ann Arbor: University of Michigan Press, 2004.

Herrera, Brian. *Latin Numbers: Playing Latino in Twentieth-Century U.S. Popular Performance*. Ann Arbor: University of Michigan Press, 2015.

Hewitt, Andrew. *Social Choreography: Ideology as Performance in Dance and Everyday Movement*. Durham: Duke University Press, 2005.

Higashiya Sakurako. "Shinsakunō 'Miikusabune' no tamondai" [The various problems of the new piece "Miikusabune"]. *Japanese Literature Bulletin*, Showa Women's University 28 (2017): 17–31.

Hing, Bill Ong. *Making and Remaking Asian America Through Immigration Policy, 1850–1990*. Stanford: Stanford University Press, 1993.

Hirasawa Nobuyasu. "Shoki bunkagakuin ni okeru buyō kyōiku jissen—Yamada Kōsaku ni yoru" [Implementation of dance education at the early Bunka Gakuin: experiments in Yamada Kōsaku's "Dance-Poem"]. *Gakujutsu Kenkyū Kiyō, Kanoya Taiiku Daigaku* 34 (March 2006): 9–29.

Hoang, Nguyen Tan. *A View from the Bottom: Asian American Masculinity and Sexual Representation*. Durham: Duke University Press, 2014.

Hokenson, Jan Walsh. *Japan, France, and East-West Aesthetics: French Literature, 1867–2000*. Madison, NJ: Fairleigh Dickinson University Press, 2004.

Homsey, Bonnie Oda, and Los Angeles Dance Foundation. *Michio Ito: Pioneering Dance-Choreographer*. Executive producer Bonnie Oda Homsey. Produced and edited by John J. Flynn. Los Angeles Dance Foundation, 2013.

Horiguchi, Noriko. *Women Adrift: The Literature of Japan's Imperial Body*. Minneapolis: University of Minnesota Press, 2011.

Hoshino Yukiyo. "Use of Dance to Spread Propaganda during the Sino-Japanese War." *Athens Journal of History* 2, no. 3 (July 2016): 193–98.

Hosley, William. *The Japan Idea*. Hartford, CT: Wadsworth Atheneum 1990.

Hotta, Eri. *Pan-Asianism and Japan's War, 1931–1945*. New York: Palgrave Macmillan, 2007.

Houwen, Andrew. "Ezra Pound's Early Cantos and His Translation of *Takasago*." *Review of English Studies* 65 (2013): 321–41.

Houwen, Andrew. *Ezra Pound's Japan*. London: Bloomsbury Academic, 2021.

Hune, Shirley. "Asian American Studies and Asian Studies: Boundaries and Borderlands of Ethnic Studies and Area Studies." In *Color-Line to Borderlands: The Matrix of American Ethnic Studies*. Edited by Johnnella Butler, 227–39. Seattle: University of Washington Press, 2001.

Ichioka, Yuji. *The Issei: The World of the First Generation Japanese Immigrants, 1885–1924*. New York: Collier Macmillan, 1988.

Imada, Adria. *Aloha America: Hula Circuits through the U.S. Empire*. Durham: Duke University Press, 2021.

Irwin, Robert McKee. *Mexican Masculinities*. Minneapolis: University of Minnesota Press, 2003.

Ishii Kan. *Buyō shijin Ishii Baku* [Ishii Baku: dance-poet]. Tokyo: Miraisha, 1994.

Isozaki Arata. *Japan-ness in Architecture*. Translated by Sabu Kohso. Cambridge, MA: MIT Press, 2006.

Itō Michio. *Amerika* [America]. Tokyo: Hata Shoten, 1940.

Itō Michio. "Amerika no kokuminsei to geinō" [America's national character and performing arts]. *Engekikai* 2, no. 11 (November 1944): 10–12.

Itō Michio. *Amerika to nihon* [America and Japan]. Tokyo: Yakumo Shoten, 1946, 1949.

Itō Michio. *Josei handobukku, echiketto* [Women's handbook: etiquette] Tokyo: Rōdōbunkasha, 1947. Library of Congress, Asian Reading Room.

Bibliography

Itō Michio. "Ānīpairu Gekijō no koto: watashi no shigoto" [About the Ernie Pyle Theatre: my work], *Nihon Engeki*, October 1947, 41–42.

Itō Michio. "Kurui heru Nijinsuki" [The mad Nijinsky]. *Geijutsu Shinchō*, July 1950: 93–100.

Itō Michio. "Sekai ni odoru" [Dancing in the world]. *Geijutsu Shinchō*, July 1955.

Itō Michio. *Utsukushiku naru kyōshitsu* [A classroom for beauty]. Tokyo: Hōbunkan, 1956.

Itō Michio. "Omoide wo kataru" [Reminiscences]. *Hikaku bunka* [Comparative literature] 2, no. 1 (1956): 57–76.

Jaques-Dalcroze, Émile. "Remarks on Arrhythmy." Translated by F. Rothwell. *Music & Letters* 14, no. 2 (April 1933): 138–48.

Kabbani, Rana. *Europe's Myths of Orient: Devise and Rule*. London: Palgrave Macmillan, 1986.

Kashima, Tetsuden. *Judgment without Trial: Japanese American Imprisonment during World War II*. Seattle: University of Washington Press, 2003.

Katagiri Yoshio. "Naruse Jinzo to joshi taiiku: Nihon Daigakkou no 'yōgi taisō'" [Naruse Jinzo and women's physical education: "yōgi gymnastics" at Japan Women's University]. *Hikaku buyō kenkyū* 26 no. 3 (2020): 1–12.

Kataoka Yasuko. "Ishii Baku—Buyōshi to tenkai" [Ishii Baku: the development of the dance poem]. *Buyōgaku* 13, no. 1 (1989): 49–50.

Kataoka Yasuko, ed. *Nihon no gendai buyō no paioniā*. New National Theatre Tokyo. Tokyo: Maruzen, 2015.

Kern, Stephen. *The Culture of Time and Space, 1880–1918*. Cambridge, MA: Harvard University Press, 1983.

Kim, John Namjun. "On the Brink of Universality: German Cosmopolitanism in Japanese Imperialism." *Positions: East Asia Cultures Critique* 17, no. 1 (Spring 2009): 73–95.

Kim, Ju Yon. *The Racial Mundane: Asian American Performance and the Embodied Everyday*. New York: NYU University Press, 2015.

Kleeman, Faye Yuan. *In Transit: The Formation of the Colonial East Asian Cultural Sphere*. Honolulu: University of Hawai'i Press, 2014.

Kojima Shigeru, "Who Are Nikkeijin?" Translated by Mina Otsuka. *Discover Nikkei* April 17, 2017. http://www.discovernikkei.org/en/journal/2017/4/21/nikkei-wa-dare-no-koto

Kopelson, Kevin. *The Queer Afterlife of Vaslav Nijinsky*. Stanford: Stanford University Press, 1997.

Koritz, Amy. "Dancing the Orient for England: Maud Allan's 'The Vision of Salome.'" *Theatre Journal* 46, no. 1 (March 1994): 63–78.

Koshy, Susan. *Sexual Naturalization: Asian Americans and Miscegenation*. Stanford: Stanford University Press, 2004.

Kosstrin, Hannah. *Honest Bodies: Revolutionary Modernism in the Dances of Anna Sokolow*. Oxford: Oxford University Press, 2017.

Kotef, Hagar. *Movement and the Ordering of Freedom: On Liberal Governances of Mobility*. Durham: Duke University Press, 2015.

Kraut, Anthea. *Choreographing Copyright: Race, Gender, and Intellectual Property Rights in American Dance*. Oxford: Oxford University Press, 2016.

Kurashige, Lon. *Japanese American Celebration and Conflict: A History of Ethnic Identity and Festival, 1934–1990*. Berkeley: University of California Press, 2002.

Kurashige, Scott. *The Shifting Grounds of Race: Black and Japanese Americans in the Making of Multiethnic Los Angeles.* Princeton: Princeton University Press, 2008.

Kushida Kiyomi. "Ānī Pairu gekijō no sutēji shō" [The Ernie Pyle Theatre's stage shows]. *Jissen joshi daigaku bungakubu kiyō dai* 35 (2021): 53–72.

Kushida Kiyomi. "Yōbu sōsō-ki no kaitakusha to tōyō buyōka Teiko Itō no 'kyōdo' to 'minzoku' wo meguru gensetsu" [Discourses of "Ethnicity" and "The Homeland" surrounding Teiko Itō, East Asian dance artist and pioneer of early 20th century Western dance]. *Jissen joshi daigaku bungakubu kiyō dai* 64 (2022): 25–46.

Kushida Kiyomi. "Itō Yūji ga buro-dowei- ni motarashita 'tōyō': 1930 nendaigohan no nihon/ajia ni okeru minzoku geinō no chōsa" [Itō Yūji brought the "Orient" to Broadway: investigating folk performance of Japan/Asia in the 1930s]. *Jissen joshi daigaku bungakubu kiyō dai* 65 (2023).

Kuwahara Noriko, "Ānīpairu gekijō wo meguru bijutsukatachi" [Concerning artists at the Ernie Pyle Theatre], *Seitoku Daigaku Kenkyū Kiyō* 18 (2007): 41–48.

Kwan, SanSan. "Performing a geography of Asian America: the chop suey circuit." *The Drama Review: TDR* 55 (2011): 120–36.

Kwan, SanSan. *Kinesthetic City: Dance and Movement in Chinese Urban Spaces.* Oxford: Oxford University Press, 2013.

Kwon, Nayoung Aimee. *Intimate Empire: Collaboration and Colonial Modernity in Korea and Japan.* Durham: Duke University Press, 2015.

LaFleur, William. "A Turning in Taishō: Asia and Europe in the Early Writings of Watsuji Tetsurō." In *Culture and Identity: Japanese Intellectuals during the Interwar Years*, edited by Thomas J. Rimer, 234–56. Princeton: Princeton University Press, 1990.

Lambert-Beatty, Carrie. *Being Watched: Yvonne Rainer and the 1960s.* Cambridge, MA: MIT Press, 2008.

Lang, Zoë Alexis. *The Legacy of Johann Strauss.* Cambridge: Cambridge University Press, 2014.

Lavery, Grace Elisabeth. *Quaint, Exquisite: Victorian Aesthetics and the Idea of Japan.* Princeton: Princeton University Press, 2019.

Lee, Josephine. *The Japan of Pure Invention: Gilbert and Sullivan's The Mikado.* Minneapolis: University of Minnesota Press, 2010.

Lei, Daphne. "Ruptures Within and Without: *Pageantry*—A Work in Progress by Denise Uyehara and Sri Susilowati." *Theatre Research International* 35, no. 2 (July 2010): 188–92.

Leiter, Samuel, ed. *Rising from the Flames: The Rebirth of Theater in Occupied Japan, 1945–1952.* Lanham, MD: Lexington Books, 2009.

Leiter, Samuel. "Wartime Colonial and Traditional Theatre." In *A History of Japanese Theatre*, edited by Jonah Salz, 251–63. Cambridge: Cambridge University Press, 2016.

Lennon, Joseph. "W. B. Yeats's Celtic Orient." In *Irish Orientalism: A Literary and Intellectual History*, 247–89. Syracuse: Syracuse University Press, 2004.

Leong, Andrew. *Roots of the Issei: Exploring Early Japanese American Newspapers.* Stanford: Hoover Institution Press, 2018.

Lepecki, André. "Inscribing Dance." In *Of the Presence of the Body: Essays on Dance and Performance Theory*, edited by André Lepecki, 124–39. Middletown, CT: Wesleyan University Press, 2004.

Bibliography

Lepecki, André. *Exhausting Dance: Performance and the Politics of Movement*. New York: Routledge, 2006.

Lepecki, André. "The Body as Archive: Will to Re-Enact and the Afterlives of Dances." *Dance Research Journal* 42, no. 2 (Winter 2010): 28–48.

Li, Sidney Xu. *The Making of Japanese Settler Colonialism*. New York: Columbia University Press, 2019.

Lowe, Lisa. *Critical Terrains: French and British Orientalisms*. Ithaca: Cornell University Press, 1991, 2018.

Lowe, Lisa. *Immigrant Acts: On Asian American Cultural Politics*. Durham: Duke University Press, 1996.

Lowe, Lisa. *Intimacies of Four Continents*. Durham: Duke University Press, 2015.

Mack, Kimberly. *Fictional Blues: Narrative Self-Invention from Bessie Smith to Jack White*. Amherst: University of Massachusetts Press, 2020.

MacNamara, Brooks. "'Something Glorious': Greenwich Village and the Theater." In *Greenwich Village: Culture and Counterculture*, edited by Rick Beard and Leslie Cohen Berlowitz, 308–19. New Brunswick, NJ: Rutgers University Press, 1993.

Maletic, Vera. *Body, Space, Expression: The Development of Rudolf Laban's Movement and Dance Concepts*. Berlin: Mouton de Gruyter, 1987.

Manning, Susan. *Ecstasy and the Demon: The Dances of Mary Wigman*. Minneapolis: University of Minnesota Press, 1993.

Manning, Susan. *Modern Dance, Negro Dance: Race in Motion*. Minneapolis: University of Minnesota Press, 2004.

Masterson, Daniel M., with Sayaka Funada-Classen. *The Japanese in Latin America*. Urbana: University of Illinois Press, 2004.

Matsumoto, Valerie J. *City Girls: The Nisei Social World in Los Angeles, 1920–1950*. Oxford: Oxford University Press, 2014.

Mayo, Marlene J. "Civil Censorship and Media Control in Early Occupied Japan." In *Americans as Proconsuls: United States Military Government in Germany and Japan, 1944–1952*, edited by Robert Wolfe, 263–320. Carbondale: Southern Illinois University Press, 1984.

Mayo, Marlene J. "To Be or Not to Be: *Kabuki* and Cultural Politics in Occupied Japan." In *War, Occupations, and Creativity: Japan and East Asia, 1920–1960*, edited by Marlene J. Mayo and Thomas J. Rimer, 269–309. Honolulu: University of Hawai'i Press, 1999.

McAndrew, Malia. "Beauty, Soft Power, and the Politics of Womanhood During the U.S. Occupation of Japan, 1945–1952." *Journal of Women's History* 26, no. 4 (Winter 2014): 83–107.

McClintock, Anne. *Imperial Leather: Race, Gender and Sexuality in the Colonial Contest*. New York: Routledge, 1995.

McLelland, Mark. *Love, Sex, and Democracy in Japan during the American Occupation*. New York: Palgrave Macmillan, 2012.

Mills, Charles W. *The Racial Contract*. Ithaca: Cornell University Press, 1997.

Miyao, Daisuke. *Sessue Hayakawa: Silent Cinema and Transnational Stardom*. Durham: Duke University Press, 2007.

Molasky, Michael. *The American Occupation of Japan and Okinawa*. London: Routledge, 1999.

Morris-Suzuki, Tessa. "Becoming Japanese: Imperial Expansion and Identity Crises in the Early Twentieth Century." In *Japan's Competing Modernities: Issues in Culture and Democracy, 1900–1930*, edited by Sharon A. Minichiello, 157–80. Honolulu: University of Hawai'i Press, 1998.

Morris-Suzuki, Tessa. "Debating Racial Science in Wartime Japan." *Osiris* 13 (1998): 354–75.

Nakamura, Jessica. *Transgenerational Remembrance: Performance and the Asia-Pacific War in Contemporary Japan*. Evanston, IL: Northwestern University Press, 2020.

Nally, Claire. *Envisioning Ireland: W. B. Yeats' Occult Nationalism*. Oxford: Peter Lang, 2010.

Nehru, Jawaharlal. *Glimpses of World History*. Bombay: Asia Publishing House, 1934, 1962.

Nohara Yasuko. "Yamada Kōsaku no Sukuriabin juyou" [Yamada Kōsaku's reception of Scriabin], *Musashino ongaku daigaku kenkyū kiyō*, no. 51 (2019): 83–108.

Nyong'o, Tavia. *The Amalgamation Waltz: Race, Performance, and the Ruses of Memory*. Minneapolis: University of Minnesota Press, 2009.

Nyong'o, Tavia. *Afro-Fabulations: The Queer Drama of Black Life*. New York: New York University Press, 2019.

Oda, Yuki. "Family Unity in U.S. Immigration Policy, 1921–1978." PhD diss., Columbia University, 2014.

Odom, Selma Landen. "Wigman at Hellerau." *Ballet Review* 14, no. 2 (Summer 1986): 41–53.

Odom, Selma Landen. "Choreographing *Orpheus*: Hellerau 1913 and Warwick 1991." In *Dance Reconstructed: A Conference on Modern Dance Art, Past, Present, Future*, 127–32. Rutgers University, New Brunswick, NJ, October 16 and 17, 1992.

Oguma Eiji. *A Genealogy of "Japanese" Self-Images*. Translated by David Askew. Melbourne: Trans Pacific Press, 2002.

Okakura Kakuzō. *Ideals of the East: With Special Reference to the Art of Japan*. London: J. Murray, 1903, reprint Tokyo: Charles E. Tuttle, 1970.

Okawa, Gail. "Putting Their Lives on the Line: Personal Narrative as Political Discourse among Japanese Petitioners in American World War II Internment." *College English* 74, no. 1 (September 2011): 50–68.

Pacun, David. "'Thus we cultivate our own World, thus we share it with others': Kosçak Yamada's Visit to the United States, 1918–1919." *American Music* 24, no. 1 (February 2006): 67–94.

Pacun, David. "Nationalism and Musical Style in Interwar 'Yōgaku': A Reappraisal." *Asian Music* 43, no. 2 (July 2012): 3–46.

Pakes, Anna. *Choreography Invisible: The Disappearing Work of Dance*. New York: Oxford University Press, 2020.

Panzer, Mary C. "The Essential Tact of Nickolas Muray." In *The Covarrubias Circle: Nickolas Muray's Collection of Twentieth-century Mexican Art*, edited by Kurt Heintzelman, 21–45. Austin: University of Texas Press, 2004.

Park, Josephine Nock-Hee. *Apparitions of Asia: Modernist Form and Asian American Poetics*. Oxford: Oxford University Press, 2008.

Park, Sang Mi. "Wartime Japan's Theater Movement." *WIAS Research Bulletin* 1 (2009): 61–78.

Bibliography

Peattie, Mark. *Nan'yō: The Rise and Fall of the Japanese in Micronesia, 1885–1945*. Honolulu: University of Hawai'i Press, 1992, 1998.

Pellecchia, Diego. "Ezra Pound and the Politics of Noh Film." *Philological Quarterly* 92, no. 4 (Fall 2013): 499–516.

Phelan, Peggy. *Unmarked: The Politics of Performance*. London: Routledge, 1993.

Poole, Janet. *When the Future Disappears: The Modernist Imagination in Late Colonial Korea*. New York: Columbia University Press, 2015.

Pound, Ezra. "How I Began." *T.P.'s Weekly*, June 6, 1913.

Pound, Ezra. "Vorticism." *Fortnightly Review* 96 (Sept. 1, 1914): 461–71.

Pound, Ezra. "Sword-Dance and Spear-Dance: Texts of the Poems Used with Michio Itow's Dances. By Ezra Pound, from Notes of Masirni Utchiyama." *Future* 1, no. 2 (December 1916). In *Ezra Pound's Poetry and Prose*, Vol. 2, edited by Lea Baechler, A. Walton Litz, and James Longenbach, 182–83. New York: Garland Pub, 1991.

Pound, Ezra. *The Pisan Cantos*, edited by Richard Sieburth. New York: New Direction Books, 1948, 2003.

Pound, Ezra, and Ernest Fenollosa. *The Classic Noh Theater of Japan*. 1917; reprint New York: New Directions, 1959.

Preston, Carrie J. *Modernism's Mythic Pose: Gender, Genre, Solo Performance*. New York: Oxford University Press, 2011.

Preston, Carrie J. *Learning to Kneel: Noh, Modernism, and Journeys in Teaching*. New York: Columbia University Press, 2016.

Preston, VK. "Baroque Relations: Performing Silver and Gold in Daniel Rabel's *Ballets of the Americas*." In *The Oxford Handbook of Reenactment*, edited by Mark Franko, 285–310. New York: Oxford University Press, 2017.

Prevots, Naima. *Dancing in the Sun: Hollywood Choreographers, 1915–1937*. Ann Arbor: UMI Research Press, 1987.

Prevots, Naima. *American Pageantry: A Movement for Art and Democracy*. Ann Arbor: UMI Research Press, 1990.

Reed, Christopher. *Bachelor Japanists: Japanese Aesthetics and Western Masculinities*. New York: Columbia University Press, 2017.

Reynoso, Jose Luis. "Choreographing Modern Mexico: Anna Pavlova in Mexico City (1919)" *Modernist Cultures* 9, no. 1 (2014): 80–98.

Reynoso, Jose Luis. *Dancing Mestizo Modernisms: Choreographing Postcolonial and Postrevolutionary Mexico*. New York: Oxford University Press, 2023.

Richards, Thomas. *The Imperial Archive: Knowledge and the Fantasy of Empire*. London: Verso, 1993.

Rimer, J. Thomas. *Toward a Modern Japanese Theatre: Kishida Kunio*. Princeton: Princeton University Press, 1974.

Riordan, Kevin. "Performance in the Wartime Archive: Michio Ito at the Alien Enemy Hearing Board." *American Studies* 55/56, no. 4/1 (2017): 67–89.

Robertson, Jennifer. *Takarazuka: Sexual Politics and Popular Culture in Modern Japan*. Berkeley: University of California Press, 1998.

Robertson, Jennifer. "Blood Talks: Eugenic Modernity and the Creation of New Japanese." *History and Anthropology* 13, no. 3 (2002): 191–216.

Robertson, Jennifer. "Ethnicity and Gender in the Wartime Japanese Revue Theatre." In

War and Militarism in Modern Japan: Issues of History and Identity, edited by Guy Podoler, 39–52. Folkestone, England: Global Oriental, 2009.

Robertson, Marta. "Floating Worlds: Japanese and American Transcultural Encounters in Dance." *Conference Proceedings* (Congress on Research in Dance) (2014): 126–35.

Rodman, Tara. "A Modernist Audience: The Kawakami Troupe, Matsuki Bunkio, and Boston Japonisme." *Theatre Journal* 65, no. 4 (December 2013): 489–505.

Rodman, Tara. "A More Humane Mikado: Re-envisioning the Nation through Occupation-Era Productions of *The Mikado* in Japan." *Theatre Research International* 40, no. 3 (October 2015): 288–302.

Rodman, Tara. "Altered Belonging: The Transnational Modern Dance of Itō Michio." PhD diss., Northwestern University, 2017.

Rodman, Tara. "Ito Michio, 'Oriental Dance,' and the Surfaces of Japanese American Modern Dance." In *Border Crossings: Exile and American Modern Dance*, edited by Ninotchka D. Bennahum and Rena M. Heinrich, 80–89. New York: The New York Public Library for the Peforming Arts, Lincoln Center / Santa Barbara: Museum of Art, Design & Architecture, UC Santa Barbara, 2024.

Rose, Jacqueline. *States of Fantasy*. Oxford: Oxford University Press, 1996.

Rosenberg, Douglas, dir. *American Dance Festival Presents Pauline Koner: Speaking of Dance*. 1998. Oregon, WI: American Dance Festival Video, 2006.

Rosenberger, Nancy. *Gambling with Virtue: Japanese Women and the Search for Self in a Changing Nation*. Honolulu: University of Hawai'i Press, 2001.

Roxworthy, Emily. *The Spectacle of Japanese American Trauma: Racial Performativity and World War II*. Honolulu: University of Hawai'i Press, 2008.

Ruoff, Kenneth J. *Imperial Japan at Its Zenith: The Wartime Celebration of the Empire's 2,600th Anniversary*. Ithaca: Cornell University Press, 2010.

Ruskola, Teemu. "Canton Is Not Boston: The Invention of American Imperial Sovereignty." *American Quarterly* 57, no. 3 (Sept. 2005): 859–84.

Saaler, Sven, and J. Victor Koschmann, eds. *Pan-Asianism in Modern Japanese History: Colonialism, Regionalism and Borders*. New York: Routledge, 2007.

Saitō Ren. *Anī Pairu Gekijō, GI wo ian shita rebyū garu* [Ernie Pyle Theatre: The revue girls who entertained GIs]. Tokyo: Bronze Shinsha, 1998.

Sakai, Naoki. "Subject and Substratum: On Japanese Imperial Nationalism." *Cultural Studies* 14, nos. 3–4 (2000): 462–530.

Samuels, Ellen. *Fantasies of Identification: Disability, Gender, Race*. New York: New York University Press, 2014.

Sato Hiroaki. "Yone Noguchi: Accomplishments and Roles." *Journal of American and Canadian Studies*, Sophia University (March 31, 1996): 105–21.

Satō Kazumichi. "Senjika no nogaku: 'Chūrei' 'Miikusabune' wo chūshin ni" [Wartime theatre: focusing on "The Faithful" "Miikusabune"]. *Theatre Studies: Journal of the Japanese Society for Theatre Research* (November 2017): 1–17.

Satō Yoshiaki. *J-Pop Shinkaron: "Yosahoi bushi" kara "automatic" e*. Tokyo: Heibonsha Shinsho, 1999.

Sawada, Mitziko. *Tokyo Life, New York Dreams: Urban Japanese Visions of America, 1890–1924*. Berkeley: University of California Press, 1996.

Bibliography

Schrank, Sarah. *Art and the City: Civic Imagination and Cultural Authority in Los Angeles.* Philadelphia: University of Pennsylvania Press, 2009.

Sekine, Masaru, and Christopher Murray. *Yeats and the Noh: A Comparative Study.* Savage, MD: Barnes and Noble, 1990.

Senda Koreya. *Mō hitotsu no shingekishi* [One more history of shingeki]. Tokyo: Chikuma Shōbō, 1975.

Senda Koreya. "Atogaki: yume to genjitsu" [Afterword: dream and reality]. In the Japanese version of Helen Caldwell, *Michio Ito: The Dancer and his Dances* [Itō Michio: hito to geijutsu]. Translated by Nakagawa Enosuke, 137–89. Tokyo: Hayakawa Shobō, 1985.

Shibusawa, Naoko. *America's Geisha Ally: Reimagining the Japanese Enemy.* Cambridge, MA: Harvard University Press, 2006.

Shimakawa, Karen. *National Abjection: The Asian American Body Onstage.* Durham: Duke University Press, 2002.

Siegel, Marcia. *At the Vanishing Point: A Critic Looks at Dance.* New York: Saturday Review Press, 1973.

Slaymaker, Douglas. *The Body in Postwar Fiction: Japanese Fiction after the War.* New York: Routledge, 2004.

Smith, Catherine Parsons. "Founding the Hollywood Bowl." *American Music* 11, no. 2 (Summer 1993).

Smith, Catherine Parsons. *Making Music in Los Angeles: Transforming the Popular.* Berkeley: University of California Press, 2007.

Snow, Mitchell K. *A Revolution in Movement: Dancers, Painters, and the Image of Modern Mexico.* Gainesville: University Press of Florida, 2021.

Snyder, Sara Christine. "Odyssey of an Archives: What the History of the Gordon W. Prange Collection of Japanese Materials Teaches Us about Libraries, Censorship, and Keeping the Past Alive." Master's thesis, University of Maryland, 2007.

Son, Elizabeth W. *Embodied Reckonings: "Comfort Women," Performance, and Transpacific Redress.* Ann Arbor: University of Michigan Press, 2018.

Sorgenfrei, Carol Fisher. "Strategic Unweaving: Itō Michio and the Diasporic Dancing Body." In *Politics of Interweaving Performance Cultures: Beyond Postcolonialism,* edited by Erika Fischer-Lichte, Torsten Jost, and Saskya Iris Jain, 201–22. London: Routledge, 2014.

Srinivasan, Priya. *Sweating Saris: Indian Dance as Transnational Labor.* Philadelphia: Temple University Press, 2011.

Stanger, Arabella. *Dancing on Violent Ground: Utopia as Dispossession in Euro-American Theater Dance.* Evanston: Northwestern University Press, 2021.

Stanley, Amy. *Stranger in the Shogun's City: A Japanese Woman and Her World.* New York: Scribner, 2020.

Stansell, Christine. *American Moderns: Bohemian New York and the Creation of a New Century.* Princeton: Princeton University Press, 2000.

Stewart, Susan. *On Longing: Narratives of the Miniature, the Gigantic, the Souvenir, the Collection.* Durham: Duke University Press, 1993.

Stoler, Ann Laura. *Carnal Knowledge: Race and the Intimate in Colonial Rule.* Berkeley: University of California Press, 2002.

Sueyoshi, Amy. *Discriminating Sex: White Leisure and the Making of the American "Oriental."* Urbana: University of Illinois Press, 2018.

Sueyoshi, Amy. *Queer Compulsions: Race, Nation, and Sexuality in the Affairs of Yone Noguchi.* Honolulu: University of Hawai'i Press, 2021.

Swain, John D. "Senda Koreya and the *Tenkō* Paradigm." In *Modern Japanese Theatre and Performance*, edited by David Jortner, Keiko McDonald, and Kevin J. Wetmore Jr., 77–90. Lanham, MD: Lexington Books, 2006.

Tadiar, Neferti. *Fantasy-Production: Sexual Economies and Other Philippine Consequences for the New World Order.* Chicago: University of Chicago Press, 2004.

Tai, Eika. "Intermarriage and Imperial Subject Formation in Colonial Taiwan: Shoji Soichi's Chin-Fujin." *Inter-Asia Cultural Studies* 15, no. 4 (2014): 513–31.

Tanaka, Michiko. "Seki Sano and Popular Political and Social Theatre in Latin America." *Latin American Theatre Review* (Spring 1994): 53–69.

Tanaka, Stefan. "Imaging History: Inscribing Belief in the Nation." *Journal of Asian Studies* 53, no. 1 (Feb. 1994): 24–44.

Tanaka, Stefan. *Japan's Orient: Rendering Pasts into History.* Berkeley: University of California Press, 1995.

Takeishi, Midori. *Japanese Elements in Michio Ito's Early Period: 1915–1924: Meetings of East and West in the Collaborative Works*, edited by David Pacun. Tokyo: Gendai tosho, 2006.

Taki Ryōichi. "Tōyō ni okeru būyō ni tsuite" [On dance in the Orient]. *Tōyō ongaku kenkyū* 2 (1937): 32–41.

Taylor, Diana. *The Archive and the Repertoire: Performing Cultural Memory in the Americas.* Durham: Duke University Press, 2003.

Taylor, Richard. *The Drama of W. B. Yeats: Irish Myth and the Japanese Nō.* New Haven: Yale University Press, 1976.

Terami-Wada, Motoe. "The Japanese Propaganda Corps in the Philippines: Laying the Foundation." In *Japanese Cultural Policies in Southeast Asia during World War 2*, edited by Grant K. Goodman, 173–211. New York: St. Martin's Press, 1991.

Thomas, Aaron C. "Infelicities." *Journal of Dramatic Theory and Criticism* 35, no. 2 (Spring 2021): 13–25.

Thornbury, Barbara E. *America's Japan and Japan's Performing Arts: Cultural Mobility and Exchange in New York, 1952–2011.* Ann Arbor: University of Michigan Press, 2013.

Tosaka, Yuji. "The Discourse of Anti-Americanism and Hollywood Movies: Film Import Controls in Japan, 1937–1941." *Journal of American-East Asian Relations* 12, no. 1/2 (Spring-Summer 2003): 59–80.

Tsuyoshi Namigata. *Ekkyō no abangyarudo* [Transgressing the avant-garde]. Tokyo: NTT Shuppan, 2005.

Uchiyama, Benjamin. *Japan's Carnival War: Mass Culture on the Home Front, 1937–1945.* Cambridge: Cambridge University Press, 2019.

Van Valkenburg, Carol Bulger. "An Alien Place: The Fort Missoula, Montana, Detention Camp, 1941–1944." Master's thesis, University of Montana, 1988.

Vincent, J. Keith. *Two-Timing Modernity: Homosocial Narrative in Modern Japanese Fiction.* Cambridge, MA: Harvard University Asia Center, 2012.

Bibliography

Vogel, Shane. *The Scene of Harlem Cabaret: Race, Sexuality, Performance.* Chicago: University of Chicago Press, 2009.

Walker, Julia. *Performance and Modernity: Enacting Change on the Globalizing Stage.* New York: Cambridge University Press, 2022.

Wilcox, Emily. "Crossing Over: Choe Seung-hui's Pan-Asianism in Revolutionary Times." *Journal of Society for Dance Documentation and History of South Korea* 51 (December 2018): 65–98.

Winther-Tamaki, Bert. *Maximum Embodiment: Yōga, the Western Painting of Japan, 1912–1955.* Honolulu: University of Hawai'i Press, 2012.

Wong, Yutian. "Toward a New Asian American Dance Theory: Locating the Dancing Asian American Body." *Discourses in Dance* 1, no. 1 (2002): 69–90.

Wong, Yutian. "Artistic Utopias: Michio Ito and the Trope of the International." In *Worlding Dance*, edited by Susan Leigh Foster, 144–62. New York: Palgrave Macmillan, 2009.

Wong, Yutian. *Choreographing Asian America.* Middletown, CT: Wesleyan University Press, 2010.

Yagishita Emi. "Itō Michio no amerika ni okeru buyō katsudō: rosanzerusu de no katsudō wo chūshin ni" [Itō Michio's dance activities in America: focusing on his activities in Los Angeles] *Waseda RILAS Journal* 4 (October 2016): 213–24.

Yamada Kōsaku. "Michio Itō no purofairu" [Profile of Michio Itō]. Foreword to Itō Michio, *Utsukushiku kyōshitsu naru.* Tokyo: Hōbunkan, 1956.

Yamada Kōsaku. *Yamada Kōsaku Collected Works*, Vol. 1, edited by Gotō Nobuko, Dan Ikuma, and Tōyama Kazuyuki. Tokyo: Iwanami Shoten, 2001.

Yano, Christine R. "Global Asias: Improvisations on a Theme (a.k.a Chindon-ya Riffs)." *Journal of Asian Studies* 80, no. 4 (Nov. 2021): 845–64.

Yoshida Yukihiko. "National Dance under the Rising Sun, Mainly from National Dance, Buyō Geijutsu and the Activities of Takaya Eguchi." *International Journal of Eastern Sports and Physical Education* 7, no. 1 (October 2009): 88–103.

Yoshihara, Mari. *Embracing the East: White Women and American Orientalism.* Oxford: Oxford University Press, 2002.

Young, Louise. *Japan's Total Empire: Manchuria and the Culture of Wartime Imperialism.* Berkeley: University of California Press, 1998.

Zarina, Xenia. *Classic Dances of the Orient.* New York: Crown Publishers, 1967.

Zheng, Guohe. "From War Responsibility to the Red Purge." In *Rising from the Flames: The Rebirth of Theater in Occupied Japan, 1945–1952*, edited by Samuel Leiter, 279–316. Lanham, MD: Lexington Books, 2009.

INDEX

Page locators in *italics* indicate illustrations.

Abbey Theatre, 74
Abdellah Hassan (imagined figure), 38–39, 41–43, 61
Abe, Marié, 252
Abel, Jonathan, 94
abjection, 34, 82, 109, 242
aestheticism, 4, 96–98
Ailey, Alvin, 256
Ainley, Henry, 88
Albéniz, Isaac, 91
alienation/loneliness, 50–51, 53–56, 111, 252
Alien Registration Act, 189, 192
Allied Occupation. *See* Occupation
America (Ito), 56, 120
America and Japan (Ito), 38–39, 43, 53–55, 185–87
American Dancer, 138
American Repertory Dance Company (ARDC), 255–56
Andante Cantabile (Tchaikovsky), 139–40, 148
Anderson, John Murray, 102
anti-Asian laws: "alien registration," 189, 192; immigration/land use, 27, 101, 125, 133, 172; marriage/citizenship, 27, 151, 168
Appia, Adolphe, 51, 207
archive, 15–16, 37, 40, 187–88, 197–98, 200, 237
Argus Bowl, 135–36
Arikawa Okura, Lily, 153, 255

arrhythmia, 51, 53–54; racial, 33, 53–56
Asahi Shimbun, 167, 180–82, 198
Asakusa Kannondō (Yoshi), 69
Asakusa Opera, 68
Asian American studies, 8, 29–32, 35, 117, 143, 188, 197
Asian studies, 29–31, 35, 188, 197
Asia-Pacific War / World War II: disarmament conference, 185–86; Japanese American military units in, 143, 149; Japanese defeat in, 2, 200, 204, 209–10, 214; Japanese imperialism in, 3–4, 25, 28, 158–59, 200, 210; Pearl Harbor, 13, 184, 187, 189, 192; theater "comfort tours" during, 206, 282n46, 283n55; total mobilization, 26, 35, 187, 201–6, 215–16, 245; US entertainments under, 231; US/Japanese relations, 81–82, 129, 160, 181–83, 190–92, 196. *See also* incarceration; internment; Occupation
Asquith, H. H., 90, 268n70
assimilation: choreographic/dance, 19, 227, 229; Ito's own, 32, 104, 125–27, 132, 150–51, 163, 172; Japan's project of, 2–3, 26, 34, 147, 168, 200; vs. *kokutai,* 148; US project of, 34, 245–46
At the Hawk's Well (Yeats): Egypt/Hawk in, 33, 61, 65, 82, 87–90, *89,* 100; in Japan/US, 99–100, 136, 179–80; in London, 11–12, 64, 69, 72, 84, 88, 100; noh and, 77, 87–88, 100, 180

305

authenticity/authentication, 31, 43, 97, 100, 105, 107, 110–11, 266n32
avant-garde, 65–67, 74, 97, 111, 278n37
Ave Maria (Ito), 47, *49*
Azuma, Eiichiro, 34, 126, 132–33, 162, 173, 279n56

backstage, 234–39, *236*, *239*
Baird, Beatrix, 136, 140
balance: integration/Japaneseness, 125, 129, 140–42; kinetic, 39, 49, 103, *118*, 119
ballet, 66, 144, 171, 176, 227. *See also Blue Danube*; *Etenraku*
Ballet Intime, 94, 105, *106*, 108
Ballets Russes, 11, 105, 120, 178, 180
Beaumont, Cyril, 121
belatedness, 40, 52–54
Bennahum, Judith, 255
Berlant, Lauren, 8, 146
Berlin. *See* Germany
Bernstein, Robin, 59
Bhabha, Homi, 53
Black Dragon Society, 192
Blue Danube (Ito), 20–22, *21*, 24, 152–53, 155–60, *156–57*, 210
Blue Flame (Yamada), 71, 99
Bluntschli, J. C., 147
body: desire and, 8, 33, 82–84, *83*, 219–20; as expressive medium, 79–82; as honest/unmediated self-expression, 250–52, *251*; *nikutai* and, 149, 242–43; self-scrutiny of, 218–19, *219*; as site of fantasy, 8, 144–46, *145*, 246
Bolm, Adolf, 94, 105, *106*, 108
Booloo, 12, 135
Borglum, Gutzon, 185–86
Borodin, Alexander, 124, 140–42
Bourdaghs, Michael, 243
Bow, Leslie, 8, 116–17
Brandon, James R., 284n65
Bright and Dark (Yamada), 69–70
Broadway, 12, 34, 96, 101, 110–15, 227, 229, 231. *See also Pinwheel Revel*
Bücher, Karl, 51, 53
Buddhism/Buddha, 2, 24, 70, 181–82

Burgess, Dana Tai Soon, 46–47, *49*, 255, 263n21
burlesque/parody, 112–13, 194–96
Bush, Christopher, 80, 97, 111
butoh, 64, 97
buyōshi undo. See dance poem

Cable Act, 27, 151, 168
Café Royal (London), 75–76
Caldwell, Helen, 4–5, 66, 88, 254–55, 263n21
California Art Club, 134
Camp, Pannill, 18
"Camp Livingston" notebooks (Ito), 85, 187–88, 193–98, 201
Candelario, Rosemary, 97–98
Cantos, The (Pound), 75
Caresse Dansée (Scriabin), 95
Carriger, Michelle Liu, 59, 107, 222
Carter, Artie Mason, 138
Cathay (Pound), 75
Cavaliera Rusticana, 10
censorship, 15, 215, 221, 237; self-, 15, 193–94, 284n66
Chandler, Harry, 190–91
Chang, Juliana, 8, 143
Cheng, Anne Anlin, 8, 54, 117, 119, 233, 249
Children of East Asia, 212
China/Chinese: ambassador of, 186; Pound's interest in, 75; racialization of, 121; in travelogues, 41–42. *See also* Second Sino-Japanese War
chindon-ya, 252
Chinese Buffoon (Ito), 95
Chinese Dance, 108–9
Chinese Spear Dance (Ito), 95
Chinese Written Character as Medium of Poetry, The (Fenollosa/Pound), 80–81
Ching-a-ling, 110
Chitra (Tagore), 69
Choe Seung-hui (Sai Shōki), 203
Chopin, Frédéric, 75, 140, 176
Chow, Rey, 119–20
Chuh, Kandice, 31, 143
Churchill, Winston, 88

Index

circulation. *See* movement/mobility

citizenship, 27, 34, 125, 133, 142–44, 151, 168

civic arts movement. *See* community arts movement

Clark, Paul J., 193

Classroom for Beauty, A (Ito), 36, 43, 71, 77

Coburn, Alvin Langdon, 33, 57, *58*, 71, *73*, 82–84, *83*, 87–89, *89*, 220

Coliseum (London), 11, 75–76, 78

collection. *See* japoniste collection

"comfort woman" system, 200, 282n46

community arts movement, 126, 137–42, 147

community dance movement, 126, 138–42, 152, 208

comportment, 20, 50, 215, 227, 240–41, 244, 247, 250

concert dance, 24, 94–95, 110, 112, 121, 149, 216, 229. *See also* modern dance; "oriental dance"

corporeal rejuvenation/remaking: dance and, 223, 227, 229, 231, 233–34, 240, 242–43; postwar necessity of, 214–19, *219*; walking and, 240–47; women and, 35, 214–16, 224–25, 226, 240, 244–50, *248*. *See also* Ernie Pyle Theatre

cosmopolitanism: artistic, 35, 44, 51–52; cultural emulsion/agglomeration, 99, 146–47, 150–51, 172–73; embodied in Western dance, 227, 229; as fantasy, 7, 20–22, *21*, 25, 28, 143; of Greenwich Village, 111–14, 117; Ito's performance of, 16, 20–22, *21*, 25–26, 36–37, 40, 151–52, 171–73; *mestizaje* and, 163–64, 171, 176–79; in postwar Japan, 215, 217, 222–23, 229, 231, 233, 243; Silk Road and, 1–3; "worldliness" vs. "foreignness" and, 163, 166–67, 180–83. *See also* imperialism; Japan's imperial project; Pan-Asianism

costume: Egyptian Hawk, 33, 82, 87–90, *89*; embodied pleasure/fantasy of, 20–25, *21*, *23*, 104; at Ernie Pyle, 223, 224–25, 227, *228*, 231, 232; for *Etenraku/Blue*

Danube, 20–22, *21*, 24, 152–58, *154*, *156–57*; female-gendered noh kimono, 33, 82–87, *83*; Latin dance, 91, *92*; modern concert dance drapery, 113; women's fashions/postwar attire, 244–47

Cowell, Mary-Jean, 5, 14, 46, 124–25, 254

Craig, Edward Gordon, 10, 198

Cullingford, Elizabeth, 74

Cunard, Maud, Lady, 11, 75, 88, 90

Daibutsu Kaigen (Ito), 179, 181–82

Dalcroze eurythmic method: ideologies of, 44–45, 50–54, 60, 138–39, 142, 203–4; Ito and, 11, 33, 44, 46–47, *48–49*, 50–52, 72, 103, 148–49, 208; sequence of poses, 44–46, 50, 89

dance criticism, 114, 126, 165–66, 169, 171, 175–79

dance drawings, 62–64, *63*, 201

dance education, 67–68, 102, 138–40, 182–83. *See also* Jaques-Dalcroze Institute for Eurythmics

Dance of the Green Pine (Ito), 75

dance poem 舞踊詩: conceptualized, 68–70; Ito's experiments with, 12, 33, 64–66, 70–72, *73*, 90, 93, 265n17; Japanese modern dance movement of, 33, 64–70, 72, 90, 98–99

dance symphony, 12–13, 34, 133, 137, 182, 208; *Blue Danube/Etenraku* pairing, 152–60, *154*, *156–57*, 210; *Prince Igor,* 124, 140–42, 180

Davis, Mike, 126

Dawn of the East, 12, 135

Debussy, Claude, 38, 40–41, 95, 176

Delibes, Léo, 62, 66, 95

Delsarte system, 250–51, *251*

Denishawn School (Los Angeles), 126, 165

desire: backstage/private, 235–37, *236*; body as setting for, 8, 33, 82–84, *83*, 219–20; circulation of, 18–19; collection as practice/object of, 94–96, 114–15, 120; Egyptian art/artifacts and, 38–39, 89–90; for exotic/

308 Index

desire (*continued*)

erotic, *83*, 84–87, 115–17, 121, 123, 231; fantasy's exploration of, 5, 7, 16, 160; fetish object/subject and, 34, 94–95, 115–20, *118*; heterosexual, *225*, 226–27, 231; homoerotic/queer, 120–23, 220; intimacy and, 109–10, 113, 120–23; Ito's own, 33–34, 64–65, 82, 93, 257; Ito's reception and, 7, 15, 64–65, 93, 163–64; for Japan, *83*, 84–87, 93; spectator's role in producing, 15–16, 59. *See also* fantasy; watching/being watched

Devi, Ratan (née Alice Richardson), 105, *106*, 108, 112

Diaghilev, Sergei, 123, 180

Diem, Carl, 3

Dohrn, Wolf, 51–52

Doi Takeo, 235

Donkey, The (Ito), 99

Dulac, Edmund, 71, *73*, 76, 87–88, 100

Duncan, Isadora, 64, 67, 69

Dvořák, Antonín, 140

earthquakes, 9, 128, 169, 265n11

East/West binaries, 103–4, 108, 146–47, 150, 175, 223, *224–25*

Eaton, Mary, 105

Ecclesiastique (Ito), 95, 112, 148–49, 165

Egypt, 4, 33, 36, 38–44, 61, 82, 87–90, *89*

Eiko & Koma, 97

Ekici, Didem, 50

Eliot, T. S., 88, 266n36

El Jarabe Tapatío (Pavlova), 171

Emperor Jones (O'Neill), 12, 111

Empire Waltz (Ito), 166

En Bateau (Ito), 95, 165

Enemy Alien Hearing Board, 184, 192

"enemy aliens," 13, 184, 187, 280n10. *See also* internment

Eng, David, 8

Enters, Angna, 102, 108

Ernie Pyle Theatre (Tokyo): backstage workers/desires, 234–39, *236*, *239*; corporeal possibility for Erniettes, 218,

222–29, 233–34, 252; foreign-centered revues at, 229–33, *230*, *232*; GI audiences of, 220–23, 224, 226, 229, 231, 233, 237; Ito's role at, 13–14, 35, 213, 215, 220–21; Japan-centered revues at, 223–27, *224–25*, *228*; staged fantasies at, 222–23, 227, 233; training at, 215, 220–21. *See also* Takarazuka Theater/ Revue; *individual revues*

escapism, 6, 14, 127, 146, 158–60, 233–34, 240, 255

Etenraku (Ito), 152–55, *154*, *157*, 158–60, 210

ethnic dance, 24, 212–13, 274n37

Etiquette (Ito), 214–15, 217–19, *219*, 238–43, 250

Etude (Ito), 165

Eubanks, Charlotte, 94

eurythmics. *See* Dalcroze eurythmic method

Ewick, David, 76, 79, 267n38, 268n70

Executive Order 9066 (incarceration), 144, 280n10

expressionism, 67–69

extraterritoriality, 162

fabulation, 18–19

Falkenstein, Waldeen, 136, 165, 170, 256

fantasy: body as site of, 8, 144–46, *145*, 246; conceptualized, 5–8, 19–20, 257; cosmopolitanism as, 7, 20–22, *21*, 25, 28, 143; FBI's view of Ito as, 184, 187, 189; of history, 153–60, *157*, 181–82, 207–9; of integration, 126–27, 142–46, *145*, 152–53, 163; of intimacy, 109–10, 113, 120–23; Ito's strands of, 6–8, 15–16, 18–19, 36–37, 120, 253, 255–58; Japan as, 31, 37, 82, 84–87, 103, 222–23, 233–34, 242, 252–53; of *kokutai*, 148–50; of liberal subjecthood, 143–46, *145*, 148; as methodology, 16–20, 43–44, 257; of orientalism, 20, 24–25, 28; of self, 16–17, 20, 43, 216–17, 220, 240–41, 247–52, *248*; of social formation, 137–43, 208; of theater's

Index

enchantment, 226–27, 233; touristic, 113, 128, 233; of US/New York, 100, 126, 143; *voyage imaginaire*/travelogue, 37, 40–43. *See also* desire; utopianism/utopic visions
Fantasy Japonica (Ito), 13, 221, 223–27, *224–25*, 233, 237
fashion models/industry, 14, 35, 133, 215, 218, 246–52, *248*, *251*
Fay, Frank, 112
FBI, 13, 35, 160, 163, 183–84, 187, 189–92
Federal Music Project (Los Angeles), 152
femininity, 46, 178
Fenollosa, Ernest, 11, 76, 80–81
Fenollosa, Mary, 76
Fessler, Susanna, 41
fetish, 34, 94–95, 115–20, *118*
flâneuse/flâneur, 247–49, *248*
Flower Drum Song, 117, 119
Fogel, Joshua, 41–42
folk practices/dances, 57–59, *58*, 105, *106*, 112, 115
Foster, Susan, 8
Fox Dance (Ito), 71–72, *73*
Fox Dance by Moonlight, A (Ito), 75, 78
Fox's Grave, The, 136
France, Anatole, 38, 40
Frontier (Graham), 64
Frueh, Alfred J., *106*
Fujita Fujio, 4, 14, 169–70, 183, 186, 205
Fujitani, Takashi, 29, 149
Fuller, Loie, 87
Funeyama Takashi, 70
Furushō, Taeko, 256
Furushō Motō, 9, 191, 256

gagaku, 152, 158, 181, 227
García, Jerry, 171
gender: "comfort women," 200, 282n46; effeminacy, 112–16, 121, 178; female kimono and, 33, 82–87, *83*; flâneuse, 247–49, *248*; of liberal subject, 240; *mestizaje* and, 178; *panpan* girl, 243; women's fashion choices and, 244–

45. *See also* corporeal rejuvenation/remaking; femininity; masculinity
Geneva Convention, 193
Gente, Arnold, 47, *48*
Gentlemen's Agreements, 27
Germany: Berlin Olympics, 1–2; Ito's later writings about, 36, 39–40, 53–56, 61; Ito's time in Berlin, 10–11, 22, 32–33, 36, 39, 42; *kokutai* and, 50–51, 147–48; National Socialism, 168, 205. *See also* Jaques-Dalcroze Institute for Eurythmics
Gershwin, George, 229
Gesamtkunstwerk, 50–51, 206
Global Asias, 29–30, 35, 188
Gluck, Christoph, 52, 60, 152
Goffman, Erving, 15
Golliwog's Cakewalk (Ito), 95
Gonzalez Peña, Carlos, 176–79
Graham, Georgia, 136
Graham, Martha, 12, 64, 102, 117, 136, 256
Greater East Asia Co-Prosperity Sphere, 13, 28, 187, 199–200, 206–7, 211
Greater East Asia Ministry, 198, 204
Greater East Asia Stage Arts Research Institute 大東亜舞台芸術研究所: planning documents for, 13, 35, 187, 198, 200–207, 213; realized imperial revue, 211–13; unrealized Philippines festival pageant, 13, 35, 142, 206–11, 257
Greenberg, Mitchell, 160
Greenwich Village, 111–14, 117
Greenwich Village Follies, 12, 111
Greenwich Village Theatre (New York), 12, 99–100
Guevara, Alvara, 86
Gypsy Dance (Ito), 95

Habanera (Wright), 165
Habima Players, 96
Hagoromo, 87, 101
haiku, 75, 81, 194
Haiyū-za (Japan), 205, 211–12

Halzack, Sarah, 47, *49*
Hanayagi Sumi, 165
Harding, Warren G., 4, 185–86
Harlan, John Marshall, 121
Harootunian, Harry, 53
Harusame (Komori), 99
Hatano Sumio, 283n64
Hattori Ryōichi, 14
Hattori Tadashi, 212
Hauptmann, Gerhart, 10
Hayakawa, Sessue, 169–70
Hayashi Kōjirō, 252
Hayot, Eric, 266n32
Hellerau. *See* Jaques-Dalcroze Institute for Eurythmics
Herndon, Richard, 111–12, 114
Herrera, Brian, 229, 231
Hewitt, Andrew, 240–42, 249, 251
Higher Normal School (Tokyo), 10, 76
Hirata Kiichi, 76
Hitchcock, Raymond, 112–14
Hitler, Adolf, 3
Hoang, Nguyen Tan, 272n61
Hobbes, Thomas, 240
Hollywood Bowl: *Blue Danube/Etenraku,* 20–22, *21*, 152–60, *154*, *156–57*, 210; community arts movement and, 137–39; dance symphonies at, 12–13; Nisei performers at, 127, 143–44, 146, 153, 158; *Prince Igor,* 124, 140–42, 180
Hollywood film industry, 12, 125, 128, 131, 134–35, 169, 191–92, 231
homogenous-nation theory, 2, 147
homosexual desire, 84–86, 111–14, 178–79
Homsey, Bonnie Oda, 255–56
Hongo-za, 69
Horton, Lester, 88, 136, 256
Hoshino Yukiyo, 203
Houwen, Andrew, 79
Humphrey, Doris, 117

Ibsen, Henrik, 9
ice-skating spectaculars, 14
Iijima Isao 飯島魁, 9

Ikuta Kizan, 60
Imada, Adria, 222
imagism, 74, 79
Immigration Act (1924), 27, 101, 125
Immigration and Naturalization Service (INS), 189, 192
imperialism: British, 74, 107; disciplinary divides and, 29, 35; German, 50–51; intimacy of, 109–10, 166, 203–4; Ito's artistic participation in, 2–4, 13, 15, 25–26, 107–10, 149, 160, 163, 188; japoniste collection and, 94; masculinity and, 169–70; nationalist retrenchment after, 159, 171–72, 179–82; orientalism and, 20, 29; racial fetishism produced by, 116–17, 120; settler colonialism and, 162, 175; Western/US, 3, 26–27, 29, 94, 171–72. *See also* cosmopolitanism; Japan's imperial project
Imperial Rule Assistance Association, 203
Imperial Theatre, 10, 24, 67, 69–70, 104, 233
Impressions of a Chinese Actor (Ito), 95
Imura Kyoko, 254
"In a Station of the Metro" (Pound), 76, 79–80
incarceration: Executive Order 9066 and, 144, 280n10; of Issei, 131; of Nisei/Ito's students, 127, 146, 149, 158, 160, 254; of Tsuyako (Ito's wife), 13, 192
India/Indian dance, 22–24, *23*, 74, 104–5, *106*, 108
industrialization, 50–51
integration: fantasy of, 126–27, 142–46, *145*, 152–53, 163; history fantasies as path toward, 153–60, *157*, 181–82, 207–9; Issei goal of, 34, 125–26, 128, 131–33, 143–44, 160; Ito as advocate for, 126–27, 138–42; Ito as successful model of, *130*, 131–32; vs. Japaneseness, 125, *130*, 131–32, 140–42; white progressive goal of, 126, 137, 143–44, 147
intermarriage/amalgamation: Japanese

Index

views on, 164, 168–69, 174; Mexican *mestizaje* and, 163–64, 171, 177–79; US fears of, 96, 150–51, 164, 168
International Club (Tokyo), 166
internationalism, 1, 11, 40, 54–56, 60, 204
internment: vs. incarceration, 280n10; internees' camp experiences, 35, 193–97; Ito's arrest/trial and, 13, 81, 127, 129, 160, 184, 187, 189–92; Ito's "Camp Livingston" notebooks, 85, 187–88, 193–98, 201
interpretive dance, 12, 22, 24, 95, 98, 102, 112, 136, 149, 161. *See also* modern dance; "oriental dance"
intimacy: of empire, 109–10, 166, 203–4; imperial hospitality as, 222, 231, 233; performances of self, 227; queer, 84–86, 111–14, 120–23
Irish myth/nationalism, 74–75, 87–88
Irwin, Robert McGee, 178
Ishibashi Katsurō, 11
Ishii Baku (Ishii Tadazumi, Ishii Rinrō) 石井漠, 10, 33, 65, 67–70, 72, 98–99, 165, 200, 203
Islington, Lord and Lady, 88
Isoda Koryūsai, 83, 84
Isozaki, Arata, 31
Issei (first-generation): incarceration/internment of, 131, 189, 192–93; integration efforts of, 34, 125–26, 128, 131–33, 143–44, 160; laborers in, 131, 279n56. *See also* Japanese Americans/immigrants; Los Angeles; Nisei
Ito, Donald, 12–13, 165, 168
Ito, Gerald "Jerry," 12–14, 165, 168, 189
Ito, Michele, 256
Ito, Teiji, 256
Itō, Teiko (née Ono), 12, 13, 109, 179–81, 256
Itō Aiko 愛子, 9
Itō Kanae 鉄衛, 9
Itō Kimie (née Iijima) 伊藤喜美栄 (飯島), 9, 85, 179–80, 189
Itō Kisaku 熹朔, 9, 13, 141, 180–82, 202, 205, 221

Itō Kōichi 晃一, 9
Ito Michio 伊藤道郎: biographical overview of, 8–14, 27, 253; dance/familial descendants of, 253–58; drawings by, 62–64, 63, 79, 201; as elusive/adaptable, 4–5, 14–15, 28–29, 32, 146–47, 161; financial situation of, 75, 84, 90, 102, 125, 189–92; marriage to Wright, 12, 27, 96, 127, 150–51, 165, 168–69, 189; memoirs of, 37–40, 43, 53–56, 61, 77, 262n1; name of, 28–29, 177; performance of self, 15, 20–22, 21, 57–59, 58, 61, 103–4, 115, 211; pictured dancing, 23, 48, 89, 92, 106, 235, 236; pictured looking away from camera, 237–38, 239; strands of fantasy of, 6–8, 15–16, 18–19, 253, 257–58; turn to fashion industry, 246–52, 248, 251. *See also* internment; *individual dances/memoirs/locations*
AFFILIATIONS: community arts/dance movement, 126, 137–42; cosmopolitanism, 25–26, 36–37, 51–52, 143, 172–73, 203–4, 209–11; imperialism, 13, 15, 25–26, 107–10, 149, 160; Japanese immigrant community, 129–32, 130; modernism, 7, 10, 52–53, 72; orientalism, 22–26, 23, 30–32, 104–5, 106; Pan-Asianism, 7, 24, 34–35; as strand of fantasy, 6–7
CHOREOGRAPHY/DANCE TECHNIQUE: balance/tension, 39, 49, 118, 119; breathwork, 46–47; compressed/internalized energy, 33, 62–64, 63, 66; Dalcrozian influence on, 44, 46–47, 50–52, 60, 138–39, 148–49; expressive individuality, 102–3, 123; mimetic/abstract in, 71–72, 73, 91–93, 92; "one-arm lead," 46–47, 48–49; pictorial nature of, 134–35, 141; rhythmic harmony, 44, 47, 50, 52, 182; series of poses, 44, 46, 50, 139, 148–49, 209, 229; vorticism's vigor/movement, 77–80; walking, 47–49

FANTASIES IN DANCE-MAKING: history incorporated into, 152–60, *157*, 181–82, 207–9; as strand of fantasy, 7; as transformative, 71–72, *73*, 91–93, *92*, 186–87

FAILED/UNREALIZED PROJECTS: international dance school exchanges, 182–83, 186; Little Tokyo revitalization, 127–29; Olympic plans, 1–4, 14, 17, 253; as strand of fantasy, 6, 188; Theatre of the Sun, 185–87, 204. *See also* Greater East Asia Stage Arts Research Institute

RECEPTION: of commercial work, 111–14; desire and, 7, 15, 64–65, 93, 163–64; New York's Japan craze and, 96–98, 101; as paradigm of success abroad, 129–32, *130*, 141, 170–75, 180; as racially ambiguous/*mestizo*, 171, 175–79; as untrustworthy/alien enemy, 184, 187; by white Los Angeles arts patrons, 131, 134–35, 138, 146–47, 153; as "worldly" vs. "foreign," 164–69, 180–83

SELF-FASHIONING: cipher/screen for desires, 7, 14–15, 65, 82–87, *83*, 91–93, *92*; "communitarian," 136–42; community-instantiating artist, 127–32, *130*; cultural mediator, 1, 16–17, 22, 60–61, 80–82, 127, 129, 174–75, 181–84, 190–91; fetish object/subject, 115–20, *118*; figure of "the Orient," 37, 42–43, 56–59, *58*, 61; individual, 103–4, 123; modernist artist/innovator, 16, 72, 77, 82, 123, 133–34, 137; postwar cosmopolitan teacher/expert, 214–15, 218–20, 222, 238, 240, 242–47, 250, *251*; self-mythologizing, 61, 65–66, 76–77, 89–90, *89*, 123

STORIES: Christmas at Jaques-Dalcroze Institute, 54–56; divorce from Wright, 150–51; imagined travels to Paris/Egypt, 37–44; London life/noh demonstration, 75–77, 90; *Pinwheel*'s origination, 112–14; *Pizzicati*'s origin, 66; plan for Theatre of the Sun, 185–87; relationship with Nijinsky, 115, 120–23; as strand of fantasy, 6, 32–33, 36–37, 120

Itō Nobuko 暢子, 9

Itō Ousuke 翁介, 9, 212

Itō Tadao 忠男, 9

Itō Tamekichi 伊藤為吉, 9, 75, 179–80, 189, 273n13

Itō Teiryō 貞亮, 9

Itō Yoshiko 嘉子, 9, 256

Itō Yūji 祐司, 9, 12–13, 109, 112, 179–81, 256

Izumida, Teru, 165

Jane, Edith, 136, 139, 141, 274n33

Japan: "borderless empire" of, 162, 171–75, 183; carefully cultivated image of, 70, 97, 159, 173–74, 222; fantasy of, 31, 37, 82, 84–87, 103, 222–23, 233–34, 242, 252–53; foundational myth of, 181–82, 197; imperial armada of, *130*, 131; Ito's dance descendants in, 254–55; Ito's postwar life in, 13–14, 35, 40, 61, 67, 77, 220; Ito's three trips to, 13, 34, 160, 161, 163–70, 179–84, 189; Ito's wartime repatriation, 13, 35, 187, 192–93, 197, 199–200, 280n16; Ito's youth/study in, 9–10, 24, 41, 49–50, 67, 98; as mixed vs. homogenous nation, 2–3, 25–27, 147–49; public morality policed in, 166–69; Tokyo Olympics, 1–4, 14, 17, 253; wartime anticommunist arrests, 182, 203, 205; Yeats/Pound and, 74–81. *See also* Japan's imperial project; *kokutai*; Occupation; Pan-Asianism; *tōyō*

Japancentrism, 188

Japanese: as exemplary vs. exceptional, 37, 41, 56–57, 59–61, 107–10; names/transliteration, 28–29, 31–32, 182; slippage with Japanese American, 127, 158; slippage with "Oriental," 41, 56–57, 61, 104, 107–10, 116, 150–51. *See also* performing Japanese

Index

Japanese American Citizens League (JACL), 132–33, 144

Japanese Americans/immigrants: achievements of, *130*, 131–32; class divides, 132, 172–73; in Los Angeles, 101–2, 124–25, 129–32, *130*; in Mexico City, 163, 171–75; New York, 98, 100–102. *See also* Issei; Nisei

Japanese-American Women's Association, 141

Japanese Lady with Umbrella and Fan (Ito), 75

Japaneseness: as commercial product, 111–14; vs. integration, 125, *130*, 131–32, 140–42. *See also* performing Japanese

Japanese universal aestheticism: commercial entertainment and, 110–15; Japanese immigrants and, 100–102; Japan's imperial project and, 94, 97, 101; in Little Tokyo revitalization plan, 127–29; white audiences and, 96–101, 103–4, 114–15, 141. *See also* japonisme

Japanism, 81

Japanophilia, 84–86, 115, 129

Japan's imperial project: as absorptive, 34, 132, 168, 231; artistic corollary to, 94, 97, 101; borderless empire, 162, 171–75, 183; cosmopolitanism of, 25–29, 34–35, 42, 53, 163, 166, 231, 258; devastation in aftermath of, 215–16, 226, 233, 243; Ito's cosmopolitan ideals and, 187, 203–4, 209–11; Ito's proposed Philippines pageant and, 13, 35, 142, 206–11, 257; Ito's wartime notebooks and, 196–99, 201; mixed-nation theory, 2–3, 147–49; Pan-Asianism as ideology of, 192, 199–200, 206, 253; violent territorial expansion and, 199–200, 210; wartime performances in support of, 201–3. *See also* imperialism; Pan-Asianism

japonisme, 82–85, *83*, 93, 176; orientalism and, 93–94, 103–4, 107–10, 115–16, 119, 153. *See also* Japanese universal aestheticism

japoniste collection: conceptualized, 31, 33–34, 93–96, 120; Ito as collector, 94–96, 108–10, 114–15, 117–20, *118*, 164; Ito as curio, 94–96, 104–5, *106*, 115–20, *118*, 164; Orient-as-collection paradigm and, 105–8, *106*; traditional and modern in, 97–100

Jaques-Dalcroze, Émile, 44–45, 51–54, 263n18

Jaques-Dalcroze Institute for Eurythmics: classes/training at, 44–47, 243; festivals/pageants at, 52, 60, 152, 207–8, 210, 263n33; goals/founding of, 28, 44, 50–51, 60, 128, 142, 203–4, 207; Ito's dance method/philosophy and, 11, 22, 33, 44, 47, 49–52, 80, 103; Ito's memories/stories of, 52–56, 60, 193, 196; performing Japanese at, 33, 36–37, 56–57, 59–61, 76; as visible strand in Ito's work, 75, 87, 142, 152, 182, 204, 210; Yamada at, 11, 36, 42, 67–68, 98

Javanese Temple Dance (Ito), 22–24, *23*

Jones, Isabel Morse, 146, 151

Jungle Drums, 221, 231

Kabbani, Rana, 42

kabuki, 85, 95, 97, 173, 202, 227

Kahlo, Frida, 117

Kamiyama Sōjin, *130*, 131–32

Kappore from Suite Japonaise (Yamada), 95, 99

Kasagi Shizuko, 14

Kenbu (Ito), 78

kikōbun, 41–43

Kikuchi, Yuriko (née Amemiya), 12

Kikyō Monogatari (Kimiyasu), 212

Kim, John Namjun, 25

Kim, Ju Yon, 15, 245

kimono, 101, 133, 152, 223, *224*, 244–45; Ito in, 33, 57, *58*, 82–87, *83*

kinesthetic awareness, 18, 119, 238, 246–49, *248*, 252, 257

Kipling, Rudyard, 146–47, 150

Kishida Kunio, 203, 205

Kitasono Katue, 81
Kitsmiller, Michiko Yoshimura, 255
Kohana, 109
Kojima, E. Gitaro, 191
kokutai: conceptualized, 34, 147–48; German parallels to, 50–51, 147–48; Ito's interpellation as, 34–35, 126–27, 148–51, 163, 166; vs. *nikutai*, 148, 242–43. *See also* national embodiment
Komai Tetsu, *130*, 131–32, 136
Komine Kumiko, 49, 254
kōminka movement, 26, 168
Komori Toshi 小森敏, 10, 12, 69, 98–100, 269n1
Koner, Pauline, 47, 125, 256
Kon Hidemi, 205
Konoe Fumimaro, 13, 159, 199
Konoe Hidemaro, 13, 152, 155, *157*, 158–59
Korean War, 221, 247
Kōri Torahiko, 11, 76
Kotef, Hagar, 240
Kowal, Rebekah, 8
Kreutzberg, Harald, 68
Krotona Theosophical Society, 137
Kubota Mantarō, 205
Kume Tamijurō, 11, 76
kuroko, 237
Kurosawa Akira, 243
Kushida Kiyomi, 32, 109
Kuwahara Noriko, 220
Kwan, Nancy, 117, 119
Kwan, SanSan, 247–49
Kwon, Nayoung Aimee, 109–10, 203
kyōgen, 95, 135–36
Kyoto School, 25

La Argentina, 165
Laban, Rudolf von, 52, 62–64
Lacan, Jacques, 7
Lambert-Beatty, Carrie, 238
La Meri, 274n37
Laplanche, Jean, 5, 7, 17, 160, 257
L'après-midi d'un faune, 120
Lavery, Grace, 84, 97

League of Nations, 199
Lebensreform, 60, 62–64
Ledoux, Louis V., 136
Leong, Andrew, 32, 132
Lepecki, André, 8, 257
Leser, Tina, 246
liberal subjecthood, 216, 233–34, 240–42, 244–46, 249, 252; fantasy of, 143–46, *145*, 148; self-possession and, 45, 241–44, 252
Life Reform Movement, 50–51, 210
Lindahl, Tulle, 98–99, 105, *106*, 108–9
L'interieur (Maeterlinck), 10
Little Shepherdess (Wright), 165
Little Theatre (New York), 114, 137
London: Ito's trajectory in, 11–12, 33, 60–61, 64–65, 71–72, 90; modernists of, 72–76, 84–85, 87–90, 137; performing Japanese in, 57–59, *58*, 75–77, 81–87, *83*; sword dances/vorticist work, 77–81, 90, 99. *See also At the Hawk's Well*; dance poem; Pound, Ezra; Yeats, W. B.
loneliness/alienation, 50–56, 193–96
Los Angeles: Ito's "communitarian" focus in, 136–42; Ito's dance descendants in, 254–55; Ito's early dance concerts in, 134–36; Ito's life in, 12–13, 20, 27, 34, 125, 150–52, 189–90, 204; Japanese American community in, 101–2, 124–25, 129–32, *130*; Little Tokyo, 127–29, 133–34, 136, 146, 255; modern dance in, 126, 136. *See also* Hollywood Bowl; Issei; Nisei
Los Angeles Dance Foundation, 255
Los Angeles Philharmonic, 138–39
Los Angeles Times, 127–28, 135–37, 141, 146–47, 159, 190–91
Lotus Land (Ito), 95, 180
Lowe, Lisa, 42, 53, 144
Luigi, 256

Madame Butterfly, 9, 12, 110, 135
Maeterlinck, Maurice, 10, 39, 41
Maihime Dariā (Nagata), 10

Maki Ryūko, 254
Manchukuo/Manchuria, 26, 28, 164, 196, 199–200, 279n56
Mandarin Ducks (Ito), 95
Manning, Susan, 17
Marco Polo Bridge Incident, 28, 158
Martin, John, 114
Martin, Randy, 8
Maruyama Masao, 243
masculinity: Asian American, 115–16; imperialism and, 169–70; Ito's, 35, 169–70, 177–79; Japanese, 169; *machismo*, 93, 178; national embodiment and, 151, 163–64, 169–70, 177–79; Nijinsky's, 121, 178; in *Pinwheel* framing, 112–13; remasculinization, 272n61; tango and, 91–93, 92
masks, 57–59, 58, 71, 73, 100, 170
Matsumoto, Valerie, 133
McClintock, Anne, 116
McLaughlin, Frank Y., 190
Mehiko Shinpō, 172–73, 179
Meiji era/Meiji Restoration, 2, 26, 101, 108, 222, 240, 246
mestizaje, 163–64, 171, 177–79
Metropolitan Opera House, 122–23
Mexican Revolution, 171, 175, 177
Mexico: *mestizaje/machismo* discourse in, 163–64, 171, 177–79; modern dance movement of, 136, 165, 170–71, 176; *Tabasco*'s fantasy of, 229, 231–33, 232
Mexico City: Ito's trip to, 13, 34, 160, 161, 163, 170–79, 183; Japanese immigrant community in, 163, 171–75; Mexican critics/cultural elite of, 163, 171, 175–79
Mezamashitai, 211
Michio Ito, Pioneering Dancer-Choreographer, 256
Michio Ito Alumni Association, 254
Michio Ito Foundation, 256
Miikusabune, 211–12
Mikado, The, 12–13, 96, 110, 221
Miki Kiyoshi, 25
mime plays, 99

Minobe Yōji, 209
Miranda, Carmen, 231
miscegenation, US anxieties of, 96, 150–51, 164, 168
Mitsuhashi Renko, 211
Miura Tamaki, 9–10, 95
mixed-nation theory, 2–3, 147–49
Miyabe Shizuko, 69
Miya Misako, 269n1
Miyao, Daisuke, 169
Miyatake, Toyo: Ito photographs, 14, 20, 21, 23, 62, 92, 254; Nisei dancers photographed, 34, 144–46, 145, 154, 156
Mobile Theatre Federation (Japan), 202, 205
"Modern and Classic Japanese Pantomimes and Dances," 99
modern dance: as art vs. entertainment, 111–15; vs. community arts, 137, 141; Japan's dance poem movement, 33, 64–70, 72, 90, 98–99; in Southern California, 126, 136; tango's popularity with, 91–93, 92, 167; terminology of, 24. *See also* Dalcroze eurythmic method; interpretive dance; "oriental dance"
modernism: high/popular culture divide, 111–15, 117, 136–37, 167, 171; Ito's fantasy of artistic kinship and, 38, 40, 52, 66; Ito's New York projects and, 98–99; Japanese, 10, 12, 22, 70, 72, 81, 93; Japanophilia of, 84–86, 129; London, 72–76, 137; modernity and, 44, 50–53, 60, 128–29; myth-making of, 65–66; poetry/dance viewed as connected, 68–70, 72, 78, 88; "unity of image," 76–79. *See also At the Hawk's Well*; Dalcroze eurythmic method; dance poem
modernity: colonial, 53–54; industrialization/ills of, 44, 50–53, 60, 128, 201–2; Mexico's, 171; urban, 38, 128–29; white/Western vs. Japanese, 3–4, 53, 104, 111, 246

Molinari, Bernardino, 140–41
Mordkin, Mikail, 117
Mori Ogai, 69, 85–86
Morrell, Ottoline, Lady, 11, 75, 82, 90, 104, 267n38
Morris-Suzuki, Tessa, 168
movement/mobility: in dance poem, 68–72, *73*; factory work/war mobilization captured in, 201–2; of Issei experience, 131–32; Ito's dancing as constitutive of, 30, 148; *suriashi* and, 49–50; of vorticism, 77–80. *See also* rhythm; walking
Mozart, Wolfgang Amadeus, 56, 153
Murata Minoru, 10
Muray, Nickolas, 34, 115, 117–19, *118*
music as essential/not, 50, 68–71
music education, 44–45, 67. *See also* Jaques-Dalcroze Institute for Eurythmics

Nagai Kafu, 281n24
Nagata Hideo, 69, 181
Nagata Mikihiko, 10
Nakamura, Cecelia, 153
namahage, 57–59, *58*
Nanjing Massacre, 200, 210
Nara, 2–3
national embodiment: Ito's embodied borderlessness and, 161–63, 183; Ito's interpellation as, 34–35, 126–27, 169–71; masculinity and, 151, 163–64, 169–70, 177–79; *mestizaje,* 163–64, 171, 177–79; Nisei community dancers and, 138–43; Occupation-era young women and, 216–18, 227, 229. *See also kokutai*
National New Theatre, 211
Nehru, Jawaharlal, 199
Neighborhood Playhouse (New York), 12, 95
Nelson, Richard, 75
netsuke, 115–16
New East Asia (dance group), 211

New Order in Asia/East Asia, 28, 107–8, 199, 204–9, 212
New Theater (Yamada/Ishii/Osanai), 68–70
New Tsukiji Theatre, 181
New World Symphony (Dvořák), 140
New York: collaborations/fellow dancers in, 67–68, 71, 98–100, 122–23, 169, 254; commercial theater work in, 95–96, 110–15; Ito's life/teaching in, 8, 12, 49, 101–3, 150–51; Ito's repertoire in, 95–96, 98, 108, 125, 148–49; Japanese immigrant community of, 98, 100–102; japonisme in, 33–34, 93–100, 175; "oriental dance" in, 12, 34, 94–95, 104–10, *106*, 112; *Rhapsody in Blue*'s fantasy of, 229–31, *230*
Nichigeki Theatre, 180, 211–12
nihon buyō, 10, 49, 67, 133
nihonjinron, 61
Nijinsky, Vaslav, 4, 11, 34, 67, 115, 120–23, 178
Nikkei, 132
nikutai, 148, 242–43
Nisei (second-generation): in *Blue Danube/Etenraku,* 153, 158; citizen-subjecthood performed by, 132–33, 142–44; in community dance movement, 127, 138–43; incarceration of, 127, 146, 149, 158, 160, 254; Ito's focus on, 12–13, 34, 129, 133, 152, 216; in Ito's studio, 131, 133, 144–46, *145*, 148, 152–53, 165; Miyatake photographs of, 34, 144–46, *145*, *154*, *156*; recruited into US military, 143, 149; tension with Issei, 125, 128, 132, 160. *See also* Issei; Japanese Americans/immigrants; Los Angeles
Nisei Week (festival), 132–33
No, No, Nanette, 12, 125, 135
Noguchi, Yone, 81, 84
noh: *At the Hawk's Well* and, 87–88, 100, 180; female-gendered kimono in, 33, 82–87, *83*; in Ito's imperial revue, 211;

Index

317

Ito's New York projects and, 12, 95, 98–99, 101; movement in, 64; Pound's interest in, 11, 71, 76–81, 85

Nohara Yasuko, 68

nostalgia, 52, 85, 93, 223, 229–31, 233

Nutcracker, The (Tchaikovsky), 108–9

Nyong'o, Tavia, 18

Nyū Yōku Shinpō, 101

Occupation, 13–14, 40, 213, 214–16; "blocked yen" policy, 234; fantasy of "Japan" staged for, 222–23; GI presence in, 221–23, 224, 226, 229, 231, 233, 237; *nikutai* discourse, 148, 242–43; paternalistic/"benevolent" framing of, 226, 237, 242–47; promise/opportunity of, 35, 216, 220–22, 233–34, 242–47, 251, 251; self-consciousness of, 217–20, 234–35, 237–39, 239, 252; as subjugation/exclusion, 216, 220–21, 234. *See also* corporeal rejuvenation/remaking; Ernie Pyle Theatre; Japan

Ochiai Namio, 69

Odom, Selma Landen, 45

Okakura Tenshin (Kakuzō), 2–3

Olympics, 1–4, 14, 17, 117, 253

O'Neill, Eugene, 12, 111

Ootomo Chiharu, 211

opera, 9–10, 22, 67, 152

Orient: as collection, 105–8, 106; as fantasy, 24, 30–31, 40–43; as inscrutable, 14, 22, 41; Ito's fascination with, 22–25, 23, 30–31, 42, 104–5, 107–8; as source of rejuvenation, 74–75, 87; terminology of, 30–31

"oriental dance": "Americanized," 180; as colonial intimacy, 109–10; ethnographic framing/research, 43, 105–7, 106, 203, 209, 212; Ito's, 12, 34, 94–95, 102, 104–10, 106, 112, 136, 153, 180; Ito's Javanese costume as emblematic of, 22–24, 23; Japanese imperial frame and, 26, 107–10, 166; referential hodgepodge of, 20, 22, 24, 108–9; *tōyō*

and, 107–8, 209; white racial frame of, 24, 26, 105–7, 153; "worldliness" of, 166

"Oriental Evenings" (Ito), 108–9, 186

orientalism: belatedness/immediacy and, 40–41, 52–54; as fantasy, 20, 24–25, 28; imperialism and, 20, 29; Ito's costumes and, 20, 22–24, 23, 85; Ito's self-construction and, 37, 42–43, 56–59, 58, 61; Japanese/"Oriental" slippage, 41, 56–57, 61, 104, 107–10, 116, 150–51; Latin exoticism and, 229, 231, 232; of London modernists, 74–75, 87–89; in mainstream press coverage of Ito, 127–28; Nijinsky's characterization and, 121, 123, 178; spirituality as trope of, 103–4, 175; stage, 24–25, 42, 104, 107, 233; terminology of, 30–31; in travelogue, 40–43; white, 25–26, 29. *See also* japonisme; *tōyō*

ornamentalism, 233–34, 238, 239, 249

Orpheus and Eurydice (Gluck), 52, 60, 152, 208, 263n33

O'Ryan, Anne Wynne, 99

Osanai Kaoru, 10, 67

Otobane Kaneko, 69

Ozawa Tsuyako, 13, 151, 187, 192

Ozawa v. United States, 27

pageant: beauty, 14, 133, 247; community arts movement and, 137–40; at Ernie Pyle, 221; Ito's planned Philippines festival event, 13, 35, 142, 206–11, 257; Japan/World Peace Festival, 95; Jaques-Dalcroze's Geneva event, 52, 207–8, 210; mass history, 13, 35, 77, 142, 181–82, 207–9

Pageant of Lights, 139–40

Pageantry (Uyehara/Susilowati), 256

Page from a Diary, A (Yamada), 69, 71, 99

Pagoda Queen (Ito), 180

Pakes, Anna, 260n18

318 Index

Pan-Asianism: Greater East Asia Co-Prosperity Sphere and, 13, 28, 187, 199–200, 206–7, 211; Ito's commitment to, 7, 24, 34–35, 186–87, 197, 203–4, 210–13, 253, 257; Japanese promotion of, 192, 199–200, 206; New Order in Asia/East Asia and, 28, 107–8, 199, 204–9, 212. *See also* Japan's imperial project

Pan Pacific Trading and Navigation Company, 190–91

panpan girl, 243

Paris, 36–38, 40, 44, 98, 120–21

Park, Josephine, 29, 266n32

Parker, H. T., 71–72

parody/burlesque, 112–13, 194–96

Passpied (Delibes), 95

Pavlova, Anna, 11, 66–67, 171, 176

Peace Preservation Law, 215

Pearl Harbor, 13, 184, 187, 189, 192

Peer Gynt Suite (Grieg), 140

Pellecchia, Diego, 80–81

performance: autobiography as, 38–40, 61, 77, 120; conceptualized, 15–16; pleasure of, 85–87; reconstruction methodology, 17–18, 43–44, 254–57, 263n21

performativity, 19

performing Japanese: assimilation/integration as, *130*, 131–32, 147; at Jaques-Dalcroze Institute, 33, 36–37, 56–57, 59–61, 76; in London, 57–59, *58*, 75–76, 81–87, *83*; in New York, 108

Perrottet, Susan, 52

Perry, Barbara, 153

Perry, Matthew, Commodore, 3, 26

Persian Impression (Ito), 180

Petipa, Marius, 178

"Petit Poem, Vision of Hope" (Yamada), 99

Pétrouchka, 120–21

Pettit, Margaret, 113

Phelan, Peggy, 260n18

Philippines, 13, 35, 142, 205–11, 257

Picasso, Pablo, 40

Pinwheel Revel (Ito), 12, 34, 96, 101, 111–15, 148

Pisan Cantos (Pound), 90

Pizzicati (Ito): body/movement in, 8, 66, 91, 255; Ito's choreography sketch of, 62–64, *63*, 79; performances of, 140, 165, 170, 173, 263n21

Pontalis, Jean-Bertrand, 5, 7, 17, 160, 257

Poole, Janet, 109–10

Postlewait, Thomas, 37

Pound, Ezra: *At the Hawk's Well* collaboration, 11, 64–65, 88; as cultural mediator, 81–82; esoteric nature of, 137; Ito's impact on, 65–66, 90; Japanese poetics/noh and, 11, 71, 74–81, 85; vorticism of, 33, 65, 72, 74, 77–80, 90

Powell, Lillian, 136, 141

Prelude (Ito), 165

Preston, Carrie, 5, 49, 76–78, 263n21, 266n36, 267n37

Preston, VK, 18

Prevots, Naima, 124

Prince Igor (Borodin), 124, 140–42, 179–80, 182

propaganda: anti-Japanese, 196, 226; Ito accused of, 15, 160, 189; total war mobilization and, 202, 204–6, 210, 281n24

Provincetown Players, 111

psychoanalysis, 7–8, 116–17

public morality, 166–69

queer expression/intimacy/freedom, 84–86, 111–14, 120–23, 178–79

racial arrhythmia, 33, 53–56

racialization: ethnic/white binary, 111, 176; of fetish object, 115–17, 120; japoniste collection and, 94–95, 103; liberal subjecthood and, 143–46, *145*, 148, 242; miscegenation fears and, 96, 150–51, 164, 168; national signification and, 127; of Nijinsky, 121, 123; "oriental dance" and, 24, 26, 105–7; "racial

Index

mundane" and, 245–46; white women dancers and, 24, 149–50, 153

Radio City Music Hall, 12–13

Rafu Shimpo, 124–25, *130*, 131–32, 136, 139–43, 149, 276n74

Rainer, Yvonne, 238

Ravel, Maurice-Joseph, 95

reconstruction as methodology, 17–18, 43–44, 254–57, 263n21

Redlands Bowl, 152

Reed, Christopher, 84, 97

"Reminiscences" (Ito), 43

revue, 109, 173, 202, 205; foreign-centered shows at Ernie Pyle, 229–33, *230*, *232*; Ito's Pan-Asian project, 211–13; Japan-centered shows at Ernie Pyle, 221, 223–27, *224–25*, *228*. *See also Pinwheel Revel*

Reynoso, Jose Luis, 171, 176

Rhapsody in Blue (Ito), 13–14, 221, 229–31, *230*, 235, *236*

rhythm: Dalcroze focus on, 44–45, 51–52, 60, 67–68, 103, 138, 182, 196, 208; of internment camp life, 194–96; Ito and, 44, 47, 50, 71, 180, 182, 193, 201–2; Yamada's focus on, 68–69. *See also* arrhythmia

Richards, Thomas, 107

Ricketts, Charles, 88

Riordan, Kevin, 5, 187

Robertson, Jennifer, 212

Rodin, Auguste, 38, 40–41

Roosevelt, Eleanor, 183

Roosevelt, Franklin D., 280n10

Rose, Jacqueline, 5–6, 8, 146

Rose Bowl, 12, 139–40

Rosenberger, Nancy, 235

Roshanara, 105, *106*, 108, 110

Rosi, Giovanni Vittorio, 67

Russo-Japanese war, 26

Ryūtani Kyoko, 49

Sadayakko, 96

Saitō Kazō, 11, 67

Saitō Ren, 235

Sakai, Naoki, 25

Sakaroffs, the, 165

Sakomizu Hisatsune, 191, 209

Sakuma Shōzan, 104

Sakura Flowers (Ito), 227, *228*

"Sakura Sakura" (Ito), 108–9

Samuel, Ellen, 177

Sano Seki, 169–70

Sato, Yoshiko, 153

Sato Hiroaki, 81

Sawada, Mitziko, 100

Schlemmer, Oscar, 62–64

Schmidt, Karl, 51

Schofield, Lemuel B., 189

Schumann, Robert, 95, 148

Scott, Cyril, 95

Scriabin, Alexander, 68, 95, 99

scriptive things, 57–59, *58*

Seated Movement, A (Ito), 75

Seckler, Beatrice, 49, 102

Second Sino-Japanese War, 28, 109, 127, 152, 158

self-censorship, 15, 193–94, 284n66

self-consciousness: "awareishness" and, 59; of backstage, 237–39, *239*; as constitutive of self, 216–19, *219*, 237–39, *239*, 252; of Erniettes, 218, 233–34, 238–40, *239*; of fashion models, 218, 247–52, *248*, *251*; of Ito in female kimono, 82–87, *83*; of Occupation years, 217–20, 234, 237–39, *239*, 252; as performance strategy, 35, 218; *tatemae/honne* and, 235, *236*; of walking/movement, 252. *See also* watching/being watched

self-making: dance as, 64, 102–3, 211, 216, 233–34, 240, 242–43; fashion model's walk as act of, 247–50, *248*; fetish as site of, 117–20, *118*; walking as foundational to, 240–47. *See also* corporeal rejuvenation/remaking

self-possession, 45, 241–44, 252

self-promotion, 4, 9, 16, 74

Senda Koreya (Itō Kunio) 千田是也 (伊藤国夫), 4, 9, 169–70, 180–82, 205, 209–13
Serova, Sonia, 109
settler colonialism, 162, 175
Shakka/Siddhartha (Welkmeister), 10, 24, 104
Shapiro, Lillian, 102
Shawn, Ted, 91, 110, 117, 126
Shimakawa, Karen, 8, 242
Shima Kimiyasu, 211–12
Shimazaki, Satoru, 5, 47, 254–55
Shimizu Kintarō, 10
shimpa, 13
Shineo Ono, 152–53
shingeki, 10, 181–82, 202–3, 205
Shingekijō, 68–70
Shōchiku, 212
Shōwa Kenkyūkai, 25
Siamese Dance (Ito), 95
Siegel, Marcia, 260n18
Silk Road, 1–3, 206
Slaymaker, Douglas, 242–43
social dance, 133–34, 166–69, 229
Soganoya Gorō, 60
Somebody-Nothing, 135–36
Sorgenfrei, Carol, 5, 149, 188, 264n1
Spawn of the North, 12, 135
Spear Dance (Ito), 176
Spectre de la Rose, 122
Spier, Lasalle, 99
Srinivasan, Priya, 105
Stanger, Arabella, 62, 143
Stanley, Amy, 18
St. Denis, Ruth, 43, 105, 110, 117, 126, 134, 256
Stein, Gertrude, 40
Stevenson, Christine Wetherill, 137
Stewart, Susan, 96
Stokowski, Leopold, 134
Stoler, Laura Ann, 110
Strauss, Johann, 152
Strindberg, August, 69
Sueyoshi, Amy, 271n43

Sumida, Kazuo, 153
Sumire Model Group, 247, *251*
Sunset Murder Case, The, 12, 135
Supreme Commander for the Allied Powers (SCAP), 216, 218, 237
suriashi, 49–50
Susilowati, Sri, 256
Sword Dance (Ito), 78
"Sword-Dance and Spear-Dance" (Pound), 71, 78–79
Sylvia (Delibes), 62
Synge, John Millington, 74

Tabasco (Ito), 13, 221, 229, 231–33, *232*
Tadiar, Neferti, 7
Tagore, Rabindranath, 69, 74
Taisho Democracy, 165, 216, 245
Takarazuka Theater/Revue (Tokyo), 13, 211–12, 220–21, 231. See also Ernie Pyle Theatre
Takeda Rintarō, 205, 212
Takeishi, Midori, 5, 98–100
Taki Ryoichi, 198
Tale, A (Yamada), 69
Tamon, Arnold, 136, 141
Tamura, 12, 95, 99, 101
Tanabe Hajime, 25
Tanaka, Fumi, 153
Tanaka, Stefan, 26, 94, 107–8
Tanaka Gunkichi, 191–92
Tango (Ito), 91–93, *92*, 165–66
tango dance/craze, 91–93, *92*
Taniguchi, Masaharu, 197–98
Taylor, Diana, 178
Tchaikovsky, Pyotr, 108–9, 139, 148
Teatro Arben (Mexico City), 170
Teatro Hidalgo (Mexico City), 170, 173, 178
temporalities, 61, 77, 79, 120, 123, 227, *228*
Te no odori (Ito), 95
Teske, Charles, 165
Tetsuo Shinohara, 141
theater: Ito's commercial New York productions, 95–96, 110–15; Japan's modernist, 10; kimono's association

with for Ito, 85–86; mobile/propaganda, 201–3, 205, 212; proletarian, 169–70, 203, 211; reality and, 5–6, 107; as site of political promise/remove, 142–46, *145*, 158–60, 209–11; stage orientalism and, 24–25, 42, 104, 107, 233; theoretical texts of, 198

Theatre Direction Center (Indonesia), 205

theatricality, *83*, 84–87, 104, 107, 110, 247

Thornbury, Barbara, 97

Tokyo Carmen, 14

Tokyo Kaikan, 166–67

Tokyo Metropolitan Police, 161, 165–69

Tokyo Music School, 9–11, 67

Tokyo Olympics, 1–4, 14, 17, 253

Tokyo Philharmonic, 158, 220

Tone Poem II (Ito), 263n21

Tootikian, Karoun, 256

Toridesha, 10

tori-oi, 82–84, *83*, 86

tōyō 東洋, 26, 30–31, 34, 42, 94, 103–4, 107–10, 209. *See also* orientalism

translation: author's note on, 28–32; Ito's "life in," 17; Pound's noh plays, 11, 71, 76; purposeful lack of, 99

travelogues, 40–42

Trio A (Rainer), 238

Tsubouchi Shoyō, 10

Tsuji Naoshirō, 205

Tsutsui Tokujirō, 13

Tsuyoshi Namigata, 278n37

"Ue o muite arukō" ("Sukiyaki"), 30

ukiyo-e, 82–84, *83*, 86, 88

Underhill, Harriette, 103

United Service Organization (USO) entertainers, 221, 231

unity: fostered through art, 158–60, 174–75, 181–82, 205; of image/music, 45, 50, 76–79, 180; of mass movement, 140–42

University of Southern California (USC), 141, 274n33

Uno Shirō, 10

Ushiyama Mitsuru, 165–66

US Signal Corps Photographers, 237

US Supreme Court, 27, 121

utamakura, 41

Utchiyama Masami, 78

utopianism/utopic visions: artistic cosmopolitanism, 143, 152, 158–60, 186–87, 209–11; artists' colony, 185–86; art's potential of, 7, 11, 81–82; citizenship-subjecthood, 133, 142–44; community arts movement, 137–42, 208; fantasy of Japan as, 84–86; internationalism, 54–56, 60, 204; social transformation, 50–52, 60, 62, 126, 203–4, 206; willfully blind/misdirected, 15–16, 18–19, 29, 209–11

Uyehara, Denise, 256

Vanderlip, Frank A., Mrs., 125, 134

Van Valkenburg, Carol Bulger, 193

Variety, 112–13

Vincent, J. Keith, 85–86

Vogel, Shane, 16, 37, 271n43

Vogue, 96–97, 102–3, 105, 115–16

vorticism, 33, 64–65, 74, 77–82, 90

voyage imaginaire, 37, 42–43

Wade, Allan, 88

Wagner, Dorothy, 136, 139–40, 149

Wagner, Richard, 52

Wakayagi Kichitoyo, 10

Waldeen. *See* Falkenstein, Waldeen

Walker, Julia, 44–45, 51

walking: *chindon-ya* and, 252; Enlightenment views on, 240–41, 245–47, 250; of fashion model/flâneuse, 247–50, *248*; Ito's dance training/rehearsal and, 47–49, 238–40, *239*, 243; Ito's postwar comportment lessons on, 215, 218, 240–47

Warrior (Ito), 78

Waseda University's Theatre Museum, 187–88, 200

Washington Square Players, 111

watching/being watched: as continuous/ circulating, 18–19; Ito's solicitation of spectator, 15–16, 31, 57–59, *58*, 82–87, *83*, 93; kinesthetic awareness as, 257; postwar Japan's experience of, 218–19, *219*, 237–39, *239*; as source of pleasure, 82–87, *83*, 104, 119; surveillance, 14, 237–38; walking and, 252. *See also* desire; self-consciousness

Watsuji Tetsurō, 2, 206

Watts, Jeff, *49*

wayang wong, 22, 23

Welkmeister, 9–10, 24, 104

Whyte, Gordon, 112

Wigman, Mary, 17, 50, 52, 68, 70, 136, 263n33

Wild Goose, The (Mori), 86

Winther-Tamaki, Bert, 148

women's magazines, 35, 215, 218, 237, 240, 244–46

Wong, Yutian, 5, 24, 105, 116, 131, 143, 188

world-making, 7, 137–43, 186–87, 208–11

World's Fairs, 105, 128

World War I, 11, 28, 52, 60, 122, 137, 159, 260n17

World War II. *See* Asia-Pacific War / World War II

Wright, Hazel, 12–13, 27, 96, 127, 136, 150–51, 165–66, 168–70, 189

Yagishita, Emi, 5

Yamada Gorō, 165

Yamada Kōsaku 山田耕作: dance poems of, 12, 33, 65–72, 98; in Japan, 75, 205; at Jaques-Dalcroze Institute, 11, 36, 42, 67–68, 98; in New York, 12, 67, 71, 95, 98–100; re-created by Ito as Egyptian sage, 38–39, 41–43, 61; writings about Ito, 29, 36, 71

Yano, Christine, 29–30

Yasashi Wuriu, 112

Yeats, W. B.: *At the Hawk's Well* collaboration, 11, 64–65, 72, 79, 87–88, *89*; esoteric nature of, 137; Ito's impact on, 65–66, 88, 90, 267n38; Japanese poetics turned to, 74–77, 180. *See also At the Hawk's Well*

"Yellow Peril," 27

Yōga, 148

yōgaku, 67

Yoro, 87

yosahoi bushi, 194–96

Yoshi Isamu, 69

Young, Louise, 199–200

Yuya, 10

Zarina, Xenia (Jane Zimmerman), 136

Žižek, Slavoj, 7